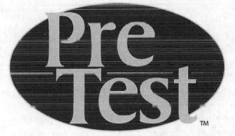

Neuroscience

PreTest™ Self-Assessment and Review

Notice

Medicine is an ever-changing science. As new research and clinical experience broaden our knowledge, changes in treatment and drug therapy are required. The authors and the publisher of this work have checked with sources believed to be reliable in their efforts to provide information that is complete and generally in accord with the standards accepted at the time of publication. However, in view of the possibility of human error or changes in medical sciences, neither the authors nor the publisher nor any other party who has been involved in the preparation or publication of this work warrants that the information contained herein is in every respect accurate or complete, and they disclaim all responsibility for any errors or omissions or for the results obtained from use of the information contained in this work. Readers are encouraged to confirm the information contained herein with other sources. For example, and in particular, readers are advised to check the product information sheet included in the package of each drug they plan to administer to be certain that the information contained in this work is accurate and that changes have not been made in the recommended dose or in the contraindications for administration. This recommendation is of particular importance in connection with new or infrequently used drugs.

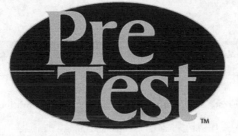

Neuroscience

PreTest™ Self-Assessment and Review
Seventh Edition

Allan Siegel, PhD
Professor of Neurology & Neuroscience and Psychiatry
University of Medicine & Dentistry of New Jersey
New Jersey Medical School
Newark, New Jersey

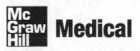 **Medical**

New York   Chicago   San Francisco   Lisbon   London   Madrid   Mexico City
Milan   New Delhi   San Juan   Seoul   Singapore   Sydney   Toronto

Neuroscience: PreTest™ Self-Assessment and Review, Seventh Edition

1 2 3 4 5 6 7 8 9 0 DOC/DOC 14 13 12 11 10

ISBN 978-0-07-162347-6
MHID 0-07-162347-7

This book was set in Berkeley by Glyph International.
The editors were Kirsten Funk and Cindy Yoo.
The production supervisor was Sherri Souffrance.
Project management was provided by Madhu Bhardwaj, Glyph International.
The cover designer was Maria Scharf.
RR Donnelly was printer and binder.

This book is printed on acid-free paper.

Library of Congress Cataloging-in-Publication Data

Siegel, Allan, 1939-
   Neuroscience : pretest self-assessment and review / Allan Siegel.—7th ed.
      p. ; cm.
   Includes bibliographical references and index.
   ISBN-13: 978-0-07-162347-6 (pbk. : alk. paper)
   ISBN-10: 0-07-162347-7 (pbk. : alk. paper)
   1. Neurophysiology—Examinations, questions, etc. I. Title.
   [DNLM: 1. Nervous System—anatomy & histology—Examination Questions.
   2. Nervous System Physiological Phenomena—Examination Questions.
   WL 18.2 S571n   2010]
   QP356.S49 2010 612.8076—dc22   2009047850

McGraw-Hill books are available at special quantity discounts to use as premiums and sales promotions, or for use in corporate training programs. To contact a representative, please e-mail us at bulksales@mcgraw-hill.com.

To Carla, whose patience, support, and understanding made this book possible, and to David Eliahu, Tzipporah Hannah, Matan Dov, Nadav David, Adi Hila, and Eden Chava.

Student Reviewers

Daniel Eskenazi
MD/PhD candidate
University of Washington School of Medicine
Class of 2012

Sarah Fabiano
SUNY Upstate Medical University
Class of 2010

Jason Margolesky
University of Miami Miller School of Medicine
Class of 2012

J. Eva Selfridge
MD/PhD candidate
University of Kansas School of Medicine
Class of 2012

Gustaf Van Acker III
MD/PhD candidate
University of Kansas School of Medicine
Class of 2012

Kelvin Young
SUNY Upstate Medical University
Class of 2010

Contents

Preface xi
Introduction xiii

High-Yield Facts

High-Yield Facts in Neuroscience I

Gross Anatomy of the Brain

Questions 57
Answers 67

Development

Questions 75
Answers 80

Anatomical and Functional Properties of Neurons and Muscle

Questions 85
Answers 93

The Synapse

Questions 105
Answers 109

Neurochemistry/Neurotransmitters

Questions 115
Answers 130

The Spinal Cord

Questions 143
Answers 159

The Autonomic Nervous System

Questions. 173
Answers. 176

The Brainstem and Cranial Nerves

Questions. 179
Answers. 225

Sensory Systems

Questions. 257
Answers. 269

Anatomy of the Forebrain

Questions. 281
Answers. 292

Motor Systems

Questions. 299
Answers. 317

Higher Functions

Questions. 329
Answers. 360

Bibliography 381
Index. 383

Preface

The study of the neurosciences has undergone remarkable growth over the past two decades. To a large extent, such advancements have been made possible through the development of new methodologies, especially in the fields of neuropharmacology, molecular biology, and neuroanatomy. Neuroscience courses presented in medical schools and related schools of health professions generally are unable to cover all the material that has evolved in recent years. For this reason, *Neuroscience: PreTest*™ *Self-Assessment and Review* was written for medical students preparing for licensing examinations as well as for undergraduate students in health professions.

The subject matter of this book is mainly the anatomy and physiology of the nervous system. Also, an attempt was made to encompass the subjects of molecular and biophysical properties of membranes, neuropharmacology, and higher functions of the nervous system. Moreover, clinical correlations for each part of the central nervous system, often using MRI and CT scans, are presented. Although it is virtually impossible to cover all aspects of neuroscience, the objective of this book is to include its most significant components as we currently understand them.

The author wishes to express his gratitude to Leo Wolansky, MD, and Alan Zimmer, MD, of blessed memory, and Michael Schulder, MD for providing the MRI and CT scans.

Introduction

Neuroscience: PreTest™ Self-Assessment and Review, Seventh Edition allows medical students to comprehensively and conveniently assess and review their knowledge of neuroscience. The 500 questions parallel the format and degree of difficulty of the questions found in Step 1 of the United States Medical Licensing Examination (USMLE). The High-Yield Facts in the beginning of the book are provided to facilitate a rapid review of the subject. It is anticipated that the reader will use these High-Yield Facts as a "memory jog" before proceeding through the questions.

Each question in the book is followed by four or more answer options to choose from. In each case, select the **one best response** to the question. Each answer is accompanied by a specific page reference to a text that provides background to the answer, and a short discussion of issues raised by the question and answer. A bibliography listing all the sources can be found following the last chapter.

To simulate the time constraints imposed by the licensing exam, an effective way to use this book is to allow yourself one minute to answer each question in a given chapter. After you finish going through the questions in the section, spend as much time as you need verifying your answers and carefully reading the explanations provided. Special attention should be given to the explanations for the questions you answered incorrectly; however, you should read every explanation even if you've answered correctly. The explanations are designed to reinforce and supplement the information tested by the questions. For those seeking further information about the material covered, consult the references listed in the bibliography or other standard medical texts.

High-Yield Facts

GROSS ANATOMY OF THE BRAIN

Lateral view of the brain (Fig. 1). The loci of key motor and sensory structures of the cerebral cortex are indicated in this figure. Anatomical definitions: anterior—toward the front (rostral end) of the forebrain; posterior—toward the back (caudal end) of the forebrain; dorsal—toward the superior surface of the forebrain; ventral—toward the inferior surface of the forebrain. Note that with respect to the brainstem and spinal cord, the terms anterior and ventral are synonymous; likewise, posterior and dorsal are also synonymous. Here, the term *rostral* means toward the midbrain, and the term *caudal* means toward the sacral aspect of the spinal cord (with respect to embryonic development and folding of the neural tissue). In Fig. 1, note that *rostral* and *anterior* mean the same as do *caudal* and *posterior*.

Midsagittal view of the brain (Fig. 2). Magnetic resonance image: T2-weighted, high-resolution, fast-spin echo image.

Horizontal (transaxial) view of the brain (Fig. 3). Magnetic resonance image: T2 weighted. Fast inversion recovery for myelin suppression image.

Frontal view of the brain (Fig. 4). Magnetic resonance image: T2 weighted. Fast inversion recovery for myelin suppression image.

  I. Cerebral cortex and adjoining structures

    A. Lateral surface of the brain

      1. Frontal lobe

        a. Motor functions

          (1) Precentral gyrus: primary motor cortex for head region and upper limbs

          (2) Premotor cortex: assists in integrating complex motor responses

          (3) Broca area: motor speech area

        b. Areas regulating cognitive and emotional behavior

          (1) Orbital (prefrontal) cortex

      2. Parietal lobe

        a. Postcentral gyrus: primary somatosensory cortex

        b. Inferior and superior parietal lobules: areas mediating complex perceptual discriminations

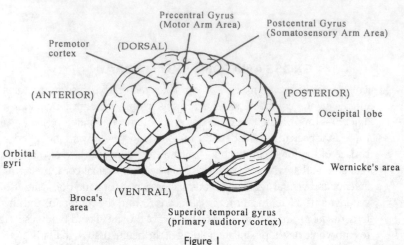

Figure 1
Lateral view of the brain.

  c. Inferior parietal lobule and adjoining aspect of the superior temporal gyrus: area mediating speech perception

  d. Spatial reasoning

 3. Temporal lobe

  a. Primary and secondary auditory receiving areas

 4. Occipital cortex

  a. Secondary visual receiving areas and region for the integration of visual signals

B. Medial surface of the brain

 1. Subcortical structures

  a. Corpus callosum: commissure connecting the hemispheres of the cerebral cortex

 2. Areas of the cerebral cortex

  a. Frontal lobe

   (1) Medial prefrontal cortex and anterior cingulate gyrus: regions regulating intellectual, emotional, and autonomic processes

   (2) Medial aspect of the precentral gyrus: region mediating motor functions of the lower limbs

  b. Parietal lobe

   (1) Primary and secondary somatosensory receiving areas for the lower limb

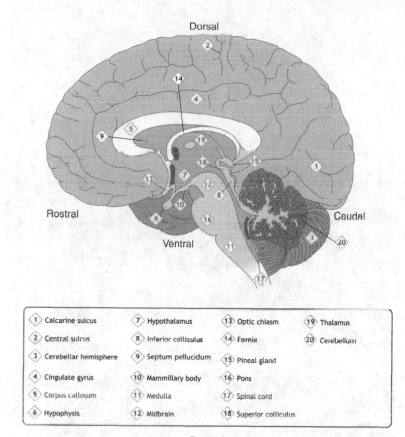

Figure 2
Medial view of the central nervous system. *(Modified, with permission, from White JS. USMLE Road Map: Neuroscience. 2nd ed. New York: McGraw-Hill; 2008:10.)*

c. Occipital lobe
(1) Primary visual cortex
C. Inferior surface of the brain
1. Frontal lobe: the part of the prefrontal cortex that relates to control of emotional and autonomic processes
2. Olfactory bulb and cortex: receiving areas for olfactory signals
3. Temporal lobe
a. Superior temporal gyrus: primary auditory receiving area

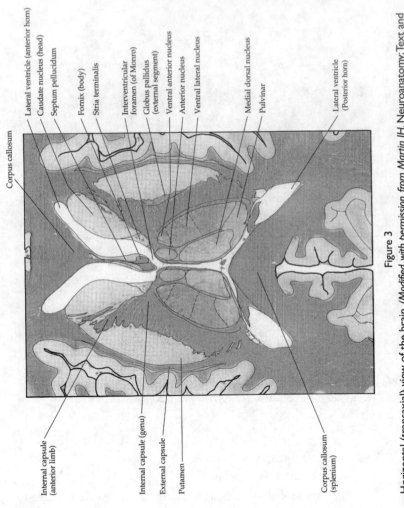
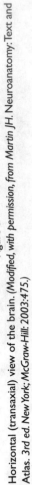

Corpus callosum

Lateral ventricle (anterior horn)
Caudate nucleus (head)
Septum pellucidum
Fornix (body)
Stria terminalis
Interventricular foramen (of Monro)
Globus pallidus (external segment)
Ventral anterior nucleus
Anterior nucleus
Ventral lateral nucleus

Medial dorsal nucleus
Pulvinar

Lateral ventricle (Posterior horn)

Internal capsule (anterior limb)

Internal capsule (genu)
External capsule
Putamen

Corpus callosum (splenium)

Figure 3

Horizontal (transaxial) view of the brain. *(Modified, with permission, from Martin JH. Neuroanatomy: Text and Atlas. 3rd ed. New York; McGraw-Hill: 2003:475.)*

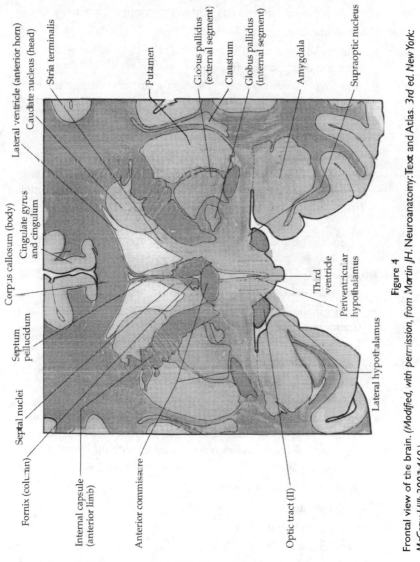

Figure 4

Frontal view of the brain. (*Modified, with permission, from Martin JH. Neuroanatomy: Text and Atlas. 3rd ed. New York: McGraw-Hill, 2003:469.*)

Septal nuclei

Fornix (column)

Internal capsule (anterior limb)

Anterior commissure

Optic tract (II)

Corpus callosum (body)

Cingulate gyrus and cingulum

Septum pellucidum

Lateral ventricle (anterior horn)

Caudate nucleus (head)

Stria terminalis

Putamen

Globus pallidus (external segment)

Claustrum

Globus pallidus (internal segment)

Amygdala

Supraoptic nucleus

Third ventricle

Periventricular hypothalamus

Lateral hypothalamus

      b. Limbic cortex: pyriform and entorhinal areas, receiving areas for olfactory signals; also serves as afferent sources of signals to the amygdala and hippocampal formation

II. Other forebrain structures

  A. Ventricular system of the brain: lateral and third ventricles; the most important function includes cerebrospinal fluid formation

  B. Septum pellucidum: membranous structure separating the lateral ventricles on each side of the hemisphere

  C. Fornix: fiber pathway that passes in a dorsomedial direction from the hippocampal formation to the diencephalon

  D. Diencephalon

    1. Thalamus: large group of nuclei that serve as relays for signals from different regions of the nervous system to the cerebral cortex

    2. Hypothalamus: structure situated below the thalamus; mediates a number of important visceral functions, such as endocrine and autonomic regulation, control of sexual behavior, aggression, and feeding and drinking behavior

  E. Anterior commissure: connects the olfactory bulbs of each side of the brain; aids in the integration of olfactory signals

  F. Basal ganglia: group of structures, seen best from horizontal and frontal sections, that serve primarily to regulate motor regions of the cortex

    1. Caudate nucleus

    2. Putamen

    3. Globus pallidus

  G. Limbic structures: important group of structures, situated mainly within the temporal lobe, that regulate emotional behavior and autonomic and visceral functions associated with the hypothalamus

    1. Amygdala

    2. Hippocampal formation

    3. Cingulate gyrus

III. Cerebellum and brainstem

  A. Cerebellum

    1. Attached to the brainstem by three pairs of peduncles (superior, inferior, and middle cerebellar peduncles) that serve primarily

as communicating links between the cerebellum and the brainstem

2. Anterior, posterior, and flocculonodular lobes: the three lobes of the cerebellum
3. Vermis: midline structure of the cerebellum, to which the cerebellar hemispheres are attached

B. Midbrain

1. Superior and inferior colliculus situated dorsally in the roof of the midbrain (tectum); mediate visual and auditory functions, respectively
2. Cerebral aqueduct: tubular portion of the ventricular system connecting the third and fourth ventricles; the aqueduct is surrounded by the periaqueductal gray, a group of compact cells that are continuous with similar cell populations surrounding the other ventricles
3. Tegmentum: part of the core of the brainstem and a continuation of the pontine and medullary tegmentum
4. Peduncular region: includes the cerebral peduncle, axons of cortical origin terminating in the brainstem and spinal cord, and the substantia nigra, a structure functionally associated with the basal ganglia

C. Pons

1. Tegmentum: core of the brainstem, functionally linked with corresponding regions of the medulla and midbrain
2. Basilar region: contains descending fiber bundles from the cerebral cortex, in addition to numerous cells and transversely oriented fibers that communicate with the cerebellum
3. Fourth ventricle: lies on the dorsal surface of the pons and upper medulla

D. Medulla

1. Open part of the medulla: rostral half of the medulla; contains many different cell groups, including some cranial nerve nuclei and ascending and descending fiber bundles
2. Closed part of the medulla: caudal half of the medulla; contains many different cell and fiber groups, including those of cranial nerves

IV. Cranial nerves

    A. Forebrain: cranial nerves I and II

    B. Midbrain: cranial nerves III and IV

    C. Pons: cranial nerves V to VII

    D. Medulla: cranial nerves VIII to X and XII (note that cranial nerve XI is mainly a spinal nerve but does have a cranial root that functions as a component of cranial nerve X)

BLOOD SUPPLY

I. Brainstem: Vertebral and internal carotid arteries are sources of blood supply to brain.

    A. Anterior spinal artery is formed as a branch of vertebral artery and supplies medial medulla; vertebral artery supplies intermediate region of medulla just lateral to region supplied by anterior spinal artery; posterior inferior cerebellar artery supplies lateral aspect of medulla and parts of cerebellum; anterior inferior cerebellar artery supplies lateral aspect of pons, including region of middle cerebellar peduncle and cerebellum; superior cerebellar artery supplies region of superior cerebellar peduncle, cerebellum, and parts of midbrain (Fig. 5).

    B. Basilar artery formed from convergence of vertebral arteries supplies much of the pons.

    C. Circle of Willis is formed by proximal branches of posterior cerebral artery, posterior communicating arteries, a part of internal carotid artery prior to its bifurcation, proximal part of anterior cerebral artery, and anterior communicating arteries.

    D. Anterior cerebral artery supplies rostral part of cerebral cortex and its medial aspect.

    E. Middle cerebral artery supplies lateral aspect of cerebral cortex.

    F. Posterior cerebral artery supplies the occipital and posterior aspects of parietal cortex and lateral aspect of midbrain.

DEVELOPMENT

The sulcus limitans divides the alar plate, from which sensory regions of the spinal cord and brainstem are formed, from a basal plate, from which motor regions of the spinal cord and brainstem are formed. (See Table 1.)

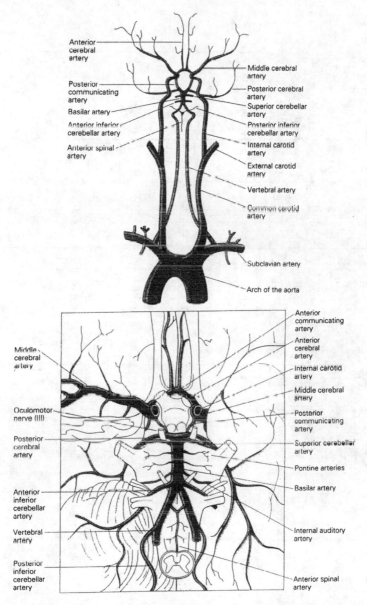

Figure 5

The blood vessels of the brain. The circle of Willis is made up of the proximal posterior cerebral arteries, the posterior communicating arteries, the internal carotid arteries, just before their bifurcations, the proximal anterior cerebral arteries, and the anterior communicating artery. Dark areas show common sites of atherosclerosis and occlusion. (*Reproduced, with permission, from Kandel E. Principles of Neural Science. 4th ed. New York: McGraw-Hill; 2000:1303.*)

TABLE I. DIFFERENTIATION OF THE NEURAL TUBE

Embryonic Derivative	Spinal Cord	Rhombencephalon (Hindbrain: Myelencephalon and Medulla) Metencephalon (Pons and Cerebellum)	Mesencephalon (Midbrain)	Prosencephalon (Diencephalon and Telencephalon)
Roof plate	Region of posterior median septum	Superior medullary velum	Commissures of the superior and inferior colliculi	Choroid tela and choroid plexus of the lateral and third ventricles.
Alar plate	Dorsal gray columns	Sensory nuclei of cranial nerves: V, VII, VIII, IX, X; cerebellum, deep pontine nuclei, inferior olivary nucleus, mesencephalic nucleus (cranial nerve V) (but displaced to midbrain)	Superior and inferior colliculi, red nucleus, substantia nigra, main sensory nucleus (cranial nerve V). Some nuclei of reticular formation	It has been suggested that diencephalon (thalamus and hypothalamus) and telencephalic structures are derived from alar plate but derivation is still unclear at this time.
Basal plate	Ventral gray columns; nucleus of cranial nerve XI	Motor nuclei of cranial nerves: V, VI, VII, IX, X, XII; nuclei of reticular formation	Motor nuclei of cranial nerves: III, IV; nuclei of reticular formation	—
Floor plate	Region of ventral median fissure	?	—	—

10

THE NEURON

I. Overview
  A. Consists of a cell body, dendrites (which extend from the cell body), and an axon
    1. Activation of voltage-gated sodium channels associated with membrane depolarization.
    2. Activation of voltage-gated potassium and chloride channels associated with membrane hyperpolarization.
    3. Temporal events: After information is received from a presynaptic neuron—depolarization of postsynaptic neuron—action potential is initiated and propagated down axon from the initial segment.
  B. Myelin formation
    1. In peripheral nervous system produced by numerous Schwann cells.
    2. In central nervous system (CNS) produced by an oligodendrocyte wrapping itself around numbers of neurons.
    3. Myelination allows for rapid conduction of action potentials by saltatory conduction (signals skip along openings in myelin called nodes of Ranvier)—eg, pyramidal tract and medial lemniscus.
    4. Damage to myelinated neurons disrupts transmission of neural signals (frequently seen in autoimmune diseases such as multiple sclerosis, sensory and motor functions severely compromised).
    5. Poorly or nonmyelinated neurons (eg, certain pain-afferent fibers to the spinal cord), slow conducting.
II. Different components of the neuron
  A. Plasma membrane—forms external boundary of neuronal cell body and its processes—consists of double layer of lipids in which proteins, including ion channels, are embedded. Inorganic ions enter and leave neuron through ion channels.
  B. Nerve cell body (soma)—consists of mass of cytoplasm, which contains the nucleus and various organelles.
    1. Soma—site of synthesis of most proteins, phospholipids, and other macromolecules.

2. Genetic material of nucleus—consists of deoxyribonucleic acid (DNA) called chromatin.

3. Nucleus contains prominent (relatively large) nucleolus—concerned with the synthesis of ribonucleic acid (RNA).

4. In female, Barr body represents one of two X chromosomes located at inner surface of nuclear membrane.

5. Cytoplasm contains
   a. Nissl substance consisting of RNA granules called ribosomes—many ribosomes are attached to membrane of rough endoplasmic reticulum (RER)
   b. Mitochondria—involved in generation of energy
   c. Golgi apparatus—site where proteins are modified, packaged into vesicles, and transported to other intracellular locations
   d. Lysosomes—membrane-bound vesicles formed from the Golgi apparatus and contain hydrolytic enzymes, serve as scavengers in neurons
   e. Cytoskeleton—determines shape of neuron, consists of microtubules, neurofilaments, and microfilaments

C. Dendrites—short processes arising from cell body, primary function is to increase surface area for receiving signals from axonal projections of other neurons.

D. Axon—a single long, cylindrical, and slender process arising usually from the soma. The axon usually arises from the axon hillock, a small, conical elevation on the soma of a neuron that does not contain Nissl substance. The first 50 to 100 μm of the axon, emerging from the axon hillock, is known as the initial segment. This segment is the site where the action potential originates. Axons are either myelinated or unmyelinated. At their distal ends, the axons branch extensively; their terminal ends, which are mostly enlarged, are called synaptic terminals.

III. Axonal transport
A. Fast anterograde transport: Precursors of peptide neurotransmitters, lipids, and glycoproteins, which are necessary to reconstitute the plasma membrane, are carried from the cell body to the terminals by this mechanism.

B. Slow anterograde axonal transport: Neurofilaments and micro-tubules are synthesized in the cell body and are transported by this mechanism to the terminals.

C. Fast retrograde axonal transport: Rapid retrograde transport carries materials from the nerve terminals to the cell body. Fast retrograde transport is involved in some pathological conditions. For example, herpes simplex, polio, and rabies viruses and tetanus toxin are taken up by the axon terminals in peripheral nerves and carried to their cell bodies in the CNS by rapid retrograde transport.

D. Neuroanatomical applications: In anterograde tracing techniques, radioactively tagged amino acids are taken up by the perikarya of the neurons for protein synthesis and are then transported anterogradely to their axon terminals. The labeled axons and their terminals are then visualized by autoradiography. Anterograde transport of carbohydrate-binding proteins, called lectins, has been used for investigating neuronal connections.

1. Retrograde tracing technique: This procedure involves the microinjection of an enzyme (eg, horseradish peroxidase [HRP]), fluorescent dyes (eg, Fluoro-Gold), cholera toxin, or virus at the desired site. The injected substance is taken up by axon terminals and transported retrogradely into the neuronal cell bodies. The labeled neurons are then visualized by a chemical reaction. Likewise, fluorescent substances such as Fluoro-Gold, microinjected at the desired site, are taken up by axon terminals and transported to the cell bodies, where they are visualized under a fluorescent microscope.

IV. Types of neurons: multipolar neurons, bipolar neurons, pseudounipolar neurons, and unipolar neurons. Neurons can also be grouped as principal or projecting neurons (also known as type I or Golgi type I) and intrinsic neurons (also known as type II or Golgi type II neurons). Principal neurons (eg, motor neurons in the ventral horn of the spinal cord) possess very long axons. Intrinsic neurons have very short axons.

V. Neuroglia (glial cells): These are supporting cells located in the CNS. They are mostly nonexcitable and more numerous than neurons. They have been classified into the following groups: astrocytes (fibrous and protoplasmic), oligodendrocytes, and microglia and ependymal cells (ependymocytes, choroidal epithelial cells, and tanycytes).

VI. Myelination: Myelinated axons are present in the peripheral nervous system as well as the CNS. In the peripheral nervous system, Schwann cells provide myelin sheaths around axons. The myelin sheaths are interrupted along the length of the axons at regular intervals at the nodes of Ranvier. The action potential becomes regenerated at uninsulated nodes of Ranvier. Therefore, the action potential traveling along the length of the axon jumps from one node of Ranvier to another (saltatory conduction). In the CNS, oligodendrocytes form the myelin sheaths around neurons. The intervals between adjacent oligodendrocytes are devoid of myelin sheaths and are called the nodes of Ranvier.

VII. Composition of peripheral nerves: Each peripheral nerve consists of epineurium, perineurium, endoneurium, and nerve fibers.

VIII. Neuronal injury: Wallerian degeneration refers to the changes that occur distal to the site of damage on an axon. Initially, the axon swells up and becomes irregular. Later, it is broken down into fragments and phagocytosed by adjacent macrophages and Schwann cells. When an axon is damaged, alterations may be restricted to the proximal segment of the axon up to the first node of Ranvier. Retrograde degeneration occurs when sectioning of an axon produces changes in the cell body. If the injury is close to the cell body, the neuron may degenerate. The cell body swells up due to edema and becomes round in appearance, and the Nissl substance gets distributed throughout the cytoplasm (chromatolysis). The nucleus moves from its central position to the periphery due to edema. Transneuronal degeneration occurs in the CNS when damage to one group of neurons results in the degeneration of another set of neurons closely associated with the same function.

IX. Recovery of neuronal injury (regeneration): If the damage to the neurons is not severe, regeneration is possible. However, complete recovery may take as long as 3 to 6 months. Although sprouting occurs in axons in the CNS, this process ceases within a short time (about 2 weeks). CNS neuronal function cannot be restored. However, in peripheral nerves, an axon can regenerate satisfactorily if the endoneurial sheaths are intact. In this situation, the regenerating axons reach the correct destination and function may be restored.

X. Neuronal membrane

   A. The neuronal membrane, like other cell membranes, consists of a lipid bilayer in which proteins, including ion channels, are embedded.

   B. The lipid bilayer determines the basic structure of the neuronal membrane. The proteins embedded in it are responsible for most of the membrane functions, such as serving as specific receptors, enzymes, and transport proteins

XI. Permeability of the neuronal membrane

   A. The neuronal membrane is permeable to all lipid-soluble substances and some polar (lipid-insoluble, water-soluble) molecules, provided they are uncharged and small in volume.

   B. The neuronal membrane is impermeable to most polar and charged molecules (even if they are very small).

   C. Cations and anions contain electrostatically bound water (waters of hydration). The attractive forces between the ions and the water molecules make it difficult for the ions to move from a watery environment into the hydrophobic lipid bilayer of the neuronal membrane.

XII. Carrier proteins (carriers or transporters)

   A. When a specific solute binds to a carrier protein, a reversible conformational change occurs in the protein, which, in turn, results in the transfer of the solute across the lipid bilayer of the membrane.

   B. When a carrier protein transports a solute from one side of the membrane to the other, it is called a uniport.

   C. A carrier protein that moves one solute in a particular direction and another solute in the opposite direction is called an antiport.

   D. A carrier protein that carries one solute in a particular direction and another solute in the same direction is called a symport.

XIII. The channel proteins: The channel proteins span the neuronal membrane and contain water-filled pores. Inorganic ions of suitable size and charge (eg, Na^+, K^+) can pass through the pore when it is in open state and thus pass through the membrane.

XIV. Simple diffusion: The substances that pass through the neuronal membrane by simple diffusion include all lipid-soluble substances and some polar (lipid-insoluble or water-soluble) molecules, provided they are uncharged and small in volume.

XV. Passive transport (facilitated diffusion): In this type of transport, solutes are transported across the neuronal membrane without requiring energy.

XVI. Active transport: Some carrier proteins transport certain solutes by active transport (ie, the solute is moved across the neuronal membrane against its electrochemical gradient). This type of transport requires coupling of the carrier protein to a source of metabolic energy.

XVII. Intracellular and extracellular ionic concentrations: The concentration of sodium ions is much greater outside the neuron as compared to that inside the neuron. On the other hand, the concentration of potassium ions is greater inside the cell than outside. (See Table 2.)

XVIII. Na^+, K^+-ATPase.

   A. The differences in intracellular and extracellular concentrations of different ions are maintained by Na^+, K^+-ATPase (also known as Na^+, K^+ pump), which is located in the neuronal membrane.

   B. It transfers three Na^+ ions out of the neuron for every two K^+ ions that are taken in. A net outward ionic current is generated because of this unequal flow of Na^+ and K^+ ions across the

TABLE 2. NEURONAL INTRACELLULAR AND EXTRACELLULAR CONCENTRATIONS OF SOME IMPORTANT IONS		
Ion	Extracellular Concentration (mM)	Intracellular Concentration (mM)
Cations (positively charged):		
Na^+	145–150	15
K^+	4–5	100
Ca^{2+}	1–2	2×10^{-4}
Cl^-	150	10–16
Anions: A^- (fixed anions; organic acids and proteins)	—	385

neuronal membrane. Because of the generation of this current, the Na^+, K^+ pump is said to be electrogenic.

XIX. Ion channels

A. Ion channels are made up of proteins and are embedded in the lipid bilayer of the neuronal membrane across which they span.

B. Nongated channels: These are always open and control the flow of ions during the resting membrane potential. Examples include nongated Na^+ and K^+ channels that contribute to the resting membrane potential.

C. Gated channels: All gated channels are allosteric proteins. At rest, these channels are mostly closed, and they open in response to different stimuli (eg, change in membrane potential, ligand binding, or mechanical forces).

D. Voltage-gated channels: They are opened or closed by a change in the membrane potential. Examples: voltage-gated Na^+ channels, voltage-gated Ca^{2+} channels, and voltage-gated K^+ channels.

E. Ligand-gated channels: Opened by noncovalent binding of chemical substances (transmitters or second messengers) to their receptors on the neuronal membrane.

F. Mechanically gated channels: These channels open by a mechanical stimulus, for example, channels involved in producing generator potentials of stretch and touch receptors.

XX. Nernst equation: Can be used to calculate the equilibrium potential of any ion that is present both inside and outside the cell where the cell membrane is permeable to that ion.

XXI. Goldman equation: This equation is used to determine the membrane potential when the membrane is permeable to more than one ion species.

$$\frac{P_k[K^+]_o + P_{Na}[Na^+]_o + P_{Cl}[Cl^-]_i}{P_k[K^+]_i + P_{Na}[Na^+]_i + P_{Cl}[Cl^-]_o}$$

where P is the permeability of the specific ion, i = inside, and o = outside the cell.

XXII. The ionic basis of the resting membrane potential.

A. When the neuron is at rest, the potential difference across its membrane is called the resting membrane potential.

B. In the resting state, a neuron has a more negative charge inside relative to outside.

C. If the neuronal membrane contained only K^+ channels, the resting membrane potential would be determined by the K^+ concentration gradient and be equal to the equilibrium potential for K^+ ions (approximately -90 mV).

D. However, neurons at rest are selectively permeable to Na^+ ions also. The Na^+ ions tend to flow into the neuron. Due to influx of Na^+ ions, the resting membrane potential deviates somewhat from that of the K^+ equilibrium potential, but it does not reach the equilibrium potential for Na^+. The reason for the inability of the neuron to attain a resting membrane potential closer to the Na^+ equilibrium potential is because the number of open nongated Na^+ channels is much smaller than the number of open nongated K^+ channels in the resting state of a neuron.

XXIII. The ionic basis of the action potential.

A. When a neuron receives an excitatory input, the neuronal membrane is depolarized, resulting in an opening of some voltage-gated Na^+ channels and influx of Na^+.

B. The accumulation of positive charges due to influx of Na^+ promotes further depolarization of the neuronal membrane.

C. When the membrane potential reaches a threshold level, a large number of voltage-gated Na^+ channels open and the permeability of Na^+ increases during the rising phase of the action potential. The depolarization continues so that the membrane potential approaches the Na^+ equilibrium potential.

D. The neuron is then repolarized by slow inactivation of voltage-gated Na^+ channels (which stops influx of Na^+ through these channels) and delayed opening of voltage-gated K^+ channels (which allows increased efflux of K^+ through voltage-gated K^+ channels-delayed rectifiers). It should be noted that influx of Na^+ and efflux of K^+ through the nongated channels continues throughout these events.

XXIV. Propagation of action potentials

A. When a region of the axonal membrane is depolarized sufficiently to reach a threshold, voltage-gated Na^+ channels open, Na^+ flows into the axoplasm, and an action potential is generated in that region.

B. The local depolarization spreads electronically (passively) to an adjacent region, where an action potential is generated by the opening of voltage-gated Na^+ channels and the influx of Na^+ into the axoplasm. The passive spread of voltage along the length of an axon results in an active regeneration process.

C. In vertebrates, nodes of Ranvier (bare segments of the axonal membrane) are present in between the segments of the myelin sheath.

D. The passive spread of current can generate an intense current at the nodes of Ranvier due to the presence of a high density of voltage-gated Na^+ channels

E. The action potential propagates along an axon by saltatory conduction without decrement (ie, the jumping of an action potential from one node to another).

THE SYNAPSE AND NEUROTRANSMITTERS

The binding of the neurotransmitter to the receptor molecule is determined by the postsynaptic receptor, which serves a gating function for particular ions. The receptor is responsible for opening or closing ligand-gated channels regulated by noncovalent binding of compounds such as neurotransmitters. The neurotransmitter is contained in presynaptic vesicles and released onto the postsynaptic terminal, causing activation of the receptor, which in turn produces postsynaptic potentials.

Sequence of events in synaptic transmission is as follows: transmitter synthesis → release of transmitter into synaptic cleft → binding of transmitter to postsynaptic receptor → removal of transmitter.

Major excitatory transmitters include substance P, acetylcholine, and excitatory amino acids; major inhibitory transmitters include GABA, enkephalin, and glycine. Disruption of neurotransmitter function can lead to different diseases of the nervous system. One such example involves the role of acetylcholine at the neuromuscular junction. When antibodies are formed against the acetylcholine receptor at the neuromuscular junction, transmission is disrupted and the autoimmune disease called myasthenia gravis occurs. This disorder includes symptoms such as weakness and fatigue of the muscles.

I. Synaptic transmission.

    A. Characteristics of electrical transmission

        1. Current generated by an impulse in one neuron spreads to another neuron through a pathway of low resistance. Such a pathway has been identified at gap junctions.

        2. Current generated by voltage-gated channels at the presynaptic neuron flows directly into the postsynaptic neuron. Therefore, transmission at such a synapse is very rapid (<0.1 ms).

        3. Electrical transmission is not very common in the CNS.

    B. Characteristics of chemical transmission

        1. At chemical synapses, the pre- and postsynaptic cells are separated by synaptic clefts, which are fluid-filled gaps (about 20-40 nm). The presynaptic terminal contains synaptic vesicles, which are filled with several thousand molecules of a specific chemical substance, the neurotransmitter.

        2. An action potential depolarizes the presynaptic nerve terminal, the permeability to Ca^{2+} increases, and Ca^{2+} enters the terminal. These events cause the vesicles to fuse with the cytoplasmic membrane and then release the neurotransmitter into the synaptic cleft (exocytosis).

II. Characteristics of receptors: They consist of membrane-spanning proteins. The recognition sites for the binding of the chemical transmitter are located on the extracellular components of the receptor. The binding of the neurotransmitter to its receptor results in opening or closing of ion channels on the postsynaptic membrane or activation of second messenger cascade.

III. Characteristics of ion channels.

    A. Indirectly gated ion channels: In this type of channel, the ion channel and the recognition site for the transmitter (receptor) are separate. This type of receptor is called a metabotropic receptor. When a transmitter binds to the receptor, a guanosine-5′-triphosphate (GTP)-binding protein (G-protein) is activated, which in turn activates a second messenger system. The second messenger can either act directly on the ion channel to open it or activate an enzyme, which in turn opens the channel by phosphorylating the channel protein. Activation of this type of channel elicits slow synaptic actions, which are long lasting (seconds or even minutes).

B. Directly gated ion channels: In this type of ion channel, several protein subunits (four or five) are arranged in such a way that the recognition site for the neurotransmitter is part of the ion channel. This type of receptor is called an ionotropic receptor. A transmitter binds to its receptor and brings about a conformational change, which results in the opening of the ion channel. Receptors of this type usually bring about fast synaptic responses lasting for only a few milliseconds.

C. Directly gated synaptic transmission at a peripheral synapse (nerve-muscle synapse): At the neuromuscular junction, the axons of motor neurons whose cell bodies are located in the CNS innervate skeletal muscle fibers. As the motor axon reaches a specialized region on the muscle membrane, called the end plate, it loses its myelin sheath and gives off several fine branches. Many varicosities (swellings), called synaptic boutons, are present at the terminals of these branches. The presynaptic boutons contain the synaptic vesicles containing acetylcholine. When the motor axon is stimulated, an action potential reaches the axon terminal and depolarizes the membrane of the presynaptic bouton, which results in the opening of the voltage-gated Ca^{2+} channels. Influx of Ca^{2+} into the terminal promotes fusion of the vesicle with the terminal membrane and subsequent release of acetylcholine by exocytosis. Acetylcholine acts on the nicotinic cholinergic receptors located at the crest of the junctional folds to produce an end plate potential (EPP). The amplitude of the EPP is large enough (about 70 mV) to activate the voltage-gated Na^+ channels in the junctional folds and generate an action potential, which then propagates along the muscle fiber and brings about muscle contraction.

D. Directly gated transmission at a central synapse: A synaptic potential that excites a postsynaptic cell in the CNS is called an excitatory postsynaptic potential (EPSP). This EPSP is generated by opening of directly gated ion channels, which permit influx of Na^+ and efflux of K^+. If the depolarization produced by the EPSP is large enough, the membrane potential of the axon hillock of the spinal motor neuron is raised to a threshold and an action potential results. A synaptic potential that inhibits a postsynaptic cell in the CNS system is called an inhibitory postsynaptic potential (IPSP). An IPSP usually hyperpolarizes the neuronal membrane.

IV. Diseases affecting the chemical transmission at the nerve-muscle synapse.

    A. Myasthenia gravis: This is an autoimmune disease in which the number of functional nicotinic acetylcholine receptors is reduced by an antibody. This results in muscular weakness. The symptoms include weakness of eyelids, eye muscles, oropharyngeal muscles, and limb muscles. Antibodies, probably produced by T and B lymphocytes, against the acetylcholine receptors are present in the serum of such patients. Acetylcholinesterase-inhibiting drugs (eg, neostigmine) can reverse the muscle weakness.

    B. Lambert-Eaton syndrome: In this disorder, antibodies are developed to voltage-gated Ca^{2+} channels on presynaptic terminals. The loss of voltage-gated Ca^{2+} channels is expected to impair the release of acetylcholine from the nerve terminals. Standard treatment consists of administration of guanidine and calcium gluconate, which elicit or facilitate acetylcholine release from the presynaptic nerve terminals.

V. Major classes of neurotransmitters (see Table 3).

    A. Small molecule neurotransmitters: acetylcholine, excitatory amino acids (glutamate, aspartate), inhibitory amino acids (GABA, glycine), catecholamines (dopamine, norepinephrine, epinephrine), indoleamines (serotonin), imidazoleamines (histamine), and purines (adenosine)

    B. Large molecule neurotransmitters: opioid peptides (eg, dynorphin, endomorphins, enkephalins, nociceptin), substance P

VI. Steps in neurotransmitter release.

    A. Depolarization of presynaptic terminal

    B. Ca^{2+} entry into the terminal

    C. Fusion of vesicles containing the neurotransmitters with the presynaptic terminal membrane

    D. Release of the neurotransmitter into the synaptic cleft

VII. Individual neurotransmitters.

    A. Acetylcholine

        1. Synthesis

            a. Choline present in the plasma enters the nerve terminal by active transport.

TABLE 3. MAJOR CLASSES OF NEUROTRANSMITTERS
Small molecule neurotransmitters:

Small molecule neurotransmitters:

    Acetylcholine

    Excitatory amino acids: glutamate, aspartate

    Inhibitory amino acids: γ-aminobutyric acid (GABA), glycine

    Biogenic amines:

        Catecholamines: dopamine, norepinephrine, epinephrine

        Indoleamine: serotonin (5-hydroxytryptamine)

        Imidazoleamine: histamine

    Purines (ATP, adenosine)

Neuropeptides:

    Opioid peptides: β endorphin, methionine enkephalin, leucine-enkephalin, endomorphins, nociceptin

    Substance P

Gaseous neurotransmitters: nitric oxide

      b. Acetylcholine is synthesized in the cytoplasm from choline and acetylcoenzyme-A by choline acetyltransferase.

      c. Acetylcholine is transported into vesicles and stored there.

  2. Release and removal

      a. Acetylcholine is released into the synaptic cleft.

      b. It is hydrolyzed by acetylcholinesterase.

  3. Distribution

      a. The basal forebrain constellation including the basal nucleus of Meynert

      b. Cholinergic neurons in the dorsolateral tegmentum of the pons

  4. Physiological and clinical considerations

      a. Cholinergic neurons have been implicated in the regulation of forebrain activity and sleep-wakefulness cycles.

      b. In Alzheimer disease, there is a dramatic loss of cholinergic neurons in the basal nucleus of Meynert.

B. Glutamate
1. Synthesis.
   a. Glucose enters the neuron, undergoes glycolysis in the cytoplasm to generate pyruvic acid, which enters into the mitochondria. In the mitochondria, pyruvic acid generates an acetyl group that combines with coenzyme-A present in the mitochondria to form acetylcoenzyme-A.
   b. The acetyl group is regenerated from acetylcoenzyme-A; it enters the Krebs cycle in the mitochondria.
   c. Alpha-ketoglutaric acid, generated in the Krebs cycle, is transaminated to form glutamate.
   d. Glutamate released into the synaptic cleft is recaptured by neuronal-type and glial-type Na^+-coupled glutamate transporters.
   e. In the nerve terminal, glutamate is repackaged into vesicles.
   f. In the glial cell, glutamate is converted to glutamine by an enzyme, glutamine synthetase. Glutamine in the glial cells is then transported into the neighboring nerve terminals and converted to glutamate, which is then packaged into vesicles.
2. Release and removal: Glutamate is taken up by a high-affinity sodium-dependent reuptake mechanism into the nerve terminals and glial cells.
3. Physiological and clinical considerations.
   a. Glutamate has been implicated as a transmitter in several circuits in the brain.
   b. Alteration in glutamate levels has been implicated in Huntington chorea and amyotrophic lateral sclerosis (ALS).
   c. Prolonged stimulation of neurons by excitatory amino acids results in neuronal death or injury. This effect is known as excitotoxicity.
C. GABA
1. Synthesis: It is formed by alpha-decarboxylation of L-glutamate. This reaction is catalyzed by L-glutamic acid-1-decarboxylase (GAD), which is present almost exclusively in GABAergic neurons.
2. Release and removal.
   a. In the brain, after its release, GABA is taken up into presynaptic terminals as well as glia.

b. Most of GABA is metabolized to yield glutamate and succinic semialdehyde by an enzyme, GABA-oxoglutarate transaminase (GABA-T).

3. Physiological and clinical considerations.
   a. GABA is found in high concentrations in the brain and spinal cord; it is an inhibitory transmitter in many brain circuits.
   b. Alteration of GABAergic circuits has been implicated in neurological disorders like epilepsy, Huntington chorea, Parkinson disease, senile dementia, Alzheimer disease, and schizophrenia.
   c. Barbiturates act as agonists or modulators on postsynaptic GABA receptors; they are used to treat epilepsy and anxiety.
   d. Valproic acid (dipropylacetic acid) is an anticonvulsant. It inhibits GABA-transaminase, an enzyme that metabolizes GABA, and increases GABA levels in the brain. Since epileptic seizures can be facilitated by lack of neuronal inhibition, increase in the inhibitory transmitter, GABA, is helpful in terminating them.

D. Glycine
   1. Synthesis.
      a. In the nerve tissue, serine is formed from glucose via the intermediates, 3-phosphoglycerate and 3-phosphoserine.
      b. Glycine is formed from serine by the enzyme serine transhydroxymethylase.
   2. Release and removal: After its release, glycine is taken up by neurons via an active sodium-dependent mechanism involving specific membrane transporters.
   3. Distribution: Glycine is found in all body fluids and tissue proteins in substantial amounts. It is not an essential amino acid, but it is an intermediate in the metabolism of proteins, peptides, and bile salts. It is also a neurotransmitter in the CNS.
   4. Physiological and clinical considerations.
      a. Glycine has been implicated as a neurotransmitter in the spinal cord, the lower brainstem, and perhaps the retina.
      b. Mutations of genes coding for some of the membrane transporters needed for removal of glycine result in hyperglycinemia, devastating neonatal disease characterized by lethargy, seizures, and mental retardation.

E. Catecholamines
  1. Dopamine
    a. Synthesis
      (1) Tyrosine enters the neuron by active transport.
      (2) Tyrosine is converted into dihydroxyphenylalanine (DOPA) by tyrosine hydroxylase enzyme. DOPA is converted to dopamine by an enzyme, aromatic L-amino acid decarboxylase (DOPA-decarboxylase). These steps occur in the cytoplasm.
      (3) Dopamine is then actively transported into the storage vesicles.
    b. Release and removal
      (1) Dopamine released into the synaptic cleft is removed by reuptake into the presynaptic terminal.
      (2) It diffuses into the circulation and is destroyed in the liver by two enzymes catechol-O-methyltransferase (COMT) and monoamine oxidase (MAO).
    c. Distribution
      (1) Substantia nigra: The axons of these neurons ascend rostrally in the nigrostriatal projection and provide dopaminergic innervation of neurons located in the corpus striatum (caudate nucleus and putamen).
      (2) Ventral tegmental area: This paired area lies adjacent to the substantia nigra, and the dopaminergic neurons located in this area project to different brain areas via the following pathways: (a) the mesolimbic pathway and (b) the mesocortical pathway. In the mesolimbic pathway, the axons of the dopaminergic neurons supply limbic structures (ie, amygdala, septal area, hippocampal formation) and the nucleus accumbens (ventral striatum). In the mesocortical pathway, the axons of the dopaminergic neurons provide innervation to the frontal and cingulate cortex.
      (3) Arcuate nucleus of hypothalamus: Dopaminergic neurons in this area project to the median eminence. They release dopamine directly into the hypophyseal portal circulation, which is then carried to the anterior lobe of the pituitary to inhibit the release of prolactin.

d. Physiological and clinical considerations
   (1) Parkinson disease: This disease is characterized by tremor at rest, slowness of movement (bradykinesia), rigidity of extremities and neck, and an expressionless face. Dopaminergic neurons located in the substantia nigra are degenerated in this disease, and the release of dopamine in the caudate putamen is decreased. Treatment: oral administration of a combination of L-DOPA and carbidopa (Sinemet). (Carbidopa inhibits DOPA-decarboxylase and reduces decarboxylation of L-DOPA in peripheral tissues, enabling greater concentrations of L-DOPA [precursor to dopamine] to reach the brain).
   (2) Psychotic disorders: Many adult psychotic disorders, including schizophrenia, are believed to involve increased activity at dopaminergic synapses. Many drugs that are effective in the treatment of these disorders are believed to mediate their action through the D_2-dopamine receptors.

2. Norepinephrine
   a. Synthesis.
      (1) In the noradrenergic neurons, dopamine stored in the vesicles is converted into norepinephrine by the enzyme dopamine-β-hydroxylase (DBH).
   b. Release and removal: Norepinephrine released into the synaptic cleft is removed by the following mechanisms:
      (1) Reuptake-1: Norepinephrine is transported back into the terminal of the noradrenergic neuron.
      (2) Reuptake-2: Norepinephrine is actively transported into the effector cells (about 10%), where it is inactivated primarily by COMT.
      (3) Norepinephrine diffuses into the circulation from the synaptic cleft and is destroyed in the liver by two enzymes, COMT and MAO.
   c. Distribution: Noradrenergic neurons are located in the locus coeruleus. These neurons project to the thalamus, hypothalamus, limbic forebrain structures (cingulate and parahippocampal gyri, hippocampal formation, amygdaloid complex), and the cerebral cortex, where norepinephrine

modulates a wide variety of functions associated with these regions.

d. Physiological and clinical considerations.

   (1) Norepinephrine is released as a transmitter from post-ganglionic sympathetic nerve terminals.

   (2) It is believed to play a role in psychiatric disorders such as depression.

3. Epinephrine

  a. Synthesis.

    (1) About 10% of norepinephrine stored in the vesicles leaks out into the cytoplasm.

    (2) In the adrenergic neuron, it is converted into epinephrine by the enzyme phenyl-ethanolamine-N-methyltransferase (PNMT).

    (3) Epinephrine thus formed is actively transported into storage vesicles in the nerve terminal (or chromaffin granules in the adrenal medulla) and stored for subsequent release.

  b. Release and removal: The mechanisms for removal of epinephrine are the same as those for norepinephrine.

  c. Distribution.

    (1) C1 neurons located in the rostral ventrolateral medulla

    (2) C2 neurons located in the nucleus tractus solitarius

  d. Physiological and clinical considerations: The function of adrenergic neurons in the CNS has not been clearly established.

F. Indoleamines

1. Serotonin (5-hydroxytryptamine [5-HT])

  a. Synthesis

    (1) Plasma tryptophan enters the brain by an active uptake process and is hydroxylated at the 5 position, by tryptophan hydroxylase, to form 5-hydroxytryptophan.

    (2) 5-Hydroxytryptophan is immediately decarboxylated to form serotonin. Serotonin is then actively taken up and stored in vesicles, where it is ready for release.

  b. Release and removal

    (1) Serotonin is removed from the synaptic cleft by reuptake mechanisms.

    (2) It is also metabolized by MAO.

   c. Distribution
      (1) Serotonin-containing neurons are located in the mid-line or raphe regions of the medulla, pons, and upper brainstem.
      (2) The rostral serotonin-containing cell groups of the dorsal, median, and central superior raphe project to the diencephalon and telencephalon.
      (3) 5-HT neurons in the caudal raphe nuclei project to the spinal cord.
   d. Physiological and clinical considerations
      (1) Serotonin-containing cells in the raphe regions of the brainstem are believed to play a role in descending-pain-control systems.
      (2) Serotonin-containing neurons may play a role in mediating affective processes such as aggressive behavior and arousal.
      (3) Serotonin synthesized in the pineal gland serves as a precursor for the synthesis of melatonin, which in turn serves as a neurohormone regulating sleep patterns.
      (4) Serotonin is also believed to play an important role in depression. Fluoxetine (Prozac) selectively blocks reuptake of serotonin and enhances 5-HT levels in the brain. It may produce beneficial effects in mental depression via enhancement of transmission through 5-HT_{1A} receptors.
      (5) Sumatriptan (Imitrex), a 5-HT_{1D} receptor agonist, is a vasoconstrictor and has proved useful in treating migraine headaches.
      (6) Some drugs of abuse mediate their effects through serotonin-containing neurons. For example, ecstasy (3,4,methylene-dioxy-methamphetamine, or MDMA) is believed to release 5-HT.
 G. Imidazoleamines
   1. Histamine
      a. Synthesis.
         (1) Histidine enters the brain by active transport.
         (2) It is then decarboxylated, by histidine decarboxylase, to form histamine.

b. Release and removal.
  (1) Histamine utilizes catecholamine uptake processes in certain tissues.
  (2) It is metabolized to 1-methylhistamine and imidazole acetic acid.

c. Distribution.
  (1) The highest density of histamine-containing neurons has been found in the median eminence and premammillary regions of the hypothalamus.
  (2) These neurons project to many areas of the brain and spinal cord.

d. Physiological and clinical considerations: Histamine has been implicated as a transmitter in the regulation of food and water intake, thermoregulation, autonomic function, and hormone release.

H. Purines

1. Recently, ATP (adenosine triphosphate) has been implicated as a neurotransmitter.
2. ATP has been implicated in pain mechanisms in the spinal cord.
3. Purinergic transmission has been demonstrated in autonomic neurons innervating the bladder, vas deferens, and muscle fibers of the heart.

I. Opioid peptides

1. Synthesis
   a. β-Endorphin: The pre-propeptide (pre-proopiomelanocortin) is present in the RER of neurons in the anterior pituitary, the intermediate lobe of the pituitary, and the arcuate nucleus of the hypothalamus. It is converted into the propeptide proopiomelanocortin, which is transported to the axon terminal by fast axonal transport. β-Endorphin is derived from proopiomelanocortin.
   b. Enkephalins: The pre-propeptide (pre-proenkephalin A) is present in the RER of neurons predominantly in the hindbrain. It is converted to the propeptide, proenkephalin A, which is transported to the axon terminal by fast axonal transport. Further, proteolytic processing in the terminal results in the generation of active peptides, methionine, and leucine enkephalin. Both of them are pentapeptides.

     c. Dynorphins (1-13): These peptides can be isolated from the pituitary and consist of C-terminally extended forms of Leu^5-enkephalin.

  2. Release and removal: In the CNS, the action of most of the peptides is terminated by their degradation due to the presence of peptidases.

  3. Physiological and clinical considerations: Opioid peptides have been implicated in regulating blood pressure, temperature, feeding, and sexual behavior.

J. Tachykinins

  1. Substance P is an undecapeptide (11 amino acids) and is present in the substantia nigra, caudate putamen, amygdala, hypothalamus, and cerebral cortex. Substance P neurons in the striatum project to the dopamine-containing neurons in the substantia nigra.

  2. Physiological and clinical considerations.

     a. Substance P has been implicated as one of the transmitters in mediating pain sensation.

     b. Substance P levels are reduced in the substantia nigra in patients suffering from Huntington chorea, which is characterized by movement and psychological disorders.

K. Gaseous neurotransmitters

  1. Nitric oxide (NO)

     a. Synthesis

       (1) Glutamate, released from a presynaptic neuron, acts on NMDA receptors located on the postsynaptic neuron; calcium ions enter the postsynaptic neuron and bind with calmodulin (calcium-binding protein), which results in the activation of nitric oxide synthase (NOS) (see Table 4).

       (2) NOS then generates NO and citrulline from L-arginine.

       (3) NO stimulates soluble guanylate cyclase, which results in the formation of cGMP from GTP. Increased levels of cGMP in the postsynaptic neuron elicit a physiological response.

     b. Physiological and clinical considerations

       (1) In the CNS, the role of NO as a transmitter is still under investigation.

TABLE 4. ISOFORMS OF NITRIC OXIDE SYNTHASE (NOS)			
Property	Isoform I	Isoform II	Isoform III
Name	cNOS or nNOS	iNOS	eNOS
Expression	Constitutive	Inducible by cytokines	Constitutive
Calcium dependence	Yes	No	Yes
Tissue	Neurons, epithelial cells	Macrophages, smooth muscle cells	Endothelial cells

   (2) The relaxation of blood vessels caused by cholinergic
       agonists may be mediated by NO.

VIII. Receptors
   A. Ligand-gated or ionotropic receptors, which consist of multi-
      meric proteins directly linked to ion channels (see Table 5).
      1. Nicotinic acetylcholine receptors (nAChR) are located at the
         neuromuscular junction NMJ as well as at central neurons.
         ACh binds to the α-subunits and opens the channel to allow
         influx of Na^+ and efflux of K^+ leading to overall depolarization
         of muscle.
      2. N-methyl-D-aspartic acid (NMDA) receptor: The activity of this
         receptor can be altered through the following binding sites:
         a. Transmitter-binding site: L-glutamate and related agonists
            bind at the transmitter binding-site and promote opening
            of a high conductance channel through which sodium and
            calcium ions enter the target cells.
         b. The strychnine-insensitive glycine modulatory site: This site
            is very important because unless it is occupied, L-glutamate
            is ineffective at this receptor.
         c. The phencyclidine-binding site: This is located within
            the channel. Noncompetitive blockers of NMDA recep-
            tor-ionophore complex (eg, ketamine) also bind at the
            same site.
         d. Voltage-dependent magnesium-binding site: The channel
            associated with an NMDA receptor is blocked by Mg^{2+} at
            normal resting potentials or when the cell is hyperpolarized.

TABLE 5. IONOTROPIC AND METABOTROPIC RECEPTORS FOR DIFFERENT NEUROTRANSMITTERS

Neurotransmitter	Ionotropic Receptor	Metabotropic Receptor
Acetylcholine	Cholinergic nicotinic	Cholinergic muscarinic
Glutamate	NMDA, AMPA, Kainate	$mGlu_1$-$mGlu_8$
GABA	$GABA_A$	$GABA_B$
Glycine	Strychnine-sensitive glycine receptor	—
Dopamine	—	D_1-D_5
Norepinephrine	—	α- and β-adrenergic receptors
Epinephrine	—	α- and β-adrenergic receptors
Serotonin	$5\text{-}HT_3$	$5\text{-}HT_1$ to $5\text{-}HT_2$, $5\text{-}HT_4$ to $5\text{-}HT_7$
Histamine	—	H_1, H_2, H_3
Adenosine	—	A_1 to A_3
Opioid peptides	—	μ, δ, κ, ORL_1

When the cell is depolarized, Mg^{2+} is dislodged and Na^+ and Ca^{2+} enter while K^+ leaves the cell through the same channel.

3. Kainate receptor: Binding of kainic acid to this ionotropic glutamate receptor results in the opening of an ion channel permitting influx of Na^+ (but not Ca^{2+}) and efflux of K^+ through the same channel and efflux of K^+ ion; the neuron is depolarized.

4. AMPA/quisqualate receptor: AMPA and quisqualic acid are agonists for this ionotropic glutamate receptor. Binding of these agonists to their receptors results in the opening of an ion channel permitting influx of Na^+ (but not Ca^{2+}) and efflux of K^+; the neuron is depolarized.

5. $GABA_A$ receptors: The following major binding sites are present on these receptors:
   a. For agonists (eg, GABA, muscimol).
   b. For antagonists (eg, bicuculline).
   c. For benzodiazepines (eg, diazepam or Valium).

    d. For barbiturates.

    e. GABA agonists open the chloride channels and thus hyperpolarize the neurons. Drugs that bind to the benzodiazepine site enhance the electrophysiological effects of GABA (eg, diazepam or Valium, an anxiolytic drug). Barbiturates bind to another site and prolong the opening of the chloride channel, also enhancing the inhibitory effects of GABA.

6. Glycine receptor: Activation of glycine receptors results in an influx of chloride ions into the neuron, which is then hyperpolarized. Strychnine blocks the glycine receptors.

7. Serotonin receptors: At least seven families of serotonin receptors have been identified. Only $5-HT_3$ receptors are ionotropic receptors. All other subtypes are metabotropic receptors.

B. Metabotropic receptors

1. They consist of a single protein (monomeric) molecule that usually has seven membrane-spanning domains.

2. G-proteins bind to an intracellular loop of these domains.

3. Binding of the neurotransmitter to the receptor results in the replacement of GDP by guanosine-5' triphosphate (GTP) on the α-subunit of the G-protein. The activated GTP-α-subunit complex can have the following results: (1) it can open the ion channels directly, or (2) they can bind to effector molecules (eg, adenylyl cyclase), generate second messengers (eg, cAMP) and, later, effectors (eg, protein kinase A), which then finally phosphorylate the ion channel to open it. Ions flow across the membrane and a postsynaptic response is elicited.

4. Some examples of metabotropic receptors are as follows:

    a. Cholinergic muscarinic receptors:

    b. Acetylcholine (ACh) binds with muscarinic receptors, a G-protein is activated, phospholipase C is generated, and two second messengers—IP_3 and diacylglycerol (DAG)—are produced.

        (1) IP_3 releases Ca^{2+} from intracellular stores, which leads to opening of Ca^{2+}-activated K^+ and Cl^- channels.

        (2) DAG activates protein kinase C, which can directly open Ca^{2+}-activated K^+ channels.

(3) These events result in hyperpolarization and then inhibition of the neuron.

c. Metabotropic glutamate receptors (mGluRs): mGluRs have been assigned to three groups. Group I mGluRs stimulate phospholipase C and phosphoinositide hydrolysis. Groups II and III mGluRs inhibit adenylyl cyclase and cAMP formation.

d. Dopamine receptors: At least five subtypes of dopamine receptors (D_1-D_5) have been identified. All of them are metabotropic receptors.

e. Adrenergic receptors
   (1) Norepinephrine and epinephrine mediate their actions via adrenergic receptors. These receptors are divided into two major classes: α and β. These classes have been further subdivided into many subtypes of adrenergic receptors
   (2) Binding of norepinephrine with β-adrenergic receptors results in the activation of a stimulatory G-protein (G_s).
   (3) Adenylyl cyclase enzyme is activated, which generates the second messenger cAMP.
   (4) The latter activates protein kinase A, which phosphorylates appropriate channels and opens them.
   (5) The neurons are depolarized, the amplitude of neurotransmitter-induced EPSPs is increased, and the neuron is made more excitable.

f. $GABA_B$ receptors
   (1) They are coupled to calcium or potassium channels via second messenger systems.
   (2) Activation of presynaptic $GABA_B$ receptors by baclofen decreases calcium conductance and reduces transmitter release.
   (3) Postsynaptic $GABA_B$ receptors are indirectly coupled to potassium channels via G-proteins, and they mediate delayed IPSPs.

g. Serotonin receptors
   (1) At least five subtypes of serotonin receptors have been identified. As stated earlier, all of them except $5-HT_3$ receptors are metabotropic.

    (2) 5-HT$_1$ receptors are located primarily in the CNS.

    (3) 5-HT$_2$ receptors are located in the CNS, gastrointestinal tract (GIT), and vascular smooth muscle.

    (4) 5-HT$_4$ receptors are located in the CNS, GIT, heart, and urinary bladder.

    (5) Identification of the function of 5-HT receptors in the CNS remains an active area of research.

  h. Histamine receptors

    (1) At least three subtypes of histamine receptors (H$_1$, H$_2$, and H$_3$) have been identified. All of them are metabotropic.

    (2) The stimulation of histamine receptors results in the formation of cyclic adenosine monophosphate.

  i. Adenosine receptors

    (1) At least three adenosine receptors (A$_1$-A$_3$) have been identified.

    (2) All of them are metabotropic receptors.

    (3) Identification of their function in the CNS is an active area of research at present.

  j. Opioid receptors

    (1) Three major classes of opioid receptors have been identified in the CNS: mu (μ), delta (δ), and kappa (κ) receptors.

    (2) Morphine and endogenous opioid peptides produce their supraspinal analgesic (pain-relieving) effect via μ-receptors.

    (3) Endomorphin-1 and endomorphin-2 are endogenous μ opiate receptor ligands. Naloxone blocks the effect of these peptides.

    (4) A new opiate receptor, called ORL$_1$ receptor, has been identified. Its endogenous ligand is nociceptin. Naloxone does not block this receptor.

SPINAL CORD

Major ascending tracts of the spinal cord and their functions include (see questions relating to pathways of spinal cord and related diagram in section entitled "The Spinal Cord"):

Dorsal columns. Includes fasciculus gracilis for lower limbs and fasciculus cuneatus for upper limbs. Mediates conscious proprioception, two point discrimination, vibration, and some tactile sensation ipsilaterally to the dorsal column nuclei and then contralaterally from the dorsal column nuclei to the postcentral gyrus from the VPL of the thalamus (Fig. 6).

Lateral spinothalamic tract. Mediates pain and temperature inputs contralaterally to the VPL and posterior complex of the thalamic nuclei and then to the postcentral gyrus (Fig. 7). Unique feature is its crossing within spinal cord at a level relatively close to where it enters the CNS.

Anterior spinothalamic tract. Mediates tactile impulses contralaterally to the VPL and then to the postcentral gyrus.

Posterior spinocerebellar tract. Mediates unconscious proprioception from muscle spindles and Golgi tendon organs of the lower limbs through the inferior cerebellar peduncle ipsilaterally to the anterior lobe of the cerebellar cortex.

Cuneocerebellar tract. Mediates unconscious proprioception from muscle spindles and Golgi tendon organs of the upper limbs from the accessory cuneate nucleus through the inferior cerebellar peduncle to the anterior lobe of the cerebellar cortex.

Anterior spinocerebellar tract. Mediates unconscious proprioception from the Golgi tendon organs of the lower limbs bilaterally to the anterior lobe of the cerebellar cortex. This tract initially crosses in the spinal cord and then crosses again through the superior cerebellar peduncle.

Major descending tracts of the spinal cord and their functions include:

Lateral corticospinal tract. Mediates voluntary control of motor functions from the contralateral cerebral cortex to all levels of the spinal cord (Fig. 8).

Rubrospinal tracts. Mediates descending excitation of flexor motor neurons at both the cervical and the lumbar levels of the contralateral spinal cord (Fig. 9).

Reticulospinal tracts. The lateral reticulospinal tract arises from the medulla and descends bilaterally to the cervical and lumbar levels of the spinal cord, mediating inhibition upon the spinal reflexes, mainly of extensors; the medial reticulospinal tract arises from the pons and descends mainly ipsilaterally to the cervical and lumbar levels of the spinal cord and facilitates extensor reflexes (Fig. 9).

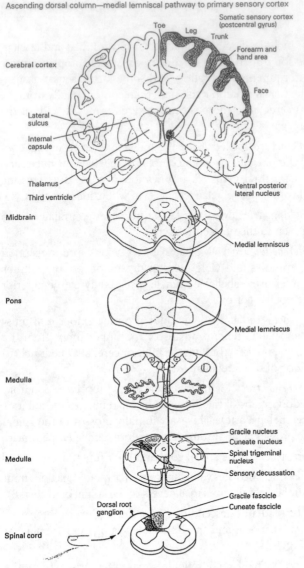

Figure 6

The medial lemniscus is a major afferent pathway for somatosensory information. Somatosensory information enters the nervous system through the dorsal root ganglion cells. The flow of information ultimately leads to excitation of the somatosensory cortex. Fibers representing different parts of the body maintain an orderly relationship to each other and form a neural map of the body surface that is maintained at each stage of information processing and ultimately in the neocortex. (*Reproduced, with permission, from Kandel E. Principles of Neural Science. 4th ed. New York: McGraw-Hill; 2000:342.*)

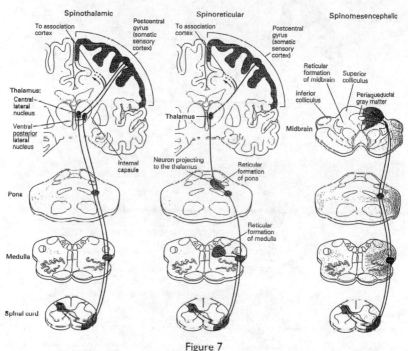

Figure 7

Three of the major ascending pathways that transmit nociceptive information from the spinal cord to higher centers. The spinothalamic tract is the most prominent ascending nociceptive pathway in the spinal cord. (*Reproduced, with permission, from Kandel E. Principles of Neural Science. 4th ed. New York: McGraw-Hill; 2000:482.*)

Vestibulospinal tracts. The lateral vestibulospinal tract arises from the lateral vestibular nucleus and descends ipsilaterally to the cervical and lumbar levels of the spinal cord, mediating powerful excitation of the extensor motor neurons; the medial vestibulospinal tract arises from the medial vestibular nucleus and descends mainly to the cervical levels of the spinal cord, mediating postural reflexes of the head and neck (Fig. 9).

Major disorders of the spinal cord include:

Brown-Séquard syndrome. Hemisection of the spinal cord often due to a bullet or knife wound—contralateral loss of pain and temperature below the level of the lesion; bilateral segmental loss of pain and

Descending lateral corticospinal pathway

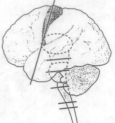

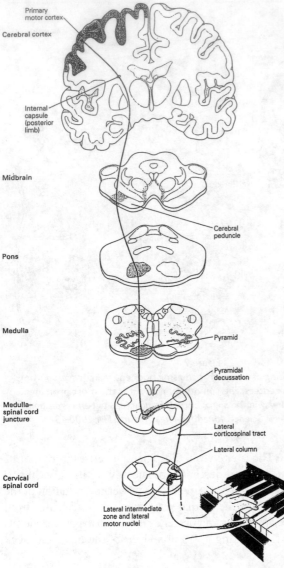

Primary motor cortex

Cerebral cortex

Internal capsule (posterior limb)

Midbrain

Cerebral peduncle

Pons

Medulla

Pyramid

Pyramidal decussation

Medulla–spinal cord juncture

Lateral corticospinal tract

Lateral column

Cervical spinal cord

Lateral intermediate zone and lateral motor nuclei

Figure 8

Fibers that originate in the primary motor cortex and terminate in the ventral horn of the spinal cord constitute a significant part of the corticospinal tract. The same axons are at various points in their projection part of the internal capsule, the cerebral peduncle, the medullary pyramid, and the lateral corticospinal tract. *(Reproduced, with permission, from Kandel E. Principles of Neural Science. 4th ed. New York: McGraw-Hill; 2000:346.)*

A Medial brainstem pathways

B Lateral brainstem pathways

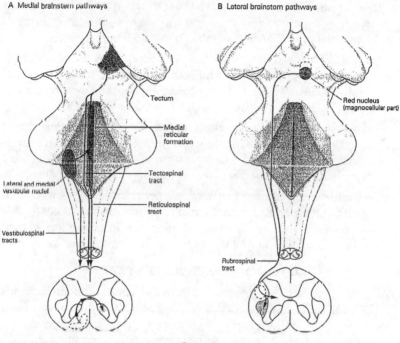

Tectum

Medial reticular formation

Lateral and medial vestibular nuclei

Tectospinal tract

Reticulospinal tract

Vestibulospinal tracts

Red nucleus (magnocellular part)

Rubrospinal tract

Figure 9

Medial and lateral descending pathways from the brainstem control different groups of neurons and different groups of muscles. **A.** The main components of the medical pathways are the reticulospinal, medical and lateral vestibulospinal, and tectospinal tracts that descend in the ventral column. These tracts terminate in the ventromedial area of the spinal gray matter. **B.** The main lateral pathway is the rubrospinal tract, which originates in the magnocellular portion of the red nucleus. The rubrospinal tract descends in the contralateral dorsolateral column and terminates in the dorsolateral area of the spinal gray matter. *(Reproduced, with permission, from Kandel E.* Principles of Neural Science. *4th ed. New York: McGraw-Hill; 2000:669.)*

temperature at the level of the lesion; ipsilateral loss of conscious proprioception, two-point discrimination, and vibration below the level of the lesion; ipsilateral upper motor neuron (UMN) paralysis below the level of the lesion; ipsilateral lower motor neuron (LMN) paralysis at the level of the lesion.

Tabes dorsalis. Damage to the dorsal root ganglion and dorsal columns resulting from syphilis—ipsilateral loss of conscious proprioception, two-point discrimination and vibration, and tendon reflexes.

Amyotrophic lateral sclerosis (ALS, Lou Gehrig disease). A disease whose etiology is not yet known destroys both corticospinal fibers and ventral horn cells (ie, UMN and LMN), causing abnormal reflexes, progressive muscle weakness, atrophy, and ultimately death.

Syringomyelia. Caused by abnormal closure of the central canal during development, by trauma, or by a tumor, the result of which is an enlargement of the central canal, causing a segmental bilateral loss of pain and temperature due to damage to the decussating spinothalamic fibers.

Combined systems disease. Results from pernicious anemia associated with a deficiency in vitamin B_{12}; there is degeneration of both the dorsal columns and the corticospinal tracts, resulting in a loss of conscious proprioception, UMN symptoms, and muscle weakness.

AUTONOMIC NERVOUS SYSTEM

The sympathetic nervous system arises from the thoracic and lumbar cords (T1-L2), and the parasympathetic nervous system arises from S2 to S4 and cranial nerves III, VII, IX, and X (see Table 6). All preganglionic neurons are cholinergic as well as parasympathetic postganglionic neurons. In addition, sympathetic postganglionic innervation of sweat glands and blood vessels in skeletal muscle is also cholinergic. Most other postganglionic sympathetic endings are noradrenergic. Examples of functions of the sympathetic nervous system include pupillary dilation, acceleration of heart rate, constriction of blood vessels of the trunk and extremities, bronchodilation, and inhibition of gastric motility. Examples of functions of the parasympathetic nervous system include pupillary constriction, decrease in heart rate, secretion of the salivary and lacrimal glands, bronchoconstriction, and stimulation of gastric motility.

    I. Divisions of the autonomic nervous system

        A. Sympathetic division: The neurons from which the outflow of the sympathetic division originates (preganglionic neurons) are located in the intermediolateral cell column (IML) of the first thoracic to second lumbar (T1-L2) spinal cord. This division of the autonomic nervous system is activated in stressful situations, and the individual is prepared for fight or flight.

TABLE 6. A COMPARISON BETWEEN SYMPATHETIC AND PARASYMPATHETIC DIVISIONS OF THE AUTONOMIC NERVOUS SYSTEM		
	Parasympathetic	**Sympathetic**
Preganglionic neurons: location	(Target organ is shown in parentheses.) Nucleus of oculomotor nerve (pupil); superior salivatory nucleus of facial nerve, inferior salivatory nucleus of glossopharyngeal nerve (salivary glands); facial nerve (lacrimal glands); dorsal motor nucleus of vagus (GIT, kidney); nucleus ambiguus (heart); intermediolateral cell column of the sacral spinal cord at S2-S4 level	Intermediolateral cell column of the spinal cord (T1-L2)
Outflow	Cranial nerves III, VII, IX, X; pelvic splanchnic nerves	Ventral roots at T1-L2
Preganglionic fibers	Myelinated, the preganglionic fibers are relatively long because the ganglia receiving them are located within the target organ or close to it	Myelinated, the preganglionic fibers are relatively short because the ganglia receiving them are located at some distance from the target organ
Transmitter at their terminals (within ganglia)	Acetylcholine	Acetylcholine
Ganglia	Ganglia located close to the organs (ciliary, otic); ganglia located within the organs (heart, bronchial tree, GIT)	Paravertebral ganglia in sympathetic chain (22 pairs); prevertebral ganglia (celiac, renal, superior, and inferior mesenteric)
Postganglionic fibers	Short, nonmyelinated	Long, nonmyelinated
Transmitter at the terminals of postganglionic fibers	Acetylcholine	Norepinephrine (acetylcholine in sweat glands)

(Continued)

TABLE 6. A COMPARISON BETWEEN SYMPATHETIC AND PARASYMPATHETIC DIVISIONS OF THE AUTONOMIC NERVOUS SYSTEM (*CONTINUED*)		
	Parasympathetic	**Sympathetic**
Ratio of preganglionic to post-ganglionic neurons and extent of action	A single preganglionic fiber may connect with only one or two postganglionic neurons. This arrangement favors localized actions	A single preganglionic fiber may connect with numerous (63-196) postganglionic neurons. This arrangement results in widespread responses

B. Parasympathetic division: Parasympathetic preganglionic neurons are located in the brainstem (Edinger-Westphal nucleus, superior salivatory nucleus of the facial nerve, inferior salivatory nucleus, nucleus ambiguus, and dorsal motor nucleus of vagus) and the sacral region of the spinal cord (second, third, and fourth segments). Activation of this division of the autonomic nervous system results in conservation and restoration of body energy.

C. Enteric nervous system: This consists of two layers of neurons that are present in the smooth muscle of the gut: the myenteric (Auerbach) and submucosal (Meissner) plexuses. The neurons of the myenteric (Auerbach) plexus control gastrointestinal motility, while the neurons of the submucosal (Meissner) plexus control water and ion movement across the intestinal epithelium.

II. Autonomic innervation of different organs

A. Eye.

1. Iris and ciliary body: The iris and the circumferential muscles of the ciliary body receive parasympathetic innervation from the preganglionic parasympathetic neurons located in the Edinger-Westphal nucleus via the oculomotor nerve (cranial nerve III) and the ciliary ganglion. Activation of the parasympathetic innervation to the eye results in contraction of circular muscles of the iris, causing constriction of the pupil (miosis) and contraction of circumferential muscles of the

ciliary body, causing the relaxation of the suspensory ligaments of the lens and making it more suitable for near vision. The preganglionic neurons providing sympathetic innervation to the radial smooth muscle fibers of the iris are located in the intermediolateral column at the T1 level. Activation of the sympathetic nervous system results in contraction of the radial muscles of the iris, which brings about pupillary dilatation (mydriasis).

2. Upper eyelid: The tarsal muscle (a small portion of the levator palpebrae superioris muscle) and the orbital muscle of M.ller receive sympathetic innervation from the preganglionic sympathetic neurons from the IML at the T1 level via the superior cervical ganglion. Interruption of the sympathetic innervation to the tarsal muscle results in pseudoptosis (partial drooping of the upper eyelid), and damage to the orbital muscle of M.ller results in enophthalmos (sinking of eyeball). These symptoms are characteristic of Horner syndrome.

B. Salivary glands.

1. Sublingual and submandibular glands: These glands receive parasympathetic innervation from the superior salivatory nucleus via the chorda tympani branch of the facial nerve and the submandibular ganglion. Activation of these parasympathetic fibers (secretomotor fibers) results in the secretion of watery saliva. They receive sympathetic innervation from preganglionic sympathetic neurons located in the T1 level of the IML via the superior cervical ganglion. Activation of the sympathetic innervation to these glands produces viscous salivary secretions.

2. Parotid glands: These receive parasympathetic innervation from the inferior salivatory nucleus via the lesser petrosal branch of the glossopharyngeal nerve and the otic ganglion. Activation of these fibers results in secretion of watery saliva from the parotid gland into the oral cavity. Sympathetic innervation to these glands is similar to that for the sublingual and submandibular glands. Activation of the sympathetic nervous system produces viscous saliva.

3. Lacrimal glands: These receive parasympathetic innervation from the superior salivatory nucleus (lacrimal nucleus) via the greater petrosal branch of the facial nerve and the pterygopalatine ganglion. Activation of these postganglionic parasympathetic fibers results in secretion of tears. Sympathetic innervation to these glands is the same as that described for the sublingual and submandibular glands.

C. Heart: The heart receives parasympathetic innervation from the preganglionic neurons located in the dorsal motor nucleus of the vagus and a region surrounding the compact zone of the nucleus ambiguus via the vagus nerve. The preganglionic sympathetic neurons innervating the heart are located in the IML at T1 to T3 spinal segments.

D. Blood vessels: Arterioles in most of the organs do not receive parasympathetic innervation. The preganglionic sympathetic neurons innervating the blood vessels are located in the thoracolumbar cord.

E. Lungs: The preganglionic parasympathetic neurons innervating the lungs are located in the dorsal motor nucleus of the vagus, and their axons travel to the thoracic cavity in the vagus nerves. The preganglionic sympathetic neurons innervating the lungs are located in the IML at T2 to T4 level.

F. Kidney: The preganglionic parasympathetic fibers descending in the vagus nerves enter the kidney along the renal artery. The preganglionic sympathetic neurons innervating the kidneys are located in the IML at the T7 to T11 level.

G. Adrenal medulla: The adrenal medulla is functionally analogous to a sympathetic ganglion; the adrenal medullary cells are directly innervated by the sympathetic preganglionic neurons, which are located in the intermediolateral column at the T7 to T11 level.

H. Gastrointestinal tract (GIT).

1. Stomach, small intestine, and proximal part of large intestine: The preganglionic neurons providing parasympathetic innervation to these organs are located in the dorsal motor nucleus of the vagus. These preganglionic fibers descend in the vagus nerves and synapse on postganglionic neurons located in the

myenteric (Auerbach) and submucosal (Meissner) plexuses. The sympathetic preganglionic neurons innervating these regions of the GIT are located in the IML at the T5 to T11 level.

2. Descending colon and rectum, parasympathetic innervation: The preganglionic parasympathetic neurons innervating these regions of the GIT are located in the intermediolateral column of the sacral spinal cord at the S2 to S4 level. The sympathetic preganglionic neurons innervating this region of the GIT are located in the IML at the L1 to L2 level.

I. Urinary bladder: The preganglionic parasympathetic neurons innervating the bladder are located in the intermediolateral column of the sacral spinal cord at the S2 to S4 level. Their axons travel via the pelvic nerves and synapse on postganglionic neurons located in the pelvic plexus and in the wall of the urinary bladder. The sympathetic preganglionic neurons innervating the urinary bladder are located in the intermediolateral column at the T11 to L2 level. The preganglionic sympathetic fibers reach the urinary bladder through the hypogastric plexuses.

1. Role of the sphincter vesicae in ejaculation: The sympathetic nerves innervating the sphincter located at the bladder neck (sphincter vesicae) play an important role during ejaculation in the male. Sympathetic activation contracts the sphincter located at the bladder neck during ejaculation and prevents seminal fluid from entering the bladder.

2. Somatic innervation: The external urethral sphincter is innervated by alpha motor neurons located in the ventral horn in the sacral segments S2 to S4 (Onuf nucleus).

3. Micturition: Urination results from activation of sacral parasympathetic neurons innervating the bladder and temporary inhibition of alpha motor neurons innervating the external urethral sphincter.

J. Male reproductive system: The preganglionic parasympathetic neurons innervating the erectile tissue in the penis are located in the IML at the S2 to S4 level. Activation of the parasympathetic nervous system results in the dilation of the arteries in the erectile tissue, causing erection of the penis. The preganglionic sympathetic neurons innervating the vas deferens, seminal vesicles, and prostate glands are located in the IML at the L1 to L2 level. Activation of the sympathetic nervous system causes ejaculation.

K. Female reproductive system: The innervation and the mechanism of vasodilation in the erectile tissue of the clitoris are similar to those described for the penis. The location of the preganglionic parasympathetic neurons and the pathways they follow to innervate the uterus are similar to those described for the penis. Parasympathetic stimulation causes relaxation of the uterine smooth muscle. The preganglionic sympathetic neurons innervating the smooth muscle of the uterine wall are located in the IML at the T12 to L1 level. Activation of the sympathetic nervous system results in contraction of the uterus.

III. Neurotransmitters in the autonomic nervous system

A. Preganglionic terminals: Within the autonomic ganglia, acetylcholine is the transmitter released at the terminals of the sympathetic as well as the parasympathetic preganglionic fibers.

B. Postganglionic terminals: At the terminals of most sympathetic postganglionic neurons, norepinephrine is the transmitter liberated with the exception of those innervating sweat glands and blood vessels of the skeletal muscles where acetylcholine is the neurotransmitter. At the terminals of all the parasympathetic postganglionic neurons, acetylcholine is the neurotransmitter liberated.

IV. Receptors

A. Cholinergic receptors

1. Muscarinic receptors: Cholinergic receptors located in the visceral effector organ cells (smooth and cardiac muscle and exocrine glands) are called muscarinic cholinergic receptors.

2. Nicotinic receptors: Cholinergic receptors located in the adrenal medulla and autonomic ganglia are called nicotinic receptors.

B. Adrenergic receptors: At the present time, adrenergic receptors are divided into two major classes: α and β. These classes have been further subdivided into α_1 and β_2 and β_1 and β_2.

V. Other autonomic functions

A. Cardiovascular regulatory mechanisms in the CNS

1. Solitary nucleus (nTS): Baroreceptor afferent fibers (sensing blood pressure changes) and chemoreceptor fibers (sensing changes in blood gases and pH) arising from the carotid sinus make their first synapse in the middle and caudal regions of the nTS.

2. Caudal ventrolateral medullary depressor area (CVLM): These neurons are located in the ventrolateral medulla and send GABAergic projections to a pressor region (RVLM) located rostral to it.

3. Rostral ventrolateral medullary pressor area (RVLM): The RVLM is located caudal to the facial nucleus. It is believed to be one of the most important sources of vasomotor tone. RVLM neurons send monosynaptic projections to the IML.

4. IML of the spinal cord: Sympathetic preganglionic neurons are located in the IML.

5. Baroreceptor reflex: The responses to stimulation of baroreceptors are hypotension and bradycardia. Activation of baroreceptors results in excitation of neurons located in the nTS and CVLM via excitatory amino acid receptors. Activation of CVLM neurons results in the release of GABA in the RVLM. Inhibition of RVLM neurons results in a decrease in the excitatory input to the sympathetic preganglionic neurons in the IML. Consequently, blood pressure and heart rate are decreased.

B. Respiratory regulatory mechanisms in the CNS

1. The ventral respiratory group (VRG).
   a. The caudal part (called the cVRG) contains mostly expiratory neurons.
   b. The part immediately rostral to the cVRG (called the rVRG) contains mostly inspiratory neurons. The neurons located rostral to the rVRG (called the Botzinger complex) are mostly expiratory.
   c. An area just caudal to the Botzinger complex, termed the pre-Botzinger complex, has been implicated as the site of respiratory rhythm generation.

d. The phrenic motor nucleus (PMN), located in the ventral horn of the cervical spinal cord (C3 to C5 level), innervates the diaphragm.

2. The dorsal respiratory group (DRG): These respiratory neurons are located in the ventrolateral nucleus of the solitary tract. The pneumotaxic center, located in the dorsolateral pontine tegmentum, is considered to be essential for maintaining a normal breathing pattern.

VI. Selected disorders of the autonomic nervous system

A. Horner syndrome: This is characterized by drooping of the ipsilateral upper eyelid (ptosis), constriction of the pupil (miosis), enophthalmos (sinking of the eyeball in the orbit), dilation of arterioles of the skin, and anhydrosis (loss of sweating) at the face. It is caused by lesions of the brainstem and upper cervical cord, which interrupt the sympathetic fibers in the reticulospinal tract and fibers descending from the hypothalamus to the IML. Such lesions are also encountered in multiple sclerosis and can be seen in tumors of the apex of the lung.

B. Argyll Robertson pupil: This condition occurs in syphilitic patients with CNS complications. In brief, the chief symptoms are that the pupils do not contract in response to light but do show constriction as part of the accommodation reflex.

C. Hirschsprung disease (megacolon): This is characterized by absence of peristalsis in the distal colon, due to absence of neural tissue associated with Auerbach plexus; consequently, impaction of feces is due to aperistalsis.

D. Frey syndrome: In this condition, the parasympathetic fibers eliciting secretory responses in parotid glands grow erroneously into the facial skin overlying these glands. Therefore, stimulation of the parasympathetic nervous system elicits sweating of this facial region.

THE BRAINSTEM AND CRANIAL NERVES

Lateral medullary syndrome (Wallenberg syndrome). Lesions of the lateral aspect of the lower half of the brainstem, due to occlusion of the inferior cerebellar arteries, produce loss of pain and temperature on the same side of the face and opposite side of the body, as well as Horner syndrome (ie, ipsilateral myosis, ptosis, and anhydrosis due to disruption of the sympathetic supply to the orbit and pupil, or, as applies in the present context, to disruption of descending sympathetic fibers through the brainstem to the spinal cord).

Medial medullary syndrome.   Lesions of the medial aspect of the medulla typically resulting from occlusion of the anterior spinal artery produce contralateral loss of conscious proprioception, contralateral hemiparesis, and weakness of tongue muscles, which are protruded to the side of the lesion. Body paralysis, which involves the side contralateral to the lesion, coupled with cranial nerve weakness, which involves the side ipsilateral to the lesion, is called alternating hypoglossal hemiplegia.

Cranial nerves mediate multiple functions in the nervous system: motor nuclei—general somatic efferent (cranial nerves III, IV, VI, and XII), special visceral efferent (cranial nerves V, VII, IX, X, and XI), general visceral efferent (cranial nerves III, VII, IX, and X), general somatic afferent (cranial nerves V, IX, and X), special sensory afferent (cranial nerves II and VIII), or special visceral afferent (cranial nerves I, VII, IX, and X).

SENSORY SYSTEMS

Loss of partial or total aspects of the visual field can be understood in terms of damage to the retinal pathways, including their targets in the lateral geniculate nucleus and visual cortex. The schematic diagram shown in Fig. 10 depicts the kinds of field deficits that occur following lesions of different aspects of the visual pathway. Key: (A) optic nerve lesion producing total blindness in the left eye; (B) lesion that disrupts the right retinal nasal fibers that project from the base of the left optic nerve, producing right upper quadrantanopia and left scotoma; (C) lesion of optic chiasm, producing bitemporal hemianopsia; (D) unilateral (left) optic tract lesion, producing a right homonymous hemianopsia; (E) interruption of left visual radiations that pass ventrally through the temporal lobe to the lower bank of the visual cortex (ie, the loop of Meyer), producing an upper right quadrantanopia; (F) interruption of left visual radiations that pass more dorsally through the parietal and occipital lobes to the upper bank of the visual cortex, producing a lower right quadrantanopia; and (G) lesion of the left visual cortex, producing a right homonymous hemianopsia.

The principles of an excitatory focus-and-surround inhibition, as well as those of a somatotropic organization, are present within a given receptor system and form the functional basis for discriminative functions in a

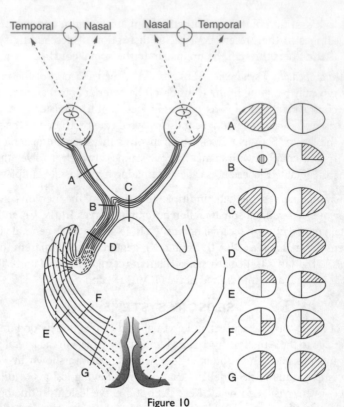

Figure 10

(Adapted, with permission, from Ropper AH, Brown RH. Adams & Victor: Principles of Neurology. 8th ed. New York: McGraw-Hill; 2005:207.)

number of the sensory systems, including the auditory circuit. The auditory pathways are complex and involve the following synaptic connections: first-order root fibers of the spiral ganglion, which originate in the cochlea (organ of Corti), synapse in the cochlear nuclei of the upper medulla; second-order neurons, which project through lateral lemnisci, terminate bilaterally in the inferior colliculus; third-order neurons project to the medial geniculate nucleus; and fourth-order neurons project to the superior temporal gyrus (primary auditory cortex).

Vestibular pathway.   First-order neurons originate from vestibular ganglia and have peripheral processes located in specialized receptors in the utricle, saccule, and semicircular canals. The central branches of this neuron reach the brain and terminate in the vestibular nuclei. Second-order neurons may pass to the cerebellar cortex (flocculonodular lobe) or project directly into the medial longitudinal fasciculus, where the fibers may run in a rostral or a caudal direction, terminating in the cranial nerves III, IV, or VI of the midbrain and pons or spinal cord, respectively. Damage to these fibers, especially within the medial longitudinal fasciculus or cerebellum, produces nystagmus (ie, involuntary movement of the eyes, in the horizontal or vertical plane, first slowly and then followed by a rapid, jerking return).

Taste pathway.   First-order neurons from cranial nerves VII, IX and X pass to the solitary nucleus. Second-order neurons project to VPM nucleus of thalamus. Third-order neurons project to lateral aspect of postcentral gyrus.

MOTOR SYSTEMS

Voluntary motor control affecting mainly the flexor system is expressed through the descending pyramidal tracts plus the rubrospinal tract, and control of functions associated with posture is mediated through such descending pathways as the vestibulo- and reticulospinal tracts. Modulation of motor functions is mediated by the basal ganglia and cerebellum. Involuntary motor disturbances at rest (called dyskinesias) are associated with the disruption of functions of the basal ganglia, and motor disturbances occurring during attempts at movement are frequently associated with damage to the cerebellum or its afferent or efferent pathways.

I. The basal ganglia consist of the neostriatum (caudate nucleus and putamen), the paleostriatum (globus pallidus), and two additional structures that are anatomically and functionally related to the basal ganglia—the substantia nigra and subthalamic nucleus.

A. Disorders of the basal ganglia

1. Parkinson disease: characterized by "pill rolling" tremor, akinesia (poverty of movement), and cog-wheel rigidity. This disorder is due to a reduction in striatal dopamine following a loss of dopamine neurons in the pars compacta of the substantia nigra, which project to the neostriatum.

2. Chorea: characterized by short, jerky movements of the distal extremities at rest. It is associated with lesions of the striatum.

One form of chorea, called Huntington chorea, is an autosomal dominant disorder that is associated with a chromosomal mutation. It results in destruction of GABAergic and cholinergic neurons in the caudate nucleus, and there is concomitant loss of neurons in the prefrontal regions of the neocortex.

3. Athetosis: characterized by slow, writhing movements of the extremities and muscles of the neck. The lesion may involve the striatum.

4. Hemiballism: characterized by wild (flailing) movements of the limbs on one side of the body. It is due to damage of the subthalamic nucleus on the contralateral side.

B. Disorders of the cerebellum

The cerebellum consists of two hemispheres and a medial region called the vermis. The cortex contains three layers, a granule cell layer, which receives most inputs from elsewhere in the CNS, a one-celled middle layer called the Purkinje cell layer, whose axon projects to deep cerebellar nuclei, and a molecular layer, which contains mainly fibers (parallel fibers of granule cell neurons) passing from one region of cerebellum to other regions. Below the cortex lies white matter and below the white matter deep cerebellar nuclei. The deep cerebellar nuclei project directly to brain stem and thalamic nuclei associated with motor functions. The deep cerebellar nuclei consist of the following:

Dentate nucleus: located laterally; it receives input from lateral aspect of hemisphere and projects via superior cerebellar peduncle to ventrolateral nucleus of thalamus

Interposed nuclei: located at midlateral position; receives input from midlateral (paravermal aspect of cerebellar cortex) and projects via superior cerebellar peduncle to red nucleus of midbrain

Fastigial nucleus: located medially; receives inputs from vermal aspect of cerebellar cortex and projects via axons (called the juxtarestiform body and uncinate fasciculus of Russell) adjacent to inferior and superior cerebellar peduncles to vestibular nuclei and reticular formation of pons and medulla

1. Anterior lobe (paleocerebellum): characterized by a wide, staggering-gait ataxia resulting primarily from damage that affects the vermal and paravermal regions of the anterior lobe.

2. Posterior lobe (neocerebellum): characterized most frequently by loss of coordination while executing voluntary movements.

3. Flocculonodular lobe (archicerebellum): characterized by a loss of equilibrium with the patient displaying a wide, staggering ataxic gait. Lesions of this region also produce eye movement disorders, including nystagmus.

HIGHER AUTONOMIC AND BEHAVIORAL FUNCTIONS

Control of autonomic and endocrine functions as well as emotional behavior are mediated by the limbic system, hypothalamus, and midbrain periaqueductal gray matter. Interrelationships among these three groups of structures are as follows:

I. For the expression of emotional behavior, such as rage and autonomic functions, these are mediated from the medial hypothalamus → midbrain periaqueductal gray → autonomic (ie, neurons in lower medulla that regulate heart rate, blood pressure, and respiration) and somatomotor neurons (ie, neurons of the trigeminal nerve that control vocalization) and autonomic and somatomotor neurons of the spinal cord. These processes are further regulated by different groups of neurons within the limbic system (ie, hippocampal formation, amygdala, septal area), which produce their effects by projecting directly or indirectly to the hypothalamus or midbrain periaqueductal gray.

II. For the regulation of endocrine functions, these are mediated from the supraoptic and paraventricular nuclei of the hypothalamus → posterior lobe of the pituitary, and from the medial hypothalamus → anterior lobe of the pituitary (via the vascular system). Limbic projections to the hypothalamus enable structures such as the hippocampal formation, amygdala, and septal area to modulate endocrine functions of the hypothalamus. Disruption of hypothalamic neurons may alter the mechanism for the expression of rage behavior and, likewise, affect temperature regulation, sexual behavior, feeding, drinking, and endocrine functions. Damage to neurons of the limbic system frequently leads to temporal lobe epilepsy and changes in the threshold for the expression of rage behavior (ie, when different groups of neurons in the amygdala are damaged, heightened aggressiveness or a reduction in aggression, such as the Klüver-Bucy syndrome, may ensue). Damage to the hippocampal formation can result in temporal lobe epilepsy and short-term memory deficits.

CEREBRAL CORTEX

Dysfunctions associated with cerebrovascular accidents and tumors can be understood in terms of the principles of cortical localization and cerebral dominance. Following is a list of common disorders, their descriptions, and the cortical regions most closely associated with each disorder.

UMN paralysis.   Damage to the precentral, premotor, and supplementary motor areas (as well as the internal capsule, crus cerebri, or corticospinal tracts), resulting in a loss of voluntary control of the upper and lower limbs, depending upon the extent of the lesion. This disorder is also associated with hyperreflexia, hypertonicity, and a positive Babinski sign.

Broca aphasia.   Damage to the inferior frontal gyrus of the dominant hemisphere. The patient cannot speak fluently but has no difficulty in comprehending spoken language.

Wernicke aphasia.   Damage to the region of the superior temporal gyrus and/or adjoining regions. The patient has difficulty in comprehending language, but speech appears fluent.

Astereognosia.   Damage to the parietal cortex of the contralateral side results in a failure of tactile recognition of objects.

Unilateral sensory (hemi) neglect.   Damage to the parietal lobe (usually of the right hemisphere) can cause this disorder. The patient typically ignores stimuli on the opposite (ie, left) side of body space, which includes visual, somatosensory, and auditory stimuli. The individual will neglect the opposite side of the body by, for example, neglecting to shave that side of the face and by denying that there is anything wrong with that side of the body, which may include a motor paralysis. The patient may further draw a picture of flowers or of a clock in which the petals on the flowers or the numbers on the clock are limited to the right side of each of the figures.

Apraxia.   Damage to the posterior parietal cortex can prevent an individual from conceptualizing the sequence of events necessary to carry out a task, even though the basic sensory and motor pathways necessary to produce the required movements are intact. In effect, the patient is thus unable to carry out the task.

Gross Anatomy of the Brain

Questions

Questions 1 to 35: Match each of the following vignettes with the region most likely affected. Each lettered option may be used once, more than once, or not at all.

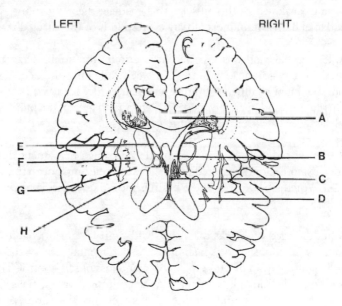

1. A 65-year-old woman is admitted to the emergency room after she was found unconscious by a family member. She is diagnosed as having had a cerebrovascular accident. A few days later, she regains consciousness but is unable to move her right leg. An MRI reveals evidence of some brain damage. Which labeled area of the brain most closely corresponds to the affected region?

2. As a result of a tumor localized to the right hemisphere of the cerebellum, a 55-year-old male patient displays abnormalities in voluntary movements. These include slowness in the initiation of movements and irregular and uncoordinated movements of the upper limbs with a distinct lack of smoothness in the overall response. Which labeled area of the brain normally supplies the cerebellum and provides important afferent information essential for the integration of smooth, purposeful movements of the upper limbs?

3. A patient admitted to a local hospital presents with difficulties in swallowing, chewing, breathing, and speaking. Further examination reveals significant weakness of the muscles that mediate these functions. Which labeled area of the brain most closely corresponds to the affected region?

4. A 25-year-old man was involved in a serious automobile accident that resulted in a major head injury. One week following the accident, the patient exhibited significant short-term memory deficit as well as heightened irritability and aggressiveness. Which labeled area of the brain is most closely associated with the affected region?

5. A 42-year-old woman was diagnosed as having a movement disorder. Further examination suggested that she was suffering from Huntington disease. Which labeled area of the brain is most likely associated with this disorder?

6. A middle-aged male was diagnosed with impairment of cognitive and personality functions such as inability to sustain mental activity, show flexibility in shifting from one task to another, and loss of self-control. The rostral aspect of the frontal lobe, including the prefrontal cortex, plays a major role in these functions, and damage to this region of the cortex produces major intellectual impairment. Which labeled area of the brain serves as a major afferent source to the frontal region of the cortex?

7. A 68-year-old man presents with a tremor at rest, slowness of voluntary movement, and upon further examination, increased resistance to passive movement of the limbs. This disorder is associated with a loss of dopamine to which labeled area of the brain?

Questions 8 to 15

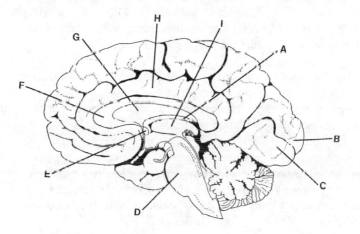

8. A 38-year-old male reports a loss of the ability to smell. Further examination reveals that this patient was suffering from a peripheral neuropathy of the olfactory nerve. Which labeled area of the brain would be most affected in terms of loss of neural transmission?

9. A 67-year-old female was admitted to a hospital after she reported to her primary care physician that she had been having very painful headaches. Further examination revealed the presence of significant increases in intracranial pressure. After viewing a magnetic resonance imaging (MRI), the neurologist concluded that the woman's condition was due to the presence of a tumor, which was developing along the rostral aspect of the medial wall of the lateral ventricle. Which labeled area of the brain would be most likely to contain this tumor?

10. A 47-year-old male who had a reputation of very friendly and quiet individual suddenly displayed marked changes in his personality. In particular, he became short-tempered, impulsive, and threatening to his colleagues in response to what most people would consider innocuous statements. He was referred to the psychiatric ward of the community hospital, and an MRI revealed a cortical tumor. Which labeled area of the brain is most likely to contain this tumor?

11. An 83-year-old woman was brought to the hospital after having received a routine eye examination, which revealed that she could not see out of the lower half of her left visual field. An MRI revealed evidence that she had experienced a cerebrovascular accident. Which labeled area of the brain was most likely affected by the stroke?

12. An investigator wishes to determine the effects of stimulation of the output neurons of the hippocampal formation upon excitability levels of the target neurons in the diencephalon. In which labeled area of the brain should he place the stimulating electrode?

13. A 69-year-old woman was admitted to the hospital after being diagnosed with a stroke. After a few days, she presented with difficulty in performing voluntary movements, she lacked coordination, and her movements were clearly jerky in appearance. Which labeled area of the brain is the most likely locus of the lesion?

14. An elderly man began to experience periods of alterations in consciousness, affective and related behavioral states, as well as hallucinations. The patient also complained of having some difficulty seeing. An ophthalmological examination revealed that he had an upper quadrantanopia. This patient was later found to have had a tumor of the temporal lobe, which disrupted axons mediating visual information. Which labeled area of the brain reflects the region that is now deprived of these visual signals?

15. A 48-year-old man had been suffering from epilepsy for a number of years. Drug treatment for this disorder had not been successful and, moreover, in recent months, seizure activity had begun to spread to other regions of the brain, including the opposite side of the brain. For this condition, surgery was indicated in order to reduce the spread of the seizures. Which labeled area of the brain would most likely be targeted by the neurosurgeon?

Questions 16 to 24

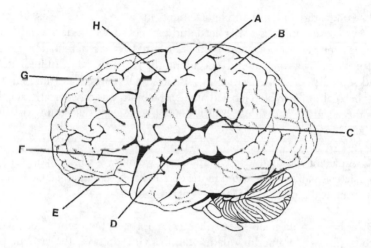

16. A patient brought into surgery for localization of a brain tumor was given an MRI and asked to move the fingers of his right hand. Which labeled area of the brain is the most likely location where the MRI would display a population response of neuronal activation?

17. A patient presented with loss of capacity to experience the feeling of a tuning fork when applied to the right leg. The diagnosis indicated that the patient suffered a stroke that affected a limited region within the cerebral cortex. Which labeled area of the brain was most likely affected by this lesion?

18. A patient experienced great difficulty in appreciating the meaning of spoken or written words. Which labeled area of the brain is the most likely locus of a lesion that would cause such a deficit?

19. After having received a head injury, a 23-year-old male complained of a partial loss of hearing. An MRI revealed evidence of brain injury. Which labeled area of the brain is the most likely locus of such damage?

20. An elderly patient, who had been diagnosed with a brain tumor, finds that he is unable to verbally express his thoughts in a meaningful way. Which labeled area of the brain is the most likely location of such a lesion?

21. Following an automobile accident in which a 23-year-old male received severe injuries to his head and parts of his body, he was admitted to the emergency room and then transferred to a rehabilitation center. Approximately a week after the accident, the patient became quite irritable and scored poorly on card sorting, delayed alternation, and measures of intellectual skills. Which labeled area of the brain was most clearly affected by the accident and direct injury could most readily account for these deficits?

22. A patient was unable to voluntarily move his eyes to the right. An MRI revealed a small tumor located in the cerebral cortex. Which labeled area of the brain is the most likely location of this tumor?

23. A 66-year-old male suffered a stroke of the right cerebral cortex that produced a right inferior quadrantanopia. In addition, the patient presented with a finger agnosia where he was unable to recognize the fingers on his or other people's hands; he had difficulty in writing and difficulty in distinguishing left from right, which led to difficulties in reading. Which labeled area of the brain is most closely associated with these deficits?

24. A 78-year-old man is found unconscious on the ground one morning and taken to the emergency room of a nearby hospital. After regaining consciousness, he is unable to move his right hand or leg. Which labeled area of the brain was most likely directly affected by the stroke?

Questions 25 to 35

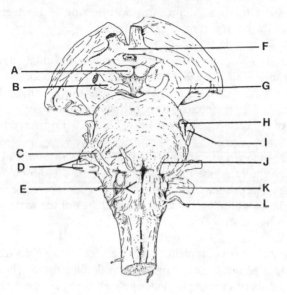

25. A 48-year-old woman complained of stomach pains. The diagnosis revealed an ulceration of the stomach wall due to overactivity of the parasympathetic input to the stomach. It was recommended that the patient have the cranial nerve, which innervates the stomach wall, partially severed. Which labeled area of the brain was most likely affected?

26. An MRI administered to a patient revealed the presence of a tumor situated in the region of the cerebellopontine angle. The patient noted considerable weakness when attempting to bite. Which labeled area of the brain was most likely affected?

27. Which labeled area of the brain shown in the illustration will likely affect the integrity of the Papez circuit, causing disruption of memory and emotional processes?

28. A 28-year-old man was exposed to very cold temperatures for several days and noted sometime afterward that he was unable to smile and display other aspects of facial expression on one side of his face. Which labeled area of the brain was most likely affected?

29. A 78-year-old woman was admitted to a local hospital after finding that she was unable to move her right arm and leg. In addition, she displayed diminution in strength of chewing, facial expression, and speech. An MRI revealed the presence of a tumor situated in the brain stem. Which labeled area of the brain would most likely be affected by the tumor?

30. A 63-year-old man was admitted to the emergency room and received an MRI, which indicated the presence of a vascular occlusion of a part of the brain stem. The patient was unable to feel any sensation on the left side of his face, chin, and forehead. Which labeled area of the brain was most likely affected by the stroke?

31. A 30-year-old man complained that he was having difficulty seeing properly and, in particular, was experiencing double vision. The ophthalmologist noted that the patient's right eye was normally abducted downward and the pupil was dilated. A subsequent MRI indicated the presence of a tumor impinging upon a cranial nerve. Which labeled area of the brain was most likely affected?

32. A neurological examination was given to a 60-year-old female because she was experiencing double vision and was unable to abduct the left eye. The examination revealed the likely presence of a small lesion of the brain stem. Which labeled area of the brain was most likely affected by this lesion?

33. An individual complained about having headaches and experiencing partial blindness, which were later identified as a bitemporal hemianopsia. A neurological examination, including an MRI, indicated that the patient had a brain tumor. Which labeled area of the brain was most likely affected by the tumor?

34. A 43-year-old female experienced dizziness, loss of balance, some nystagmus, and ringing in the ear. A neurological examination suggested damage to a cranial nerve, perhaps associated with a small peripheral tumor. Which labeled area of the brain was most likely affected?

35. Following her admission to the emergency room of a local hospital, a 71-year-old female received a diagnosis of having had a small brain stem stroke. After 2 weeks, the patient appeared normal, with the exception that her tongue deviated to the left side when she was asked to protrude it. Which labeled area of the brain was most clearly affected by the stroke?

36. A young boy was admitted to the emergency room after having experienced severe nausea, headache, and fever. The neurologist concluded that he was suffering from a form of bacterial meningitis. His cerebrospinal fluid (CSF) would most likely indicate which of the following?

a. Increased protein, decreased glucose, decreased neutrophils
b. Increased protein, decreased glucose, increased neutrophils
c. Increased protein, normal glucose, normal neutrophils
d. Decreased CSF pressure, decreased protein, decreased glucose
e. Decreased protein, normal CSF pressure, increased glucose

37. Following an automobile accident, a teenage boy was admitted to the emergency room and diagnosed as having a subarachnoid hemorrhage. Which of the following CSF findings would be expected in this individual?

a. Increased CSF pressure, bloody appearance of CSF, increased red cells, increased protein, decreased glucose
b. Decreased CSF pressure, bloody appearance of CSF, decreased red cells, decreased protein, decreased glucose
c. Normal pressure, normal red cells, increased protein, increased glucose, normal color of CSF
d. Clear CSF, normal pressure, decreased protein, increased red cells, increased glucose
e. Cloudy CSF, increased CSF, increased neutrophils, normal protein, normal glucose

38. A 70-year-old male was brought to the emergency room after experiencing headaches, nausea, and dizziness. An MRI revealed the presence of a brain tumor, which had produced a noncommunicating hydrocephalus. Which of the following is the most likely location of the tumor?

a. Cerebral subarachnoid space
b. Cistern of the lamina terminalis
c. Interventricular foramen
d. Pontine cistern
e. Cisterna magna

39. A fundamental basis underlying the application of drugs for the treatment of emotional and related disorders includes which of the following properties associated with the blood-brain barrier?

a. It has well-developed capillary pores that allow for selective diffusion of substances.
b. It is selectively permeable to certain compounds such as biogenic amines.
c. It is found within all structures enclosed by the meninges, including the pineal gland.
d. It contains junctions associated with the blood-brain barrier, which are formed exclusively by neuronal or glial processes.
e. It is restricted to highly vascular regions of the brain, such as those present at the level of the ventromedial hypothalamus.

Gross Anatomy of the Brain

Answers

1 to 7. The answers are 1-F, 2-H, 3-G, 4-B, 5-D, 6-E, 7-D. *(Ropper, pp 436-437. Siegel and Sapru, pp 6-12, 327-339, 450-452.)* This figure is a horizontal view of the brain at the level of the head of the caudate nucleus and the internal capsule. The posterior limb of the internal capsule (F) contains fibers that arise from the leg region of the cerebral cortex and project to lumbar levels of the spinal cord, thus serving as upper motor neurons (UMNs) for the elicitation of voluntary movement of the contralateral leg (because the corticospinal tract crosses in the lower medulla as the pyramidal decussation). Fibers in the anterior limb of the internal capsule (H) project in large numbers to deep pontine nuclei and represent first-order neurons in a pathway linking the cerebral cortex with the cerebellum. These fibers comprise a part of the reciprocal feedback circuit, linking the cerebellar and cerebral cortices. These fibers form part of a disynaptic pathway (through synaptic contacts in the deep pontine nuclei) that supply those regions of the cerebellar hemisphere essential for the expression of smooth, coordinated movements of the limb. Pseudobulbar palsy is characterized in part by a weakness of the muscles controlling swallowing, chewing, breathing, and speaking. It results from a lesion of the UMNs associated with the head region of the cortex, which pass through the genu of the internal capsule (G) en route to brain stem cranial nerve nuclei upon which they synapse. The descending column of the fornix (B), situated along the midline of the brain, contains fibers that arise from the hippocampal formation and project to the septal area and medial hypothalamus, including the mammillary bodies. This pathway plays an important role in the regulation of emotional behavior and short-term memory functions. Disruption of the hippocampal formation or its output pathway, the fornix, would affect levels of emotionality and short-term memory.

The head of the caudate nucleus (D) is part of an important element of the motor systems called the *basal ganglia*. Together with the putamen (not shown in this figure), it receives significant inputs from several regions associated with motor functions. These include the cerebral cortex and the dopamine-containing region of the substantia nigra (ie, the pars compacta). Loss of dopaminergic input to the neostriatum is associated with Parkinson disease. Loss of dopaminergic inputs to the neostriatum from the substantia nigra results in Parkinson disease. Huntington disease is associated with a loss of γ-aminobutyric acid (GABA) levels within the neostriatum and, in particular, the caudate nucleus. The mediodorsal thalamic nucleus (E) projects large quantities of axons to extensive regions of the rostral half of the frontal lobe, including the prefrontal cortex. It also receives significant projections from the prefrontal region of the cortex.

8 to 15. The answers are 8-E, 9-G, 10-H, 11-B, 12-A, 13-D, 14-C, 15-F. (*Afifi, pp 27-38. Siegel and Sapru, pp 8-13, 287-289, 312-315.*) This figure is a midsagittal section of the brain. A major portion of the anterior commissure (E) contains fibers mediating olfactory signals that arise from the olfactory bulb and decussate to the contralateral olfactory bulb. The septum pellucidum (G) forms the medial wall of the lateral ventricle, which in fact separates the lateral ventricle on one side from that on the opposite side. The cingulate gyrus (H) is a prominent structure on the medial aspect of the cerebral cortex and constitutes a component of the limbic lobe. As part of the limbic system, its functions relate in part to the regulation of emotional behavior. Accordingly, tumors of this region have resulted in marked changes in emotionality. The primary visual cortex lies on both banks of the calcarine fissure. Cells located on the upper bank of this fissure (B) receive inputs from the lateral geniculate nucleus that relate to the contralateral upper retina, corresponding to the lower visual field. Therefore, a lesion of this region would result in a lower visual field deficit.

The major output pathway of the hippocampal formation is the fornix system of fibers (A), which arises from cells in its subicular cortex and adjoining regions of the hippocampus. These fibers are then distributed to the anterior thalamic nucleus, mammillary bodies, and septal area. Accordingly, the most effective way of activating the output pathways of the hippocampal formation would be to stimulate these fibers of the fornix. The basilar portion of the pons (D) lies in the ventral half of this region of the brain stem. It receives inputs from each of the lobes of the cerebral cortex, which it then relays to the cerebellar cortex. As noted in the answer to Question 2, this circuit mediates functions associated with the regulation of voluntary movements of the limbs. Disruption of any part of this circuit, whether at the level of the internal capsule or basilar pons, would affect inputs from the cerebral cortex to the hemispheres of the cerebellar cortex, thus eliminating key inputs necessary for the expression of smooth, coordinated movements (thus, resulting in an "action tremor"). With respect to the neurons located on the lower bank of the calcarine fissure (C), they receive inputs from the lateral geniculate nucleus that pass through the temporal lobe and relate to the lower retinal (or upper temporal) visual fields. Therefore, a tumor of this region would produce behavioral and electrophysiological manifestations of epilepsy, resulting in an upper quadrantanopia (ie, loss of one quarter of the visual field). The corpus callosum (F) constitutes the major channel by which the cerebral cortex on one side can communicate with the cortex of the opposite side. In order to stop the spread of seizures from one hemisphere to the other (when the seizures are severe), cutting of the corpus callosum is carried out.

16 to 24. The answers are 16-H, 17-A, 18-C, 19-D, 20-F, 21-E, 22-G, 23-C, 24-H. (*Nolte, pp 55-60, 69-75. Ropper, pp 446-449. Siegel and Sapru, pp 6-8, 331-335, 475-491.*) This figure is a lateral view of the cerebral cortex. Cells in the "arm" area of the primary motor cortex (H) project their axons to the cervical level of the spinal cord and are activated at the time when a response of this limb occurs. The stroke affected the leg region of the left primary somatosensory cortex (A). It lies immediately caudal to the central sulcus, is almost devoid of pyramidal cells, is referred to as a *granulous cortex*, and receives inputs from the right leg. Damage to this region would result in loss of vibration sensibility (as well as tactile sensation and two-point discrimination) from the right leg. Damage to the cells situated in the region of the dorsal border of the superior temporal gyrus and the adjoining area of the inferior parietal lobule (Wernicke area [receptive aphasia]); (C) causes impairment in the appreciation of the meanings of written or spoken words.

The primary, secondary, and tertiary auditory receiving areas in the cortex are located mainly in the superior temporal gyrus (D). It is the final receiving area for inputs from the medial geniculate nucleus, which represents an important relay in the transmission of auditory signals to the cortex. Damage to this region of the cortex would result in some hearing loss. An additional area of the cortex governing speech (F) is called the *motor speech area*, or *Broca (expressive aphasia) area*. It is situated in the inferior aspect of the frontal lobe immediately rostral and slightly ventral to the precentral gyrus. Lesions of this region produce impairment of the ability to express words in a meaningful way or to use words correctly. The orbital frontal cortex (E) lies in a position inferior and rostral to Broca motor speech area. This region governs higher order intellectual functions and some aspects of emotional behavior. Damage to this region often results in personality changes and emotionality. The caudal aspect of the middle frontal gyrus (G) contains cells that, when activated, produce conjugate deviation of the eyes. This action is believed to be accomplished, in part, by virtue of descending projections to the superior colliculus, pretectal region, and horizontal gaze center of the pons. A lesion of this region would result in loss of capacity to produce voluntary horizontal movement of the eyes in one direction. Lesions of the inferior parietal lobule (C) can produce a homonymous inferior quadrantanopia (in the case shown on the diagram where the left side of the brain is displayed, it would be a right homony-mous quadrantanopia where there is loss of bilateral vision in the inferior quadrant of the visual field). In addition, lesions of inferior parietal lobule can also result in Gerstmann syndrome, in which the patient is unable to recognize different fingers on his or other people's hands and is unable to write, distinguish left from right, or read effectively. The precentral gyrus (H) constitutes the primary motor cortex. Lesions of this region produce a UMN paralysis involving a contralateral limb.

25 to 35. The answers are 25-K, 26-H, 27-A, 28-C, 29-G, 30-I, 31-B, 32-J, 33-F, 34-D, 35-L. *(Nolte, pp 266-293. Siegel and Sapru, pp 13-15, 223-250, 280-285, 330-339, 447-453.)* This figure is a ventral view of the brain stem. Fibers that arise from the dorsal motor nucleus and nucleus ambiguus (in part) exit the brain on the lateral side of the medulla as part of the vagus nerve (K) and innervate the myenteric plexus and smooth muscles of the stomach, which normally function to produce gastric secre-tions. Cutting some of these fibers would result in a reduction in gastric secretions. The tumor affected the motor component of the trigeminal nerve. (H) The motor root lies medial to the sensory root and innervates the muscles of mastication. The mammillary bodies (A), which lie on the ventral surface of the brain at the caudal aspect of the hypothalamus, receive many of their inputs from the hippocampal formation and project to the anteroventral thalamic nucleus as the mammillothalamic tract, which in turn send their axons to the cingulate gyrus and then back to the hippocampal formation, forming what is referred to as the Papez circuit. This circuit has been associated with memory functions and the regulation of emotional behavior. The facial nerve (C) exits the brain at the level of the ventrolateral aspect of the caudal pons, and its special visceral efferent component innervates the muscles of facial expression. Damage to this nerve causes loss of facial expression on the side of the face ipsilateral to the affected nerve.

The cerebral peduncle (G) is situated in the ventrolateral aspect of the midbrain and contains fibers of cortical origin that project to all levels of the neuraxis of the brain stem and spinal cord. A lesion in this region would affect UMNs that control motor functions associated with both the body and the head region, producing diminution in strength of the muscles of the ipsilateral head and paralysis of the contralateral leg and arm. Note that the selection of choice E, the pyramids, would not have been correct, since the fibers present at this level can only terminate within the medulla or spinal cord, and therefore could not account for the loss of muscle strength associated with the head. First order somatosensory fibers from the region of the face enter the brain laterally at the level of the middle of the pons as the sensory root of the trigeminal nerve (I). Damage to this nerve would cause loss of sensation associated with the face. The oculomotor nerve (B) exits the brain at the level of the ventromedial aspect of the midbrain, and some fibers of the general somatic efferent component of this nerve innervate the medial rectus. Damage to this component results in a loss of ability for medial gaze, and the eye will additionally be directed downward because of the unopposed action of cranial nerve IV. Another component of the oculomotor nerve, the general visceral efferent, constitutes the preganglionic parasympathetic neuron in a disynaptic pathway whose postganglionic division innervates the pupillary constrictor muscles. Accordingly, damage to the preganglionic division results in loss of pupillary constriction, which would normally occur in the presence of light as well as in accommodation. In this case, the eye will dilate following damage to preganglionic neurons of CN III because of the unopposed action of the sympathetic fibers. The abducens nerve (J) exits the brain at a ventromedial position at the level of the medulla-pontine border, and its fibers innervate the lateral rectus muscle. Damage to this nerve results in an ipsilateral gaze paralysis.

The optic chiasm (F) contains fibers that cross over to reach the lateral geniculate nucleus on the side contralateral to the retina from which they originated. Such fibers are associated with the nasal retinal (ie, temporal or lateral) visual fields. Therefore, damage to the optic chiasm will cause blindness in the lateral half of each of the visual fields. Such a deficit is referred to as *bitemporal hemianopsia*. First-order neurons from the labyrinth organs (D) (ie, semicircular canals, saccule, and utricle) convey information concerning the position of the head in space along the vestibular component of the eighth nerve into the central nervous system (CNS). This nerve enters the brain laterally at the level of the upper medulla. Damage to this nerve could result in symptoms such as ringing in the ear, nystagmus, loss of balance, and dizziness. The hypoglossal nerve (L) exits the brain at the level of the middle of the medulla between the pyramid and the olive. These fibers innervate muscles that move the tongue toward the opposite side. For this reason, a lesion of the hypoglossal nucleus or its nerve will result in a deviation of the tongue to the side of the lesion because of the unopposed action of the contralateral hypoglossal nerve, which remains intact.

36. The answer is b. (*Aminoff, pp 33-365. Afifi, pp 255, 379, 574.*) In individuals suffering from bacterial meningitis, the CSF is under increased pressure. Glucose levels are low relative to serum levels because of one or more of the following: glucose utilization by the bacteria, reduced glucose transport at the choroid plexus, increased glucose transport out of the CSF by breakdown of the blood-brain barrier, and edema; neutrophils are increased in response to the bacteria, and protein is also increased, possibly because of a subarachnoid block, loss of tight junctions, and leaky capillaries.

37. The answer is a. (*Afifi, pp 255, 379. Siegel and Sapru, pp 39-43.*) As a result of a subarachnoid hemorrhage, the CSF is bloody. Due to bleeding into the subarachnoid space, there is an increase in CSF pressure as a result of a rupture of an intracranial artery. The presence of blood will increase protein levels and red cells, while glucose levels will be reduced.

38. The answer is c. (*Siegel and Sapru, pp 42-43.*) A noncommunicating hydrocephalus is the result of an obstruction of one of the channels connecting one ventricle to the next, or the outflow of the fourth ventricle through its foramina, resulting in an enlargement of one or more of the ventricles. In the choices given for this question, the interventricular foramen, connecting the lateral with the third ventricle, is the only possible correct answer. A blockade of the interventricular foramen would lead to an enlargement of the lateral ventricle.

39. The answer is b. (*Kandel, pp 1288-1294. Siegel and Sapru, p 42.*) The blood-brain barrier is selectively permeable to certain types of substances, such as biogenic amines, and not to others, due mainly to such factors as the size, polarity, and charge of the molecules. The barrier is formed by tight junctions consisting of capillary endothelial cells that are frequently in contact with the glial end-feet of astrocytes. The barrier does not contain well-developed capillary pores. It is not found within circumventricular organs, such as the subfornical organ and the pineal gland, but it is applied to all other brain tissues.

Development

Questions

40. Upon examination of a 3-month-old infant, it is discovered that the anterior neuropore had failed to close. Which of the following deficits is most likely to appear?

a. Mental retardation
b. Loss of tactile sensation
c. Problems in ability to swallow
d. Loss of reflex activity
e. Respiratory difficulties

41. A 4-year-old child has marked difficulties in learning and also had difficulties in motor functions. Magnetic resonance imaging (MRI) reveals the presence of brain damage resulting from the failure of closure of the anterior neuropore. Which of the following regions is most likely to be affected by this disorder?

a. Medulla
b. Pons
c. Midbrain
d. Diencephalon
e. Cerebral cortex

42. A parent brings her son to a pediatric neurologist because he exhibits a number of serious neurological signs. These included lack of coordination, especially around the region of the trunk, vomiting, lack of ability to develop new motor skills, and headaches. An MRI reveals an enlarged cranium, a large cyst which appears to replace much of the cerebellum, and reduction in the size of the corpus callosum. Which of the following is the most likely diagnosis?

a. Pyramidal tract syndrome
b. Spina bifida
c. Anencephaly
d. Dandy-Walker syndrome
e. Meningomyelocele

43. A 15-month-old girl was brought to a pediatrician after her mother realized that the child did not respond to any kind of sensory stimulation of any of her limbs. Careful examination of the baby also revealed that she expressed significant lack of autonomic control. It was concluded that the child suffered from a rare disorder in which neural crest cells failed to develop. Which of the following cell types is most clearly affected by this abnormality?

a. Dorsal horn cells
b. Ventral horn cells
c. Dorsal root ganglion cells
d. Hypoglossal neurons
e. Intermediolateral cell column neurons

44. A 5-month-old boy was seen by a pediatric neurologist after his parents noted that he showed few signs of limb movement such as grasping and holding a bottle or attempts at crawling. In addition, the infant showed few signs of crying or expressing other sounds or facial expressions. It was concluded that a developmental abnormality occurred that selectively affected neurons derived from the basal plate. Which of the following cell groups would be preserved from such an abnormality?

a. Hypoglossal nucleus
b. Alpha motor neurons
c. Gamma motor neurons
d. Proper sensory nucleus
e. Abducens nucleus

45. A teenage girl complains about a loss of pain and temperature sensation around the region of her arms on both sides. A further analysis reveals that this dysfunction represents a congenital defect. Which of the following is the most likely diagnosis?

a. Arnold-Chiari malformation
b. Syringomyelia
c. Dandy-Walker syndrome
d. Anencephaly
e. Spina bifida

46. A developmental malformation was discovered in a 3-year-old boy. It presented as sensory and motor deficits of lower extremities as well as some back pain and bladder difficulties. Which of the following is the most likely diagnosis?

a. Dandy-Walker syndrome
b. Tethered cord
c. Spina bifida
d. Syringomyelia
e. Encephalocele

47. A 9-year-old girl was seen by an endocrinologist after it became apparent that her weight and height were below average and that her growth rate was also quite slow. Further analysis revealed the likelihood of the presence of a congenital malformation involving incomplete growth of the anterior pituitary. Which of the following is the most probable source of the developmental defect?

a. Basal plate
b. Alar plate
c. Sulcus limitans
d. Rhombic lips
e. Rathke pouch

48. A neonate was brought to a child neurologist at 3 months and displayed sensory-motor abnormalities and what appeared to be the presence of cognitive deficits as well. A neonatal developmental abnormality was discovered, possibly as the result of a cyst adjoining the choroid plexus of the lateral ventricle, causing reduced production of cerebrospinal fluid (CSF). Which of the following developmental zones is most likely associated with this dysfunction?

a. Basal plate
b. Alar plate
c. Neural crest
d. Roof plate
e. Floor plate

49. A neurological examination of a 6-month-old baby boy reveals that the cerebellum has failed to develop properly. It is concluded that the abnormality is related to a defect in the formation of which of the following?

a. Neural crest cells
b. Rhombic lips
c. Mesencephalon
d. Sulcus limitans
e. Telencephalon

50. A young child was admitted into the hospital emergency room with a history of episodes of vomiting, headaches, problems in acquisition of motor skills, cranial nerve dysfunction, and problems in breathing. To which of the following disorders does this combination of syndromes most closely relate?

a. Cleft palate
b. Hydrocephalus
c. Anencephaly
d. Syringomyelia
e. Congenital aneurysm

51. A brain MRI scan taken from a 6-month-old baby reveals that while the overall size of the cerebral cortex is normal, the size of the pyramidal tracts is considerably smaller than normal. Which of the following is the most likely explanation for this defect?

a. Reduction in the numbers of cortical neurons giving rise to pyramidal tract fibers
b. Reduction in the numbers of synaptic contacts made by cortical granule cells
c. Reduction in the extent of myelin found on pyramidal tract neurons
d. Reduction in the amount of neurotransmitter released by pyramidal tract neurons
e. Reduction in the numbers of glial cells attached to pyramidal tract neurons

52. A laboratory developed an animal model whose basic feature was that it caused selective neuronal death as a function of apoptosis. The most likely mechanism underlying this form of cell death is associated with which of the following?

a. Stimulation of an afferent nerve fiber
b. Loss of acetylcholine released at nerve endings
c. The beginning of myelin formation
d. Elimination of nerve growth factor
e. Reduction in brain serotonin levels

53. A 23-year-old girl reported having headaches and later presented with cerebellar ataxia and spastic quadriparesis, all of which became progressively worse over time. What is the most likely diagnosis?

a. A stroke involving the cerebral cortex
b. Spina bifida
c. Arnold-Chiari malformation
d. Medial pontine tumor
e. Dandy-Walker syndrome

54. A 44-year-old male was seriously injured in an automobile accident and was admitted to a local hospital for diagnosis and treatment. The patient presented over time with gait disturbances, some dementia, and urinary incontinence. Measurement of CSF pressure was initially slightly above normal and then gradually fell down, reaching approximately normal levels but would occasionally rise above normal values. Further examination revealed that the patient had a subarachnoid hemorrhage. This patient is most likely suffering from which of the following?

a. Parkinson disease
b. Overt tension hydrocephalus
c. Occult hydrocephalus
d. Normal pressure hydrocephalus
e. Dandy-Walker syndrome

Development

Answers

40 and 41. The answers are 40-a, 41-e. *(Afifi, pp 337-343. Nolte, pp 46-51. Siegel and Sapru, pp 18-31.)* When the anterior neuropore fails to close, there are protrusions of CSF, glia, meninges, and neighboring brain tissue. This results in damage to the cerebral hemispheres and cerebellum. Accordingly, the damage to the cerebral hemispheres is directly related to the onset of mental retardation as well as motor dysfunctions. The other choices are more closely related to processes associated with the lower brain stem and spinal cord.

42. The answer is d. *(Afifi, pp 386-387. Nolte, pp 37-49. Siegel and Sapru, p 42.)* The constellation of neurological signs seen in this child is characteristic of the Dandy-Walker syndrome. It involves the presence of hydrocephalus and significant damage and reduction in the size of the cerebellum with its consequent loss of motor coordination and related functions. The other choices constitute developmental disorders affecting other regions of the central nervous system (CNS), such as the spinal cord or cerebral cortex, which do not produce the syndromes in this case.

43. The answer is c. *(Nolte, pp 37-48. Siegel and Sapru, pp 19-22.)* A number of structures, such as the dorsal root ganglia, sympathetic ganglia, and chromaffin cells of the adrenal medulla, are derived from neural crest cells. Failure in development of neural crest cells will affect, in part, dorsal root ganglia cells. Loss of these cells will principally eliminate first-order sensory neurons and the associated somatosensory information that normally is transmitted in relation to the body and limbs. In addition, failure of development of autonomic ganglia will seriously disrupt autonomic functions.

44. The answer is d. *(Nolte, pp 37-48. Siegel and Sapru, pp 19-22.)* Structures associated with sensory functions, such as the proper sensory nucleus of the dorsal horn of the spinal cord, are derived from the alar plate. In contrast, structures related to motor functions, and in particular, lower motor neurons controlling the limbs, including the hypoglossal and abducens nuclei and alpha and gamma motor neurons, are derived from the basal plate. Loss of these lower motor neurons would clearly account for the absence of movement of the limbs, inability to cry, and absence of facial expression.

45. The answer is b. *(Siegel and Sapru, pp 30-31.)* Syringo (hydro) myelia is a cavitation around the central canal of the spinal cord and is filled with CSF. Damage to this region is usually segmental in nature and would affect those fibers that cross in the spinal cord and include principally the spinothalamic tracts. Damage to these tracts because of the cavitation around the central canal would result in segmental loss of pain and temperature sensations.

46. The answer is b. *(Afifi, pp 337, 310. Siegel and Sapru, p 31.)* A tethered cord syndrome is characterized by a shortened and/or thickened filum terminale, resulting in the spinal cord becoming anchored to the subcutaneous tissue. This results in sensory and motor deficits in the lower extremities as well as bladder difficulties, back pain, and scoliosis.

47. The answer is e. *(Martin, p 364.)* The anterior lobe of the pituitary is formed as an in-pocket derivative of the ectodermal stomodeum, called Rathke pouch.

48. The answer is d. *(Nolte, pp 43-49. Siegel and Sapru, pp 27-28.)* The choroid plexus, which is associated with the production of CSF, is attached to the roof of the ventricles and is thus derived from the roof plate. Blockade of this region would reduce the production and flow of CSF and thus be a likely factor or cause of neonatal brain damage.

49. The answer is b. *(Nolte, pp 41-46. Siegel and Sapru, pp 24-26.)* The cerebellum is formed from the dorsolateral aspects of the alar plates, which bend medially and posteriorly to form the rhombic lips.

50. The answer is b. *(Afifi, pp 380-382)* The symptoms described are characteristic of hydrocephalus. Hydrocephalus may come about as a result of defects such as the failure of formation of the cerebellar vermis, the foramens of Magendie and Luschka, or the corpus callosum. There is an enlarged cranium as a result of the buildup of CSF, causing brain damage.

Several of the symptoms may also be caused by a compression of the posterior fossa and the absence of a cerebellar vermis. Cleft palate is a fissure of the medial aspect of the lip and would not result in the symptoms described previously. Anencephaly is the complete or partial absence of the brain and is not compatible with life. Syringomyelia is associated with bilateral segmental loss of pain and temperature. A congenital aneurysm can occur in a variety of places within the CNS and is typically associated with stroke in the adult.

51. The answer is c. (*Afifi, p 332. Siegel and Sapru, pp 69-70.*) Extensive myelination occurs in postnatal development. The failure of the pyramidal tracts to form myelin would account for the reduction in their size. In this particular situation, the size of the cerebral cortex was approximately normal, suggesting that there was no significant decrease in cortical cells. Variations in the transmitter formation and glial cells would not account for a reduction in the size of the pyramidal tract. Cortical granule cells do not contribute to the pyramidal tract.

52. The answer is d. (*Purves, pp 600-605.*) When nerve growth factor is eliminated, cell death results and involves fragmentation, shrinkage, and ultimate phagocytosis of the cell. Apoptosis is believed to be triggered by a biochemical process that causes transcription of a variety of genes. Nerve growth factor blocks the activation of this process. It should also be noted that this form of cell death differs from that occurring after nerve injury or trauma to the nerve. The other choices listed are unrelated to the process of apoptosis.

53. The answer is c. (*Ropper, pp 597, 972-974. Siegel and Sapru, pp 30-31.*) The Arnold-Chiari malformation with or without a meningomyelocele is characterized by a cerebellomedullary malformation that may not develop until adolescence or adult life. The results, in addition to producing severe headaches, cause cerebellar dysfunction and weakness and impaired movement of the limbs. Other choices are incorrect. A cortical stroke would not produce cerebellar signs; spina bifida would affect spinal cord functions; a medial pontine lesion would most clearly produce an upper motor neuron paralysis of the limbs and possible fifth nerve paralysis, but not cerebellar dysfunction; and a Dandy-Walker syndrome occurs typically at an earlier period of development rather than in adolescence or early adulthood.

54. The answer is d. *(Aminoff, pp 243-245. Ropper, pp 598 599.)* In normal pressure hydrocephalus, the patient may show gait disturbances, some dementia, and urinary incontinence, but does not display marked increases in CSF pressure. It can follow a head injury and intracranial hemorrhage, which indeed, occurred with respect to this patient. Overt tension hydrocephalus, occult hydrocephalus, and the Dandy-Walker syndrome typically occur in the first few years of life. Parkinson disease is not generally the result of head injury and this disorder is also associated with hypokinesia and rigidity.

Anatomical and Functional Properties of Neurons and Muscle

Questions

55. A 48-year-old male complains of pronounced shaking in both his left and right hands and arms (4-8 Hz) and the shaking also extends to his head. The patient also reports that the tremor of the hands and head subsides during walking, after taking an alcoholic drink, and after treatment with the β-adrenergic antagonist, propranol, but is exaggerated during states of anxiety. Which of the following is the most likely diagnosis?

a. Parkinson disease
b. Essential tremor
c. Dystonia
d. Cerebellar ataxia
e. Huntington disease

56. A 68-year-old female is examined by a neurologist after she experiences difficulties when attempting to walk. When the tendon in the right arm is passively stretched, it results in repetitive, involuntary, and rhythmic contractions of the muscles of that limb at an approximate rate of 5 to 7 Hz. The neurologist concluded that she had a lesion in which of the following area?

a. Cerebral cortex
b. Gray matter of spinal cord
c. Peripheral nerve in the right arm
d. Vermis of the flocculonodular lobe
e. Dorsomedial pontine tegmentum

57. A 32-year-old woman gave birth to a healthy 8.5 lb boy. After 2 months, she suddenly experienced "pins and needles" feeling in the fingers of her right hand, which she normally used to hold the baby. A neurological examination indicated that she was suffering from carpal tunnel syndrome. The anatomical site most commonly involved in this disorder is which of the following?

a. White matter of right cervical spinal cord
b. Right radial nerve
c. Right median nerve
d. Gray matter of right cervical spinal cord
e. Right axillary nerve

58. A 72-year-old male who had been suffering with diabetes for approximately 20 years was seen by a neurologist because of complaints about discomfort around his leg and difficulty in walking. The neurologist reported that the patient displayed weakness of extension of the leg, fixation of the knee, and some wasting of the quadriceps muscle. Which of the following is the most likely anatomical structure that was injured and responsible for these symptoms?

a. Sciatic nerve
b. Tibial nerve
c. Peroneal nerve
d. Femoral nerve
e. Lateral cutaneous nerve

59. An individual sustained a severe knife wound, damaging a spinal nerve adjoining its entry to the spinal cord. If one could examine this peripheral nerve and its cell body, which of the following events would most likely be observed?

a. A displacement of the nucleus toward the periphery of the cell
b. A mitotic division of the neuronal cell body
c. A more intense staining of the Nissl granules
d. Degeneration of processes along the axon proximal but not distal to the lesion
e. An initial loss of mitochondria in the axoplasm at nodes of Ranvier

60. A 65-year-old man is diagnosed with a form of a peripheral neuropathy. Which of the following effects will this disorder have upon the patient?

a. A loss in motor function, but sensory functions will remain largely intact
b. A reduction in conduction velocity of the affected nerve
c. An increase in the number of nodes of Ranvier
d. Degeneration of myelin but the axon will typically remain intact
e. Signs of an upper motor neuron (UMN) paralysis

61. Which of the following statements best characterizes a property of nerve cells?

a. Typically, one copy of the same peptide is cut from the same precursor molecule.
b. It is generally recognized that the cytosol provides the source of selective protein synthesis limited to neurotransmitters.
c. Cytosolic proteins show significant modification or processing following their translation.
d. Nuclear and mitochondrial proteins that are encoded by the cell's nucleus are targeted to their proper organelle by a process called *posttranslational importation*.
e. Secretory proteins undergo little or no modification or processing after translation.

62. Following an injury in the workplace that affected the right arm, causing loss of movement of that limb, it was determined that the injury disrupted axoplasmic transport in the sensory and motor nerves of that limb. Which of the following statements accurately reflects a basic property of axoplasmic transport?

a. Large membranous organelles are transported by slow axonal transport.
b. Cytosolic proteins are transported by fast transport.
c. Retrograde transport is generally limited to a fixed rate of movement of particles.
d. Anterograde transport is dependent upon microtubules.
e. The motor protein, kinesin, specifically governs slow axonal transport.

63. Which of the following statements correctly characterizes ion channels?

a. The passage of ions through ion channels typically requires an active mechanism.
b. A common stimulus serves as the basis for opening ion channels.
c. Exposure of a ligand-gated channel to continuous high concentrations of its ligand is the necessary and sufficient stimulus for opening that channel.
d. The opening or closing of an ion channel may be affected by the use of drugs.
e. The neuronal membrane is permeable to most polar and charged molecules.

64. The resting membrane potential is characterized by which of the following?

a. Passive fluxes of Na^+ and K^+ are balanced by an active pump that derives energy from enzymatic hydrolysis of adenosine $5'$-triphosphate (ATP).

b. A membrane is depolarized when the differences between the charges across the membrane are increased.

c. As the inside of the cell is made more negative with respect to the outside, the cell becomes depolarized.

d. In a cell whose membrane possesses only K^+ channels, the membrane potential cannot be determined.

e. The resting membrane potential is unrelated to the separation of the charge across the membrane.

65. Which of the following statements accurately characterizes a basic property of the length constant of a nerve fiber?

a. The length constant is the distance along a dendrite where the change in membrane potential produced by a current becomes stable.

b. The length constant increases as the membrane resistance increases.

c. The length constant increases as the axial resistance increases.

d. The length constant is greater in unmyelinated than in myelinated fibers.

e. As the length constant increases in a postsynaptic neuron, the efficiency of electronic conduction of synaptic potentials (at that synapse) decreases.

66. Ligand gating of neuronal membrane channels is a common mechanism following the binding of a neurotransmitter to a postsynaptic neuron. This mechanism is best characterized by which of the following?

a. The normal triggering mechanism for gating involves nonspecific binding by large classes of molecules.

b. Channels are opened when a given molecule selectively binds with the gating molecule.

c. Ligand gating is triggered by changes in the electrical potential across the membrane.

d. The channels are constructed of a mixture of proteins and lipids.

e. The gating molecule shows no conformational change during the gating process.

67. After the occurrence of an action potential, there is a repolarization of the membrane. Which of the following is the principal explanation for this event?

a. Potassium channels have been opened.

b. Sodium channels have been opened.

c. Potassium channels have been inactivated.

d. The membrane becomes impermeable to all ions.

e. There has been a sudden influx of calcium.

68. During an in vitro experiment, the membrane potential of a nerve cell is hyperpolarized to −120 mV. At that time, a transmitter, known to be inhibitory in function, is applied to the preparation and results in a depolarization of the membrane. Which of the following is the most likely reason for this occurrence?

a. Inhibitory transmitters normally depolarize the postsynaptic membrane.
b. The normal response of the postsynaptic membrane to any transmitter is depolarization.
c. The inhibitory transmitter activates ligand-gated potassium channels.
d. Sodium channels become inactivated.
e. Calcium channels become activated.

Questions 69 and 70

69. The neurophysiologist Kuffler conducted a study on the electrophysiology of glial cells, using the optic nerve and its surrounding glial sheath. It was found that the mean value of the resting potential of these cells, as recorded by intracellular microelectrodes, was 89.6 mV. The potassium concentration in the bathing solution was 3 mEq/L. Assume that $RT/F - 61$ and that the resting potential is equivalent to the potassium equilibrium potential, which of the following is the approximate intracellular potassium concentration (in mEq/L)?

a. 11
b. 33
c. 88
d. 140
e. 155

70. Which of the following concentrations of potassium (mEq/L) in the bathing fluid would depolarize the membrane potential to zero?

a. 11
b. 33
c. 88
d. 140
e. 155

71. Stimulation of the optic nerve with a volley of impulses caused a slow and long-lasting depolarization of the associated glial cells. The mean value of the depolarization was 12.1 mV. If this depolarization was due solely to an increase in potassium ion concentration in the intracellular clefts, which of the following is the change in the concentration of potassium in the extracellular environment (in mEq/L)?

a. 1.79
b. 36.30
c. 137.00
d. 140.50
e. 5.35×10^{-6}

72. Which of the following is the most likely explanation for the depolarization of glial cells following stimulation of nerve fibers?

a. A delayed increase in potassium conductance
b. An early sodium influx
c. A large efflux of sodium ions
d. A temporal summation that results in a long-lasting depolarization
e. An influx of chloride ions

73. Where is the trigger zone that integrates incoming signals from other cells and initiates the signal that the neuron sends to another neuron or muscle cell?

a. Cell body
b. Dendritic trunk
c. Dendritic spines
d. Axon hillock and initial segment
e. Axon trunk

74. Which of the following statements most accurately characterizes the "time constant" of a neuron?

a. The time constant is a function of the membrane's resistance and capacitance.
b. The time constant is unrelated to the membrane's capacitance.
c. The time course of the rising phase of a synaptic potential is specifically dependent upon the time constant for that cell.
d. The falling phase of a synaptic potential is dependent upon active and passive membrane properties.
e. The integration of synaptic potentials is unrelated to the length of the time constant.

75. Which of the following statements best characterizes a basic function of sodium channels?

a. They are opened when the membrane is hyperpolarized.
b. They display a high conductance in the resting membrane.
c. They open rapidly following depolarization of the membrane.
d. They are rapidly inactivated by tetraethylammonium.
e. They are rapidly activated by tetrodotoxin.

76. The equilibrium potential for potassium, as determined by the Nernst equation, differs from the resting potential of the neuron. Which of the following best accounts for this difference?

a. An active sodium-potassium pump makes an important contribution to the regulation of the resting potential.
b. The membrane is selectively permeable only to the potassium ion.
c. The Nernst equation basically considers only the relative distribution of potassium ions across the membrane.
d. The resting potential is basically dependent upon the concentration of sodium but not potassium ions across the membrane.
e. The Nernst equation fails to account for local changes in temperature that influence the resting membrane potential.

77. Based upon the typical distribution of ions across a cell membrane, which of the following values best represents the appropriate resting membrane potential?

a. $+70$ mV
b. $+30$ mV
c. 0 mV
d. -70 mV
e. -100 V

78. If a membrane is permeable only to sodium ions and the concentration of sodium ions on one side of the membrane is the same as that on the other side, then which of the following statements best characterizes the resting membrane potential for that cell?

a. A pump mechanism will cause the cell to become hyperpolarized.
b. The membrane potential would be zero.
c. The tendency would be for current to be directed inward.
d. The membrane potential could not be predicted from the Nernst equation.
e. There would be an initial decrease followed by an increase in membrane potential.

79. Which of the following items best characterizes this description: A graded, fast potential, lasting from several milliseconds to seconds, resulting from a chemical transmitter binding to a receptor to produce either an excitatory postsynaptic potential (EPSP) that depends upon a single class of channels for sodium and potassium or an inhibitory postsynaptic potential (IPSP) that is dependent upon chloride or potassium conductance.

a. Receptor potentials
b. Electrical postsynaptic potentials
c. Increased-conductance postsynaptic potentials
d. Decreased-conductance postsynaptic potentials

80. To which of the following does the term *all-or-none response* most closely relate?

a. The resting potential
b. Increased-conductance presynaptic potentials
c. Increased-conductance postsynaptic potentials
d. The generator potential
e. The action potential

81. The passive spread of a presynaptic current across a gap junction is activated by changes in voltage, pH, or calcium ion levels. To which of the following does the passive spread of current most closely relate?

a. The resting potential
b. The action potential
c. Electrical presynaptic potentials
d. Electrical postsynaptic potentials
e. Receptor potentials

82. A young woman in her early twenties experiences loss of sensation in her legs and weakness in her limbs. A neurological examination further indicated some spasticity of the limbs as well. The neurologist provided a preliminary diagnosis of onset of multiple sclerosis (MS). Assuming that this diagnosis is correct, which of the following best accounts for the diminution of sensory and motor functions?

a. Loss of Schwann cells in peripheral neurons
b. An overall loss of dopaminergic release throughout the brain and spinal cord
c. Loss of peripheral cholinergic neurons
d. Demyelination of CNS neurons
e. Proliferation of oligodendrocytes

Anatomical and Functional Properties of Neurons and Muscle

Answers

55. The answer is b. (*Aminoff, pp 243-245. Ropper, pp 89-94.*) Essential tremor is characterized by a relatively low frequency of 4 to 8 Hz that involves both arms which may extend to the head. The tremor is reduced as a function of movement, such as walking, intake of alcohol, and treatment with a β-adrenergic antagonist (eg, propranolol) and is exaggerated during states of anxiety. In Parkinson disease, the face and lips are preferentially affected and the tremor is typically not symmetrical with respect to both hands. In Huntington disease, chorea and dementia are prominent characteristics. Cerebellar ataxia (sometimes called intention tremor) occurs during an act of movement at the time when fine adjustments of the movement are required. Dystonia refers to persistent posture of the extremes of athetoid movement in which the axial muscles are typically involved and the limb is placed in an unnatural position and may further involve retroflexion of the head or torsion of the spine.

56. The answer is a. (*Ropper, pp 46-53, 96-98. Siegel and Sapru, pp 338-339.*) Repetitive, rhythmic, involuntary contractions at a rate of approximately 5 to 7 Hz that occur following passive stretch of the tendon describe the pathological reflex of clonus. Clonus occurs as part of a hyperreflexic state that is characteristic of spasticity in an upper motor neuron disorder. Lesions of motor regions of the cerebral cortex result in a hyperreflexic state. Lesions of the vermal region of the flocculonodular lobe of cerebellum would result in motor dysfunctions related principally to balance such as ataxia as well as well as nystagmus, but not signs of an upper motor neuron disorder, especially involvement of the upper limbs. A lesion of the gray matter of the spinal cord or peripheral nerve would likely produce a lower motor neuron disorder (ie, flaccid paralysis). Lesions of the dorsomedial pontine tegmentum would more primarily produce eye movement deficits, such as a lateral gaze paralysis, but would not induce an upper motor neuron paralysis of the limbs.

57. The answer is c. (*Ropper, pp 1314-1315.*) Carpal tunnel syndrome results from compression of the median nerve. The median nerve, which is formed by lateral and medial aspects of the brachial plexus, innervates, in part, pronator muscles of the fingers and thumb, and serves as a sensory nerve to the palm of the hand. Therefore, compression of this nerve would cause paresthesia of the fingers and hand. The radial nerve innervates the triceps, brachioradialis, and extensor muscles of the wrist and fingers and abductor of the thumb. A lesion of this nerve would produce loss of extension of the elbow, wrist, and fingers. A lesion of the spinal cord gray matter would cause a lower motor neuron paralysis, while a lesion of the white matter of spinal cord would produce either an upper motor neuron paralysis, or loss of pain and temperature sensation, depending upon the locus of the lesion. The axillary nerve supplies the deltoid and teres minor muscles. Lesions of this nerve would affect sensation around the shoulder and ability to abduct the arm.

58. The answer is d. (*Ropper, pp 1316-1317.*) Diabetes can result in a femoral neuropathy. The femoral nerve conducts sensation from the anterior medial aspect of the thigh and provides motor innervation to the quadriceps and sensation to the medial side of the leg, mainly around or below the knee. The lateral cutaneous nerve supplies sensation to the anterolateral aspect of the thigh. When this nerve is compressed, there is typically a burning sensation around the areas which the nerve innervates. The peroneal nerve innervates the lower part of the leg and lesions of this nerve would produce weakness in dorsiflexion of the foot. The sciatic nerve innervates the hamstrings and muscles below the knee. Damage to this nerve would not affect the quadriceps. The tibial nerve (a division of the sciatic nerve) innervates the plantar flexors and inverters of the foot (ie, calf muscles). Damage to this nerve produces loss of sensation over the plantar aspect of the foot and plantar flexion and inversion are lost. Thus, a lesion of this nerve could not account for the symptoms described in the patient reported in this case.

59. The answer is a. (*Afifi, pp 18-21. Nolte, pp 12-29. Siegel and Sapru, pp 73-74.*) Damage to a nerve fiber proximal to its cell body will cause, among other changes, retrograde degeneration of the cell body. A number of changes occur in the neuron during the process of retrograde degeneration. The cell body initially shows some swelling and becomes distended. At the beginning of the degenerative process, there is an accumulation of mito-chondria in the axoplasm at nodes of Ranvier. The nucleus is then dis-placed toward the periphery of the cell. The Nissl granules break down, first in the center of the cell; later, the breakdown spreads outward. In addi-tion, the axonal process distal to the site of the lesion will undergo degen-eration. It should be noted that retrograde degeneration procedures were used experimentally prior to the advent of histochemical methods for iden-tifying cell bodies of origin of given pathways in the CNS.

60. The answer is b. (*Kandel, pp 82-83, 700-704.*) In a peripheral neu-ropathy, there may be damage to either the myelin or the axon directly, although more often there is damage to the myelin. Because of myelin (or axonal) damage, there is a reduction (or loss) of conduction velocity. The disorder may affect both sensory and motor components of the peripheral nerve, thereby causing dysfunction in both the sensory and the motor processes associated with that nerve. Because there is peripheral neuronal damage, the motor loss will be reflected in a weakness, paralysis, or reflex activity associated with the affected muscle, as well as impairment of sen-sation. The neuropathy typically does not affect one type of function over the other (ie, sensory vs motor). Nodes of Ranvier do not increase as a result of the disorder. Myelin degeneration clearly affects axonal responses. A peripheral neuropathy affects lower motor neurons, not upper motor neurons.

61. The answer is d. (*Kandel, pp 88-98.*) Nuclear and mitochondrial pro-teins are encoded by the nucleus and are formed on free polysomes. The mechanism by which they are targeted to their proper organelle is called *posttranslational importation*. Specific receptors bind and translocate these proteins, and it is the recognition of the structural features of these proteins that allows for transport into the nucleus from the cytoplasm. In the pro-cessing of large proteins such as opioid peptides, more than one copy and different peptides are produced from the same precursor molecule. This precursor is referred to as a *polyprotein* because more than one active pep-tide is present. All protein synthesis begins in the cytosol. Cytosolic pro-teins are the most extensive type of proteins in the cell and include those that make up the cytoskeleton and enzymes that catalyze the different metabolic reactions of the cell. Messenger RNAs (mRNAs) for these pro-teins pass through nuclear pores, become associated with ribosomes, and ultimately form free polysomes in the cytoplasm of the cell. Cytosolic proteins display little modification or processing compared with proteins that remain attached to the membranes of the endoplasmic reticulum or the Golgi apparatus. Messenger RNA that encodes proteins that will become a constituent of organelles or secretory products is formed on polysomes that are attached to the endoplasmic reticulum. Such sheets of membrane in association with ribosomes are called *rough endoplasmic reticulum*. Secretory products typically undergo significant modification after translation. For example, neuropeptide transmitters are cleaved from polypeptide chains, in part, in the endoplasmic reticulum and the Golgi apparatus.

62. The answer is d. *(Kandel, pp 100-104. Siegel and Sapru, pp 65-66)* Transport in either direction utilizes microtubules (kinesin, an ATPase associated with fast anterograde transport and dynein with retrograde transport) as a vehicle or track by which the particles are transported. Among the particles transported down the axon from the cell body are newly synthesized membranous organelles, including synaptic vesicles or their precursors, which ultimately reach the axon terminals. In retrograde transport, the particles transported include endosomes generated from the nerve terminal, mitochondria, and components of the endoplasmic reticulum. Large membranous organelles are transported along the axon both anterogradely and retrogradely by fast axonal transport. In contrast, cytosolic proteins and components of the matrix of the cytoskeleton are transported by slow axonal transport. There are different rates of retrograde transport in which the faster component is approximately twice as fast as the slow component.

63. The answer is d. *(Kandel, pp 107-116. Siegel and Sapru, pp 77-88.)* Ion flux through ion channels is considered to be passive in nature and functions in the absence of any mechanism that requires energy metabolism. Cation channels are generally associated with membranes that are semipermeable to selective ions such as Na^+, K^+, or Cl^-. The electrochemical gradient is a function of two forces: (1) the chemical concentration gradient, which is derived from the relative differences in the distributions of ions across the membrane, and (2) the electrical potential difference between the two sides of the membrane as a function of the distribution of the ionic charges. When ions may flow through channels, current varies as a function of concentration. However, at high ionic concentration differences, a saturation phenomenon is observed that is due to resistance to flow through the channels. It is believed that different kinds of stimuli can function to open or close channels. For example, mechanical activation may lead to the opening of channels. Some channels (ligand gated) are regulated by the noncovalent binding of chemical ligands such as neurotransmitters; others (electrically gated) are affected by changes in membrane voltage that cause a change in the conformation of the channel. Alternatively, relatively long-lasting changes may result when second messengers bind to the channel, at which time there is protein phosphorylation mediated by protein kinases. Such modification of the channel can be reversed by dephosphorylation. In contrast, when a ligand-gated channel is exposed to prolonged, high concentrations of its ligand, it tends to become refractory (ie, desensitized to the presence of that ligand). The neuronal membrane is *impermeable* to most polar and charged molecules for the following reason: since cations and anions contain electrostatically bound water, the attractive forces between ions and water molecules reduce or eliminate movement from a watery environment into the hydrophobic lipid bilayer of the neuronal membrane. Examples include convulsant drugs, blocking agents, neurotoxins, and lidocaine (affecting Na channels).

64. The answer is a. (*Kandel, pp 125-138. Siegel and Sapru, pp 84-86.*) The potential difference across the membrane is a result of the separation of charge and is called the *resting membrane potential*. Accordingly, the potential difference across the membrane is a direct function of the numbers of positive and negative charges on either side of the membrane. As the separation of charge (ie, differences between the charges) across the membrane is reduced, the membrane is said to be depolarized. Conversely, as the difference between the charges is increased, the membrane becomes hyperpolarized. In the latter case, the inside of the cell is made more negative with respect to the outside. If a cell has only a single channel in its membrane (such as for K^+), the gradients for the other ions become irrelevant and the membrane potential will approach the equilibrium potential for the single ion (K^+ in this example). There is a tendency for ions to leak down their electrochemical gradients from one side of the membrane to the other. For there to be a steady resting membrane potential, the gradients across the membrane must be held constant. Changes in ionic gradients are avoided, in spite of the leak, by the presence of an active Na^+, K^+ pump (a membrane protein) that moves Na^+ out of the cell and at the same time brings K⁺ into the cell. Such a pumping mechanism requires energy because it is working against the electrochemical gradients of the two ions. The energy is derived from the hydrolysis of ATP.

65. The answer is b. *(Kandel, pp 222-223.)* The length constant is defined as R_m/R_a, where R_m equals membrane resistance and R_a equals axial resistance. It is the distance along a fiber where a change in membrane potential produced by a given current decays to a value of approximately one-third of its original value (ie, the distance covered by an impulse before it is reduced to 36% of its initial value). As can be seen from the definition, the length constant is directly proportional to the membrane resistance and inversely related to the axial resistance (ie, the resistance of the cytoplasm within the fiber). The membrane resistance is increased significantly through the process of myelination, which thus produces an increase in the value of the length constant. When the length constant along a dendrite is relatively large, it has the effect of increasing the efficiency of electronic conduction along the dendritic process as compared with a similar dendrite with a smaller length constant. In this manner, the synaptic potential along the dendrite distal to the synapse will be relatively larger in a dendrite that has a larger length constant than one that has a smaller length constant.

66. The answer is b. *(Kandel, pp 105-119, 185, 196, 240. Siegel and Sapru, pp 82-84.)* The triggering mechanism for ligand gating involves the selective binding of a particular molecule with the protein channel. This binding causes a conformational change of the channel protein that results in the movement of the channel back and forth, which, in effect, opens or closes the channel. Neurotransmitters can regulate channels as a result of their binding properties. An example is the action of acetylcholine (ACh) at the neuromuscular junction, which is capable of activating channels in the membrane of skeletal muscle. Most cation channels are selective for sodium, potassium, or calcium. Ion channels are composed of large-membrane glycoproteins that vary widely in their molecular weights. In contrast to ligand gating, other types of channels may be activated by changes in the electrical potential across the cell membrane, a process referred to as *voltage gating*.

67. The answer is a. *(Kandel, pp 150-164. Siegel and Sapru, pp 86-88.)* In the late phase of the action potential, potassium channels become opened and potassium efflux produces a hyperpolarization of the membrane. During the repolarization of the membrane, sodium channels are closed (sodium inactivation). Recall that activation of sodium channels is associated with the generation of the action potential. Calcium has a strong electrochemical gradient that drives it into the cell; this coincides with the upstroke of the action potential. A number of different types of calcium-gated potassium channels have been described that are activated during the action potential. Thus, it would appear that calcium influx during the action potential could generate opposing effects. On the one hand, calcium influx carries a positive charge into the cell, which contributes to the depolarization of the membrane. On the other hand, calcium influx may help to open up more potassium channels, which contributes to an outward ionic flow of potassium that causes repolarization of the membrane.

68. The answer is c. *(Kandel, pp 125-138. Siegel and Sapru, pp 82-88)* To understand how an inhibitory transmitter can actually cause a partial depolarization of the membrane, refer to the Goldman equation. The release (or application) of an inhibitory transmitter will serve to open specific ion channels, notably those of potassium. If the membrane is artificially hyperpolarized to −120 mV, the opening of the potassium channel will lead to a redistribution of the ions across the membrane to a normal level. If the normal equilibrium potential for potassium is approximately −75 mV, then application of an inhibitory transmitter (that typically functions by opening potassium channels) will result in a redistribution of potassium ions toward the potassium equilibrium potential (ie, −75 mV). Consequently, the membrane potential will be reduced (ie, depolarized) from −120 mV to a value close to −75 mV. Other possible answers are clearly incorrect. Inhibitory transmitters normally function to hyperpolarize the membrane. Postsynaptic membranes may either be depolarized or hyperpolarized, depending upon the nature of the transmitter and receptor complex present at the synapse. Since the influx of calcium during the depolarization phase of the action potential leads to opposing effects, activation of this channel cannot account for the observed effects. Inactivation of sodium channels would not result in a depolarization of the membrane, but, instead, may contribute to the hyperpolarization of the membrane.

69. The answer is c. *(Kandel, pp 132-138. Siegel and Sapru, p 85.)* To solve the problem, use the Goldman equation, which reduces to the Nernst equation:

$$\text{Equilibrium potential} = (RT/F) \times \ln{(K_i)/(K_o)}$$
$$-89.6 = 61 \, [\ln{(K_i)} - \ln{(3)}]$$
$$-89.6/61 = \ln{(K_i)} - 0.48$$
$$1.47 = \ln{(K_i)} - 0.48$$
$$1.95 = \ln{(K_i)}$$
$$88.54 = K_i$$

70. The answer is c. *(Kandel, pp 132-138. Siegel and Sapru, pp 84-88.)* If the bathing solution is brought to 88 mEq/L, the ionic concentrations outside and inside the membrane would be equal and, therefore, the membrane potential would be depolarized to zero.

71. The answer is a. *(Kandel, pp 132-138. Siegel and Sapru, pp 84-88.)* Use the Goldman equation reduced to the Nernst equation. The resting membrane potential is −89.6 mV, $RT/F = 51$, the potassium concentration is 3 mEq/L, and K_i is calculated to be 88.54 mV.

$$\text{Equilibrium potential} = (RT/F) \times 61 \ln{(K_o/K_i)}$$
$$-89.6 - 12.1 = 61 \times \ln{(K_o - 88.54)}$$
$$-77.5 = 61 \times (\ln{K_o} - \ln{88.54})$$
$$-1.27 = \ln{K_o} - \ln{88.54}$$
$$-1.27 - (-1.95) = \ln{K_o}$$
$$+0.68 = \ln{K_o}$$
$$4.79 \text{ mEq/L} = K_o$$

Therefore, the change in extracellular potassium would be

$$4.79 - 3.00 = 1.79 \text{ mEq/L}$$

72. The answer is a. *(Kandel, pp 132-138. Siegel and Sapru, pp 84-88.)* In this situation, the roles of sodium and chloride ions were not of central importance. Temporal summation also cannot account for these findings and is thus irrelevant to the question at hand. The depolarization of 12.1 mV can be attributed to an increase in the concentration of potassium in the intracellular cleft.

73. The answer is d. *(Kandel, pp 222-223. Siegel and Sapru, pp 86-87.)* The trigger zone for the initiation of impulses from a neuron includes a specialized region of the cell body—the *axon hillock*—together with the section of the axon that adjoins this region—the *initial segment*. Other components of the neuron, such as the dendrites and cell body, receive inputs from afferent sources but are not capable of initiating impulses at these sites. The same is true concerning more distal aspects of the axon over which the impulse is conducted.

74. The answer is a. (*Kandel, pp 140-149.*) The time and space constants represent passive properties of a neuron. The electrical equivalent circuit utilizes the concept that a membrane has both capacitive and resistive properties in parallel, in which case, the rising phase of a potential change is governed in part by the product of the resistance and capacitance of the membrane. The rising phase of a synaptic potential is governed by both active and passive properties of the membrane; however, the falling phase is regulated solely by the passive properties. As the time constant is increased, the probability of integration of converging synaptic signals is increased because such signals will be more likely to overlap in time (temporal summation).

75. The answer is c. (*Kandel, pp 105-123, 154-169. Siegel and Sapru, pp 84-88.*) Sodium channels are rapidly opened following depolarization of the membrane. The rapid influx of ions results in a further depolarization of the membrane, which, in turn, can lead to an action potential. When the membrane is hyperpolarized, sodium channels are closed. Moreover, in the resting membrane, sodium channels are not activated. Tetraethylammonium is a drug that selectively blocks only potassium channels. Tetrodotoxin blocks sodium channels.

76. The answer is a. (*Kandel, pp 125-148. Siegel and Sapru, pp 84-88.*) Because the membrane is a leaky one, the sodium-potassium pump assists in actively transporting ions from one side of the membrane to the other. The membrane is permeable to ions other than potassium, such as sodium and chloride. This fact is taken into consideration in the Goldman equation. This equation includes the distribution of all of these other ions in its formula for determining the value of membrane potential. Accordingly, the resting membrane potential is dependent upon the concentration of these other ions as well as potassium. While it is true that the Nernst equation considers the relative distribution of potassium ions across the membrane, this statement in itself does not explain why the equilibrium potential for potassium differs from the resting potential of the neuron. The statement that the Nernst equation does not take into account differences in temperature is false. But, again, even if that statement were true, it would nevertheless not account for the differences between the equilibrium potential for potassium and the resting potential of the neuron.

77. The answer is d. (*Purves, pp 30-35.*) At rest, the cell typically generates a constant voltage across the membrane. The voltage is negative (inside), varying from approximately −40 to −90 mV, which is determined by the relative concentrations of the different ions inside and outside the membrane.

78. The answer is b. (*Kandel, pp 175-295. Purves, pp 30-35.*) If the cell membrane is permeable to only one ion such as sodium, and the concentration of this ion is equal on both sides of the membrane, then there will be no membrane potential recorded across the membrane. This is intuitively so, as determined from the Nernst equation where both the numerator and denominator are the same, therefore generating the logarithm of 1, whose value is 0.

79. The answer is c. (*Kandel, pp 175-295. Purves, pp 30-38. Siegel and Sapru, pp 99-101.*) Increased-conductance postsynaptic potentials are fast, graded potentials, lasting from several milliseconds to several seconds. If the potential is an EPSP, it depends upon a single class of ligand-gated channels for sodium and potassium. If the response is an IPSP, then it depends upon ligand-gated channels for potassium and chloride. Decreased-conductance postsynaptic potentials are mediated by a chemical transmitter or intracellular messenger to produce a graded, slow potential, lasting from seconds to minutes. This response is related to a closure of sodium, potassium, or chloride channels. Receptor potentials result from the application of a sensory stimulus that produces a fast, graded potential that involves a single class of channels for both sodium and potassium.

80. The answer is e. (*Purves, pp 30-38. Siegel and Sapru, pp 99-101.*) The action potential is characterized by an all-or-none response in which the overshoot may reach an amplitude of up to 100 mV. The mechanism involves separate ion channels for sodium and potassium. The resting potential is characterized by a relatively steady potential, usually in the region of 270 mV, but which may range from 235 to 270 mV. This potential is mainly dependent upon potassium and chloride channels.

81. The answer is d. (*Kandel, pp 140-148.*) Electrical postsynaptic potentials involve the passive spread of current across a gap junction that is permeable to a variety of small ions. The stimulus for such activation may be a change in either voltage, pH, or intracellular calcium. Answers and explanations for Questions 74 to 77 relate to the other choices presented.

82. The answer is d. (*Aminoff, pp 164–167.*) Multiple sclerosis is a demyelinating disease. The lesions may also involve some reactive gliosis and axonal degeneration as well. It occurs mainly in the white matter of the spinal cord and brain as well as in the optic nerve. Choices (a) and (c) are incorrect because they refer to the peripheral nervous system while multiple sclerosis is a disorder affecting the CNS. Proliferation of oligodendrocytes (unless cancerous) would presumably not significantly affect CNS neurons. Loss of dopaminergic neurons is not a correct choice because many of the neurons in the CNS affected by multiple sclerosis are not dopaminergic.

The Synapse

Questions

83. Gap junctions are characteristically associated with which of the following?

a. Axodendritic synapses
b. Axoaxonic synapses
c. Axosomatic synapses
d. Dendrodendritic synapses
e. Electrical synapses

84. In treating a patient with a movement disorder, you administer a newly developed drug whose functions were mediated at axosomatic synapses. Which of the following statements best characterizes axosomatic synapses?

a. It is referred to as a type I synapse.
b. They have an electrical continuity linking the pre- and postsynaptic cells.
c. They are typically inhibitory.
d. Synaptic transmission is mediated by glutamate.
e. They form the predominant synapse of cortical projections to the neostriatum.

85. In a typical chemical synapse, which of the following constitutes the correct sequence of events involved in neurotransmission?

a. The action potential stimulates the presynaptic terminal → the presynaptic terminal is depolarized, opening voltage-gated Ca^{2+} ion channels, causing an influx of these ions into the presynaptic terminal → release of the transmitter into the synaptic cleft by exocytosis → a postsynaptic current produces an EPSP or an IPSP, changing the excitability of the postsynaptic cell.

b. Release of the transmitter into the synaptic cleft by exocytosis → an influx of Ca^{2+} through channels, causing the vesicles to fuse with the presynaptic membrane → opening of the postsynaptic channels → binding of the transmitter to the receptor molecules in the postsynaptic membrane.

c. The vesicular membrane is retrieved from the plasma membrane → release of the transmitter into the synaptic cleft by exocytosis → the action potential stimulates the presynaptic terminal → binding of the transmitter to the receptor molecules in the postsynaptic membrane.

d. Opening or closing of the postsynaptic channels → depolarization of the presynaptic terminal causing an opening of Ca^{2+} ion channels → release of the transmitter into the synaptic cleft by exocytosis → synthesis and storage of the transmitter in the presynaptic terminal.

e. The presynaptic terminal is depolarized, opening voltage-gated Ca^2 ion channels, causing an influx of these ions into the presynaptic terminal → opening or closing of the postsynaptic channels → release of the transmitter into the synaptic cleft by exocytosis → the vesicular membrane is retrieved from the plasma membrane.

86. Which of the following best describes a basic property of synapses in the central nervous system (CNS)?

a. Synaptic vesicles constitute important features for transmission in both chemical and electrical synapses.

b. A postsynaptic neuron typically receives input from different presynaptic axons that are either excitatory or inhibitory, but it cannot receive inputs from both types.

c. Synaptic delay is approximately the same for both chemical and electrical synapses.

d. Receptors can provide a gating function with respect to a given ion channel.

e. The mechanism of indirect gating of ions normally does not involve the activation of G-proteins.

87. A neurologist selects a drug that has properties similar to that of γ-aminobutyric acid (GABA) for the treatment of temporal lobe epilepsy. This neurotransmitter serves important functions within the CNS. Which of the following accurately characterizes a basic property of this neurotransmitter?

a. GABA is known to have inhibitory as well as excitatory properties.
b. The associated channel is permeable to charged chloride ions
c. GABA is formed from serine.
d. GABA is associated with the generation of seizure activity.
e. GABA is present mainly in spinal cord.

88. A patient with a history of depression is treated with a novel compound that acts mainly upon N-methyl-D-aspartate (NMDA) receptors. Which of the following best describes a basic property associated with the N-methyl-D-aspartate (NMDA) receptor?

a. It controls a high-conductance anion channel.
b. The NMDA channel is blocked by the presence of magnesium.
c. NMDA is selective for metabotropic receptors.
d. Insufficient amounts of glutamate, acting through NMDA receptors, may cause neuronal cell death.
e. Current flow is blocked in the presence of glutamate, leading to hyperpolarization of the cell.

89. A noradrenergic drug that binds to β-adrenergic receptors was recommended for use in an acutely depressed patient. Which of the following second-messenger systems are directly activated as a function of the binding of norepinephrine to these receptors?

a. Inositol 1,4,5-triphosphate (IP$_3$)
b. Adenosine 3′,5′-cyclic monophosphate (cAMP)
c. Diacylglycerol (DAG)
d. Arachidonic acid
e. Prostaglandins

90. A drug designed to hyperpolarize neurons was recommended for use in the treatment of a movement disorder associated with the basal ganglia. Hyperpolarization of a neuron is governed by the actions of which of the following ions?

a. Chloride and sodium
b. Chloride and potassium
c. Potassium and sodium
d. Sodium and calcium
e. Sodium only

91. Which of the following events determines the release of a neurotransmitter from the terminals of a presynaptic neuron?

a. Sodium influx
b. Sodium efflux
c. Potassium influx
d. Potassium efflux
e. Calcium influx

92. A patient was treated with a drug whose basic mechanism involves the activation of second messengers. Which of the following statements is appropriate to second messengers within neurons?

a. They most frequently generate a marked hypersensitization of most types of receptors.
b. They regulate gene expression causing neuronal growth and synthesis of proteins.
c. They generally do not interact in the opening or closing of ion channels.
d. Glutamate typically generates inhibitory effects upon metabotropic receptors.
e. They are directly involved in the gating of sodium channels by NMDA receptors.

93. An experimental drug that acts upon NMDA, kainate, and α-amino-3-hydroxy-5-methyl-4-isoxazole propionic acid (AMPA) receptors was employed for the treatment of schizophrenia. Which of the following transmitters is associated with these receptors?

a. GABA
b. Glutamate
c. Norepinephrine
d. Opioid peptides
e. Dopamine

The Synapse

Answers

83. The answer is e. (*Kandel, pp 178-180. Purves, pp 85-87. Siegel and Sapru, pp 95-96.*) Electrical synapses are less common than chemical synapses but can be found in the nervous systems of different species. A unique feature of electrical synapses is that two neurons communicate with each other by having the membranes of each neuron lie very close together. The contact between the neurons is called a *gap junction*. These junctions contain aligned paired channels so that each paired channel forms a pore larger than those observed in ligand gated channels and which allows for the bidirectional transmission.

84. The answer is c. (*Kandel, pp 209-217. Purves, pp 5-9, 85, 117.*) Axon terminals that make synaptic contact with the soma of postsynaptic cells are frequently observed to be inhibitory and are referred to as *type II synapses*. A classic example of this is in the cerebellar cortex, where an interneuron (basket cell) makes synaptic contact with the soma of the Purkinje cell. These are chemical and not electrical synapses, and their actions are frequently mediated by GABA. Activation of the basket cell results in subsequent inhibition of the Purkinje cell. The overwhelming number of excitatory synapses are observed to be axodendritic. They are referred to as *type I synapses* and are frequently characterized by specialized extensions of the dendrites called spines. These synapses also display a dense basement membrane and a prominent presynaptic density. Cortical projections to the neostriatum have been shown to be excitatory and their functions mediated by glutamate.

85. The answer is a. (*Purves, pp 85-101. Siegel and Sapru, pp 96-99.*) The sequence of events that occur in the transmission of a chemical synapse is as follows: The transmitter is synthesized and stored in the presynaptic vesicles. The action potential is propagated down the presynaptic axon to its presynaptic terminal. The presynaptic terminal is then depolarized, which causes the opening of voltage-gated Ca^{2+} channels. Then there is Ca^{2+} through these channels, causing the vesicles to fuse with the presynaptic membrane. The transmitter is then released into the presynaptic cleft (by exocytosis) and binds to receptor molecules in the postsynaptic membrane. This leads to the opening or closing of postsynaptic channels. The resultant current results in an EPSP or IPSP, which causes a change in excitability of the postsynaptic cell. The vesicular membrane is then retrieved from the plasma membrane.

86. The answer is d. *(Kandel, pp 207-219. Purves, pp 115-117, 156-164. Siegel and Sapru, pp 127-130.)* Perhaps the most significant feature of the receptor is that it serves a gating function for particular ions. It can do this either directly, if it is part of the ion channel, or indirectly, by activating a G-protein that, in turn, activates a second-messenger system. This process results in a modulation of the ion channel's activity. In particular, the G-protein stimulates adenylate cyclase, converting ATP to cAMP. In turn, cAMP induces activation of cAMP-dependent protein kinase, which modulates channels by phosphorylating the channel protein or some other protein that works on that channel. The synaptic vesicles may be round or flat, and filled or empty. They are typically filled with a neurotransmitter that is released onto the synaptic cleft. The receptive process on the postsynaptic region (ie, the postsynaptic receptor) takes on a very important function. The binding of the transmitter to the receptor molecule is determined by this receptor, which is a membrane-spanning protein. When the transmitter is released onto the postsynaptic membrane, it leads to an action potential in the postsynaptic neuron (see the answer to Question 81 for further details). In contrast, transmission at electrical synapses are mediated through gap junctions. Because the presynaptic and postsynaptic membranes of (gap junctions of) electrical synapses are connected by gap junction channels, electrical synapses function by means of the passive flow of ionic current through the gap junction from one neuron to the next. Postsynaptic neurons can receive both excitatory and inhibitory inputs. A classic example is a ventral horn motor neuron, which may receive an excitatory sensory input emanating from the same side of the body and an inhibitory input from the contralateral side. (See the chapter entitled "The Spinal Cord" for further discussion of this point.) Because of the nature of the difference in mechanisms for synaptic transmission and the relative sizes of the synaptic gaps, which are much smaller for electrical synapses, the synaptic delay for electrical synapses is much shorter than that for chemical synapses.

87. The answer is b. (*Kandel, pp 214-221. Purves, pp 133-135. Siegel and Sapru, pp 126-127.*) GABA is an inhibitory transmitter found in the spinal cord and throughout the brain. It acts on the chloride channel, which, when activated, permits this ion to enter the cell and makes it more negative (ie, hyperpolarize the cell). Since GABA is inhibitory, it is assumed that its actions would be to inhibit seizure activity. GABA is formed from decarboxylation of glutamate and not from serine (from which glycine is formed).

88. The answer is b. (*Kandel, pp 212-215. Purves, pp 126-133. Siegel and Sapru, pp 124-126.*) The NMDA receptor is an ionotropic receptor that regulates a channel permeable to several cations, which include calcium, sodium, and potassium. This channel, however, is easily blocked by magnesium. In fact, it requires a significant depolarization of the membrane in order for magnesium to be exuded from the channel so that sodium and calcium can enter the cell. Glutamate receptors can be divided into two categories: (1) metabotropic receptors that gate channels indirectly through second messengers and (2) ionotropic receptors that gate channels directly. One of the unusual features of this transmitter-gated channel is that it is also gated by voltage. Thus, conductance reaches its peak when both glutamate is present and the cell is depolarized. High concentrations of glutamate could result in death of the cell. This may be due to an unusually large influx of calcium through NMDA-activated channels. The calcium might activate proteases, resulting in the formation of free radicals that could be toxic to the cell.

89. The answer is b. (*Kandel, pp 181-185, 281-294. Purves, pp 137-140, 156-166. Siegel and Sapru, pp 124-129.*) When norepinephrine reaches a β-adrenergic receptor, a G-protein activates adenyl cyclase, which generates a second messenger, cAMP, from ATP. cAMP activates a cAMP-dependent kinase that alters the conformation of regulatory subunits of other kinases. This frees catalytic subunits to phosphorylate specific proteins, which in turn leads to the cellular response. IP$_3$ and DAG are associated with the transmitter acetylcholine (ACh), which binds to muscarinic receptors, and arachidonic acid is linked to histamine, which binds to histamine receptors. Prostaglandins are metabolites of arachidonic acid.

90. The answer is b. (*Kandel, pp 181-185, 281-294. Purves, pp 133-135. Siegel and Sapru, p 126.*) In neurons within the CNS, an inhibitory transmitter will open chloride channels. In addition, second messengers may also mediate inhibition. It is likely that they do so by opening potassium channels. When a chloride channel is opened, it will lead to movement of this ion down its concentration gradient and into the cell. This will make the cell more negative (ie, hyperpolarized). At the same time, there will be an efflux of potassium, which will also produce hyperpolarization of the cell because positive charges are now being removed. On the other hand, sodium and calcium influx are associated with depolarization of the cell.

91. The answer is e. (*Kandel, pp 208-226, 253-276. Purves, pp 61-70.*) Experimental methods permit evaluation of the relative contributions of different ions in the regulation of transmitter release. Neither tetrodotoxin, which blocks voltage-gated sodium channels, nor tetraethylammonium, which blocks voltage-gated potassium channels, will block the generation of a postsynaptic potential when the presynaptic cell is artificially depolarized. In contrast, presynaptic calcium influx triggers the release of the transmitter and results in a postsynaptic potential. Moreover, when presynaptic calcium influx is blocked, no postsynaptic potential is produced. Action potentials at the presynaptic axon terminals open up calcium channels, permitting calcium influx. This event helps move synaptic vesicles to active sites as actin filaments (which anchor the vesicles) are dissolved.

92. The answer is b. (*Kandel, pp 182-185, 208-226, 253-276.*) Second-messenger kinases can lead to the phosphorylation of ion channel proteins. Such a process can lead to either the closing of a previously open ion channel or the opening of a previously closed channel. For example, norepinephrine acts through cAMP to close the potassium channel, resulting in an increase in excitability. Second messengers can phosphorylate transcriptional regulatory proteins and thus alter gene expression. In particular, existing proteins may be altered and new proteins may be synthesized. Moreover, such effects may generate other alterations, such as the induction of neuronal growth. Second messengers can also interact directly with an ion channel to cause it to open or close (in the absence of a protein kinase). They also can produce a level of desensitization in receptors, which is a function of the extent of phosphorylation. While glutamate excites ionotropic receptors, it has a more diverse modulatory effect upon metabotropic receptors, which could be expressed in either receptor excitation or inhibition. The direct gating of ion channels by NMDA receptors is an example of a process that does not immediately involve a second messenger.

93. The answer is b. *(Kandel, pp 212-214. Purves, pp 126-136. Siegel and Sapru, pp 124-126.)* NMDA, kainate, and AMPA receptors are activated by glutamate. The NMDA receptor differs from the other types of receptors in that it is blocked by Mg^{2+} and controls a cation channel permeable to calcium, sodium, and potassium. Pharmacologically, NMDA receptors can be blocked by 2-amino-5-phosphonovaleric acid. The AMPA receptor is activated by quisqualic acid; it has a high affinity for L-glutamate and AMPA. The kainate receptor is activated by kainic acid. It regulates a channel that is permeable to sodium and potassium, binds AMPA, and is important in the process of excitotoxicity. Other neurotransmitters, including GABA, opioid peptides, dopamine, and norepinephrine do not activate excitatory amino acids.

Neurochemistry/ Neurotransmitters

Questions

94. A middle-aged man is brought to the hospital for a neurological examination after displaying uncontrollable movements of his upper limbs. He is diagnosed with a rare genetic disorder affecting dopamine synthesis in brainstem neurons. However, there is some controversy concerning at what step in the biosynthesis of dopamine this failure took place. If the failure lay in the immediate precursor stage in the biosynthesis of dopamine, which of the following is the precursor?

a. Tyrosine
b. Tyrosine hydroxylase
c. Tryptophan
d. L-dihydroxyphenylalanine (L-DOPA)
e. Dopamine β-hydroxylase

95. If a patient is suffering from a genetic disorder affecting the rate-limiting step in the biosynthesis of dopamine, which of the following is the rate-limiting step?

a. Tryptophan hydroxylase
b. Tyrosine hydroxylase
c. Dopamine β-hydroxylase
d. Phenylethanolamine-N-methyltransferase
e. Choline acetyltransferase

96. A baby is born with an inherited autosomal recessive trait in which there was a delay in development, resulting in the occurrence of seizures and mental retardation. The child is diagnosed with phenylketonuria (PKU). Which of the following is the most likely neurochemical locus of this genetic defect?

a. Tyrosine
b. Tryptophan
c. Tryptophan hydroxylase
d. Dopamine
e. Phenylalanine (Phe) hydroxylase

97. Your patient is suffering from a disorder of unknown etiology that blocks neural transmission at the neuromuscular junction. You recommend a drug whose specific action is believed to modulate the end-plate potential. Which of the following best describes a basic feature of the end-plate potential?

a. It is dependent upon the release of dopamine from the nerve ending.
b. The amplitude of this potential is much higher than central nervous system (CNS) postsynaptic potentials.
c. It is an all-or-none response.
d. It is unrelated to the concentration of transmitter released from the presynaptic terminals.
e. It is selectively associated with the opening of chloride channels.

98. The channel at the neuromuscular junction associated with the end-plate potential is which of the following?

a. Blocked by a noradrenergic β-receptor antagonist
b. Blocked by an N-methyl-D-aspartate- (NMDA-) receptor antagonist
c. Blocked by an α-amino-hydroxy-5-methyl-4-isoxazolepropionic acid- (AMPA-) receptor antagonist
d. Nicotinic gated
e. Muscarinic gated

99. A patient is admitted to the hospital because of a variable weakness of cranial nerve and limb muscles, which worsen significantly following exercise, but shows no clinical signs of denervation from tests, which includes electromyogram (EMG) recordings. This disorder is partially reversed by the administration of drugs that inhibit acetylcholinesterase. Which of the following is the most likely diagnosis?

a. Multiple sclerosis (MS)
b. Amyotrophic lateral sclerosis (ALS)
c. Myasthenia gravis
d. Lambert-Eaton syndrome
e. Muscular dystrophy (MD)

100. A 62-year-old male diagnosed with lung cancer displays weakness in his arms and legs. A battery of tests are administered to the patient, including those involving nerve conduction. The nerve conduction test reveals a reduction in the compound motor action potential relating to muscles of the hand. However, the amplitude of this potential improves significantly following exercise involving the relevant muscles. Which of the following is the most likely diagnosis?

a. MS
b. ALS
c. Myasthenia gravis
d. Lambert-Eaton syndrome
e. MD

101. A patient receives a diagnosis of myasthenia gravis. Which of the following most likely constitutes the basis for this disorder?

a. The production of excessive quantities of acetylcholine (ACh)
b. The production of antibodies that act against nicotinic ACh receptors
c. A reduction in brain catecholamines
d. Reduction in presynaptic Ca^2 channels
e. Viral encephalitis

102. A patient complains of weakness in the proximal muscles of the limb as well as dryness of the mouth and constipation. On the basis of a neurological examination, it is concluded that the patient is suffering from the Lambert-Eaton syndrome. Which of the following best characterizes the basic defect underlying this disorder?

a. The production of excessive quantities of ACh
b. The production of antibodies that act against nicotinic ACh receptors
c. A reduction in brain catecholamines
d. Reduction in presynaptic Ca^2 channels
e. Viral encephalitis

103. A 10-year-old boy accidentally swallowed a toxic substance that contained a neurotoxin, whose actions mimic those of curare. This resulted in a neuromuscular blockade, partial respiratory failure, and paralysis. To which of the following receptors does this toxin bind?

a. γ-Aminobutyric acid-A (GABA$_A$) receptor
b. GABA$_B$ receptor
c. Nicotinic receptor
d. NMDA receptor
e. Histamine receptor

104. A patient who complains about disruption in limb muscle function is diagnosed with a disorder in which the transmitter released at the neuromuscular junction was not removed from the synaptic cleft. Which of the following is the primary mechanism involved in removal of the transmitter at the neuromuscular junction?

a. Enzymatic degradation
b. Diffusion
c. Reuptake
d. Actions of antibodies
e. Distribution of sodium and potassium ions along muscle membrane

105. It was discovered that a patient who was suffering from muscle weakness in his limbs had developed a deficiency in the availability of the enzyme required for the metabolism of the neurotransmitter present in the synapse at the neuromuscular junction. Which of the following enzymes was deficient in this patient?

a. Choline acetyltransferase
b. Glutaminase
c. Glutamine synthetase
d. Acetylcholinesterase
e. Serine hydroxymethyltransferase

106. A patient is admitted to the emergency room after taking a drug of abuse that destroyed selective groups of neurons in the brainstem. After the patient became ambulatory, he was chronically depressed. Which of the following neuronal groups in the brainstem is most likely related, either directly or indirectly, to this patient's condition?

a.   Vestibular nuclei
b.   Nucleus ambiguus
c.   Trigeminal spinal nucleus
d.   Dorsal column nuclei
e.   Raphe nuclei

107. A study utilizing peripheral measures of a variety of neurotransmitters in patients suffering from chronic depression was conducted over a 4-month period. It was discovered that there was a significant decrease in one of these neurotransmitters. Which of the following neurotransmitters was most significantly reduced in these patients?

a.   Enkephalin
b.   Dopamine
c.   Norepinephrine
d.   Serotonin
e.   Glycine

108. A patient is diagnosed with clinical depression and is administered a drug to treat this disorder. Which of the following properties best characterizes the drug given to the patient?

a.   A selective serotonin reuptake inhibitor (SSRI)
b.   A CNS depressant
c.   A dopaminergic antagonist
d.   A noradrenergic antagonist
e.   An NMDA blocker

109. A patient is diagnosed as having elevated levels of glucose and lactate in blood, due in part to the actions of epinephrine. In order to improve the condition of this patient, a drug was applied that could reduce epinephrine levels. At what step in the biosynthetic pathway for epinephrine would such a drug act to selectively block the synthesis of epinephrine?

a. Tyrosine hydroxylase
b. Dopamine β-hydroxylase
c. Phenylethanolamine-N-methyltransferase
d. 5-Hydroxy-indole-O-methyltransferase
e. Tryptophan hydroxylase

110. In response to a form of sleep disorder in which individuals tend to suffer from excessive sleep, a pharmaceutical company undertakes to develop a drug that selectively alleviates this problem by blocking the rate-limiting step in the biosynthesis of serotonin. Which of the following would represent the rate-limiting step?

a. Tyrosine hydroxylase
b. Tryptophan hydroxylase
c. Phenylethanolamine-N-methyltransferase
d. Dopamine β-hydroxylase
e. Glutamic acid decarboxylase

111. An elderly male is brought to his physician by his family after increasing incidences of disorientation coupled with memory loss. The patient is diagnosed with Alzheimer disease. A few years later, after further physical and mental deterioration, the patient dies. An autopsy is taken of his brain and regional brain chemistry and neuropathology identified. Which of the following structures represents the most likely site where the neuropathology could be identified?

a. Cerebellar cortex
b. Substantia nigra
c. Vestibular nuclei
d. Basal nucleus of Meynert
e. Subthalamic nucleus

Questions 112 to 114

112. A patient was recently diagnosed with Alzheimer disease and is placed on a drug treatment program. Which of the following are the drugs of choice for this disorder?

a. Carbamazepine and neurontin (Gabapentine)
b. Haloperidol and clonidine
c. Memantine and donepezil (Aricept)
d. Paroxetine and sertraline
e. Levodopa and lithium

113. An analysis was undertaken of the histological, pathological, and neurochemical alterations in the brains of patients who died of Alzheimer disease. Following examination of the brain, which of the following would most likely be present in the affected regions?

a. A decrease in substance P in the hypothalamus and brainstem reticular formation
b. Marked degeneration of most myelinated pathways
c. Amyloid deposits and neurofibrillary tangles
d. Marked retrograde degeneration in sensory neurons of the brainstem
e. Glial loss associated with the medial lemniscus and spinothalamic pathways

114. A clinical study was conducted to develop a promising therapeutic strategy for treatment of Alzheimer disease. Which of the following strategies was utilized in this study?

a. Surgical removal of selective regions of the cerebral cortex
b. Administration of serotonergic agonists that act specifically on cerebral cortical neurons
c. Administration of cholinergic antagonists directed against nicotinic receptors in the cerebral cortex
d. Administration of noradrenergic agonists directed against α_2 receptors in the cerebral cortex
e. Administration of compounds that slow aggregation of amyloid-β peptide into its fibrillar form

115. In their attempts to develop drugs that specifically act upon a given neurotransmitter system, pharmaceutical companies are beset with the problem that the neurotransmitter in question may have widespread presence throughout the CNS. Consequently, drugs aimed at blocking the biosynthesis or release of the neurotransmitter may generate unwarranted side effects by acting on neural systems unrelated to the neural systems the drug is designed to modulate. Which of the following neurotransmitters would appear to be the most difficult to work with because of its ubiquity within the CNS?

a. ACh
b. Glutamate
c. Norepinephrine
d. Dopamine
e. Substance P

116. A patient admitted to the emergency room is diagnosed with cortical damage and resultant neuronal degeneration due to an ischemic insult. The neurologist concludes that the brain damage involved neurotoxicity of those cells. Which of the following neurotransmitter changes associated with neurotoxicity is most likely to have occurred?

a. Extracellular accumulation of norepinephrine
b. Extracellular accumulation of ACh
c. Extracellular accumulation of glutamate
d. Extracellular loss of serotonin
e. Extracellular loss of GABA

117. A 73-year-old female suffered an injury involving the left middle cerebral artery and affecting mainly the pre- and post-central gyri. Characteristically, there were neurotoxic effects of cortical ischemia resulting from a stroke that were noted. Which of the following is a likely mechanism underlying the phenomenon of cortical neurotoxicity?

a. Entry of Ca^{2+} into the cell
b. Reduction of extracellular chloride
c. Delayed removal of norepinephrine from the synapse
d. Hypersensitivity of the postsynaptic membrane to the GABA
e. Failure of degradation of the ACh

118. A 50-year-old man suffers from anxiety attacks. A general medical, neurological, and psychiatric evaluation indicates that the patient is in good physical health, and, likewise, no neurological signs can be detected. Further analysis suggests that the anxiety attacks are brought on because of recent events at his place of employment, which led him to believe that his position might be terminated. Which of the following is the most appropriate drug to treat this patient?

a. Picrotoxin
b. Naloxone
c. Chlordiazepoxide
d. Bicuculline
e. Dopamine

119. A 17-year-old male, who was suffering from repeated anxiety attacks, was selected for a study for the treatment of this disorder. The study involved a determination of the efficacy of an experimental drug whose mechanism of action specifically attempts to reduce anxiety levels. Which of the following is the most likely mechanism underlying the action of this drug?

a. Blockade of chloride channel permeability
b. Opioid receptor blockade
c. Binding of the drug to the GABA benzodiazepine site
d. Activation of muscarinic cholinergic receptor
e. Competitive binding of the $GABA_A$-receptor site

120. A 55-year-old female patient is admitted to the hospital for treatment of hypertension. Prior to her admission to the hospital, her blood pressure was slightly above normal, but in recent weeks, her blood pressure appeared to rise significantly. A general medical and neurological examination indicates that she is otherwise in acceptable health, and no medical or neurological signs can be detected. Which of the following is the drug of choice to treat this patient?

a. Sumatriptan (Imitrex)
b. Clonidine
c. Topiramate
d. Valproic acid
e. Butorphanol

121. A 67-year-old male was under treatment for hypertension and was given prazosin for the treatment of this condition. The antihypertensive effect of prazosin is mediated by which one of the following receptors?

a. Cholinergic muscarinic receptors
b. Dopaminergic receptors
c. α_2-Adrenergic receptors
d. Serotonergic receptors
e. α_1-Adrenergic receptors

122. As a result of a leg injury, a 30-year-old male develops chronic pain and is subsequently treated with morphine. Consequently, he develops an addiction to morphine. On which of the predominant receptor sites is this effect mediated?

a. Opioid nociceptin receptor
b. Opioid μ-receptor
c. Opioid δ-receptor
d. Opioid κ-receptor
e. Dopamine D_2-receptor

123. A patient was treated for a disorder of unknown etiology which also caused severe and chronic pain. Part of the treatment involved administration of drug whose actions targeted the region of the brain containing the highest densities of opioid receptors. Which of the following regions of the brain would likely contain heavy concentrations of this receptor?

a. Mammillary bodies
b. Precentral gyrus
c. Midbrain periaqueductal gray
d. Inferior olivary nucleus
e. Deep pontine nuclei

124. A 76-year-old woman was diagnosed as having had a cortical stroke. Concern was expressed in part because of the hypoxic and ischemic effects of the stroke. Recent evidence has suggested that the deleterious effects of the stroke were due in part to excitotoxicity of neurons situated in the region of the stroke. Based on this evidence and reasoning, which of the following drugs would most likely be given to the patient to reduce the deleterious effects of the stroke?

a. GABA antagonist
b. Dopamine antagonist
c. Norepinephrine antagonist
d. NMDA antagonist
e. Serotonin antagonist

125. A 71-year-old male was taken to the emergency room after having been found unconscious in his home. After it was determined that he suffered a cortical stroke, pharmacological treatment was immediately administered. In applying a drug for the treatment of the stroke, which of the following would likely be the primary objective of this approach?

a. Raise blood pressure
b. Decrease disruption of the blood-brain barrier
c. Reduce cortical seizure activity
d. Stabilize body temperature
e. Reduce cortical brain serotonin levels

126. A patient is admitted to the hospital after experiencing increasing episodes of temporal lobe seizure activity. Which of the following drugs should be administered to treat this disorder?

a. Physostigmine
b. Bicuculline
c. Pilocarpine
d. Kainate
e. Gabapentin

127. A 36-year-old male was diagnosed with temporal lobe epilepsy. In attempting to treat this condition, the neurologist recommended a drug that would activate which one of the following receptors?

a. NMDA receptors
b. Noradrenergic receptors
c. GABA receptors
d. Cholinergic receptors
e. Dopamine receptors

128. A 29-year-old male was severely hurt in an automobile accident which resulted in a brain injury affecting the prefrontal region. Recent studies have revealed that nitric oxide may be a deleterious factor in brain injury, in particular, because nitric oxide is a source of reactive oxygen species in producing toxic compounds. In order to reduce or eliminate the effects of nitric oxide, which one of the following compounds would have to be blocked as part of a drug treatment plan recommended by a neurologist in order to reduce or inactivate its deleterious effects?

a. Glutamate
b. Choline
c. L-arginine
d. Tyrosine
e. Tryptophan

129. Which of the following best explains how nitric oxide differs from other "classical" neurotransmitters?

a. Nitric oxide is a gaseous transmitter.
b. Nitric oxide has both excitatory and inhibitory functions.
c. Nitric oxide occurs only in response to injury.
d. The distribution of nitric oxide is limited to the peripheral nervous system.
e. Nitric oxide is packaged in vesicles.

130. A 60-year-old male has high blood pressure, and the diagnosis indicates that it is due in part to retention of water. Which of the following compounds would most likely relate to this process?

a. Oxytocin
b. Serotonin
c. Histamine
d. Vasopressin
e. Somatostatin

131. A 65-year-old man is experiencing considerable pain due to a chronic back problem and is administered morphine to alleviate the problem. Which of the following constitutes a possible mechanism by which morphine provides effective action?

a. Release of somatostatin
b. Release of histamine
c. Release of vasopressin
d. Release of ACh
e. Release of substance P

132. A 16-year-old boy took the recreational drug of abuse phencyclidine (PCP or "angel dust"), resulting in an initial feeling of euphoria but followed by ataxia, sweating, seizures, and respiratory depression. To which of the following mechanisms are the deleterious effects of the drug in part due?

a. Blockade of NMDA receptors
b. Blockade of AMPA receptors
c. Blockade of cholinergic receptors
d. Blockade of GABA$_A$ receptors
e. Blockade of GABA$_B$ receptors

133. A patient is diagnosed with a form of epilepsy. One approach to treating this disorder is to give the patient a drug that would have a selective blocking action upon neurotransmitter receptors. Which of the following receptors would such a drug block in order to serve as an effective treatment procedure?

a. GABA receptors
b. Glutamate receptors
c. Nicotinic receptors
d. Serotonin receptors
e. Glycine receptors

134. A patient with severe anxiety attacks was administered an experimental drug for the treatment of this disorder. Which of the following was the most likely drug administered to this individual?

a. An opioid peptide antagonist
b. A cholinergic agonist
c. A cholecystokinin receptor antagonist
d. A serotonin 1-A receptor antagonist
e. A noradrenergic α_2 receptor agonist

135. A teenage boy attempted to make his own drug of abuse. In doing so, he developed a drug which had general hyperexcitable effects upon his behavior, such as prolonged periods of wakefulness. He was taken to the emergency room and recovered over the next 24 hours. Blood samples were taken and sent for analysis. It was determined that the drug developed had the capacity to block the enzyme directly responsible for the degradation of norepinephrine. Which of the following enzymes was blocked by this drug?

a. Tryptophan hydroxylase
b. Tyrosine hydroxylase
c. Dopamine β-hydroxylase
d. Catechol-O-methyltransferase
e. Choline acetyltransferase

136. A 50-year-old woman has been treated over the past 6 months with lithium for an ongoing emotional disorder. From which of the following disorders is this patient most likely suffering?

a. Panic attacks
b. Schizophrenia
c. Obsessive-compulsive disorder
d. Bipolar disorder
e. Anxiety

137. A patient was admitted to a local hospital after it was determined that she was suffering from low blood pressure. In attempting to treat the patient, a resident administered a catecholamine agonist to increase blood pressure to more normal levels. However, in doing so, a most unusual response took place in that blood pressure continued to drop somewhat. It was concluded that the catecholamine agonist served to attenuate catecholamine release rather than to increase it. Which of the following could best account for this result?

a. The presence of a GABAergic neuron at the catecholaminergic synapses
b. Postsynaptic inhibition in regions containing catecholamine synapses
c. The presence of presynaptic catecholaminergic autoreceptors
d. Destruction of the catecholamine cell body
e. Collateral inhibition at catecholamine synapses

138. A group of neuropharmacologists attempted to develop an experimental drug for research purposes that would selectively block the removal of norepinephrine from the region of the synaptic cleft. Which of the following mechanisms would be selectively blocked by this experimental drug?

a. Reuptake
b. Enzymatic degradation
c. Diffusion
d. A combination of enzymatic degradation and diffusion
e. A combination of enzymatic degradation, diffusion, and reuptake

Neurochemistry/ Neurotransmitters

Answers

94. The answer is d. (*Kandel, pp 282-284. Siegel and Sapru, pp 115-118.*) The biosynthesis of catecholamines includes the following steps: Tyrosine is converted into L-DOPA by tyrosine hydroxylase. L-DOPA is then decarboxylated by a decarboxylase to form dopamine (and CO_2). The conversion of dopamine to norepinephrine comes about by the action of the enzyme dopamine β-hydroxylase. The rate-limiting enzyme in the biosynthesis of serotonin is tryptophan hydroxylase. In this process, tryptophan is converted to 5-hydroxytryptophan by tryptophan hydroxylase and by 5-hydroxytryptophan decarboxylase into serotonin.

95. The answer is b. (*Kandel, pp 282-284. Siegel and Sapru, pp 115-117.*) As indicated in the answer to Question 90, the rate-limiting step in the biosynthesis of dopamine is tyrosine hydroxylase, which converts tyrosine into L-DOPA. The rate-limiting step in the biosynthesis of serotonin is tryptophan hydroxylase. The enzyme dopamine β-hydroxylase converts dopamine to norepinephrine. Phenylethanolamine-*N*-methyltransferase is involved in the conversion of norepinephrine to epinephrine. Choline acetyltransferase is involved in the biosynthesis of ACh.

96. The answer is e. (*Kandel, pp 36-37. Siegel, pp, 212, 647-648, 672-673.*) Phenylketonuria results in severe mental retardation and is caused by a defect in the gene that provides the code for Phe hydroxylase, the enzyme that converts Phe to tyrosine. As a result of this defective gene, there is an abundance of Phe in the brain, which produces a toxic metabolite, thus interfering in brain development and maturation. Note that patients suffering from this disorder must avoid aspartame (which contains Phe) in their diets.

97. The answer is b. (*Kandel, pp 187-197. Siegel and Sapru, p 99.*) The amplitude of the end-plate potential differs from that of postsynaptic potentials observed in the CNS in that end-plate potentials can be as great as 70 times larger than CNS postsynaptic potentials. The end-plate potential is dependent upon the release of ACh from the nerve endings. Dopamine is not released at the neuromuscular junction. The end-plate potential is a graded potential and is not an all-or-none response. Another important feature of this potential is that it is directly related to the quantity of neurotransmitter (ACh) released from the presynaptic terminals. The release of ACh onto the muscle membrane is associated with the opening of sodium and potassium channels, and not chloride channels.

98. The answer is d. *(Kandel, pp 196-198. Siegel and Sapru, p 99.)* The transmitter at the neuromuscular junction is ACh, and its actions are mediated by the nicotinic ACh-gated channel. As noted, it produces the end-plate potential by permitting the passage of both sodium and potassium ions. Noradrenergic, muscarinic, and excitatory amino acid receptors are not known to function at the neuromuscular junction.

99. The answer is c. *(Kandel, pp 298-304. Siegel and Sapru, pp 101-102.)* Myasthenia gravis is an autoimmune disease that causes cranial nerve and limb muscle weakness by producing antibodies that act against the nicotinic receptor at the neuromuscular junction. See explanation to Question 101 for mechanism underlying myasthenia gravis. MS and ALS (see the chapter entitled "The Spinal Cord") involve damage to axons and/or nerve cells within the CNS, producing much more profound damage to motor functions. The Lambert-Eaton syndrome (see explanation to Question 102) bears a resemblance to myasthenia gravis, but the mechanism underlying dysfunction differs—the Lambert-Eaton syndrome involves a reduction in presynaptic Ca^+ channels. MD is typically characterized, in part, by progressive weakness of muscles and degeneration of the muscle fibers. The other disorders listed all affect the CNS, and thus the symptoms associated with these disorders differ significantly from those described in this case.

100. The answer is d. *(Siegel and Sapru, pp 88, 102).* This disorder is usually associated with small cell carcinoma and results in muscle weakness. There is a reduction in size of the compound action potentials in affected muscles, but such effects can be partially reversed with exercise. (See explanations to Questions 99, 101, and 102 for further details concerning why other possible answers were not correct.)

101. The answer is b. (*Siegel and Sapru, pp 101-102*). As noted above, myasthenia gravis is an autoimmune disease that causes cranial nerve and limb muscle weakness (and a reduction in the size of the muscle action potential) by producing antibodies that act against the nicotinic receptor at the neuromuscular junction. The net result disrupts the function of the nerve fibers that innervate the muscles in question because ACh released at the neuromuscular junction is now less effective than in a healthy individual. This disorder can be reversed by administration of drugs that inhibit the enzyme, acetylcholinesterase, which degrades ACh. Excessive release of ACh is not a realistic event that is likely to occur (except from the bite of a black widow spider). In theory, if it were to occur, there is no reason to believe that muscular weakness would be a symptom. Instead, there would be some rigidity and muscle spasms. Reductions in brain catecholamines are more closely associated with behavioral (and psychiatric disorders) but are not likely to produce muscle weakness characteristic of myasthenia gravis. A reduction in Ca^2 channels is associated with the Lambert-Eaton syndrome (see explanations to Questions 100 and 102). Viral encephalitis is more likely to have a more generalized effect on many brain functions, which can be fatal.

102. The answer is d. (*Siegel and Sapru, p 102*). The mechanism underlying the Lambert-Eaton syndrome involves a reduction in presynaptic Ca^2 channels, causing a reduction in release of ACh from these terminals at the neuromuscular junction. Evidence supporting this view includes the presence of antibodies to Ca^2 channels in these patients. Thus, this mechanism differs from that underlying myasthenia gravis (see explanation to Question 101 above, ie, production of antibodies acting against the nicotinic ACh receptor). The other choices involve events unrelated to the Lambert-Eaton syndrome.

103. The answer is c. (*Kandel, pp 190, 299. Siegel, 186-203.*) Curare blocks neuromuscular transmission by binding to the ACh nicotinic receptor, thus rendering the release of ACh at the neuromuscular junction ineffective. The other choices are incorrect because the transmitter at the neuromuscular junction is ACh, and the receptors for the other neurotransmitters listed as possible answers play no role at this synapse.

104. The answer is a. (*Kandel, pp 107-112, 294-295. Siegel and Sapru, pp 109-111. Siegel, pp 186-203.*) There are three basic mechanisms by which the transmitter is removed from the synaptic cleft: (1) enzymatic degradation, (2) reuptake, and (3) diffusion. In the case of the neuromuscular junction, ACh (and not glutamate) is the neurotransmitter and the primary mechanism involves enzymatic degradation. Glutamate's primary mechanism of removal involves reuptake.

105. The answer is d. (*Kandel, pp 280-295. Siegel and Sapru, pp 109-111. Siegel, pp 172, 195-196, 720.*) The enzyme involved is acetylcholinesterase, which helps break down ACh into acetate and choline. Choline is then taken up by the presynaptic terminal. Concerning the other choices, choline acetyltransferase is the enzyme involved in the synthesis of ACh; glutaminase and glutamine synthetase are involved in the formation of glutamate from glutamine and glutamine from glutamate, respectively. Serine hydroxymethyltransferase is the enzyme that converts serine into glycine.

106. The answer is e. (*Kandel, pp 280-295. Siegel and Sapru, pp 119-120. Siegel, pp 227-247.*) There is an increasing body of evidence that shows reductions in serotonin levels play an important role in depressive disorders. The raphe neurons, located along the midline of the brainstem, provide the basic sites of serotonergic neurons that project to all parts of the brain and spinal cord. The other choices refer to structures that concern motor and/or sensory functions mainly associated with cranial nerves. Since the raphe neurons were damaged, the neurotransmitter most likely responsible for the onset of depression in this instance is serotonin. It is possible that other transmitter systems, such as the catecholamines, may also play a role in this disorder; however, they would not be chiefly responsible for the disorder in this instance because of the restricted locus of the lesion. Recent practice has been to treat depression with serotonin reuptake inhibitors such as fluoxetine (Prozac), which has been found to be effective after several weeks of treatment. The other choices for Question 106 would be inappropriate because they would likely have a depressant effect on CNS functions.

107. The answer is d. (*Kandel, pp 280-295. Siegel and Sapru, pp 119-120, 512-514. Siegel, pp 227-247.*) As noted in the explanation to Question 106 above, reductions in serotonin levels have been more closely associated with depressive disorders than the other choices provided in this question. It should be noted, however, that some recent drugs utilized combinations of agonists, which may include catecholamines as well. But the drugs of choice for the treatment of depression include serotonin agonists.

108. The answer is a. (*Kandel, pp 280-295. Siegel and Sapru, pp 512-514. Siegel, pp 227-247.*) Recent practice has been to treat depression with serotonin reuptake inhibitors such as fluoxetine (Prozac), which has been found to be effective after several weeks of treatment. The other choices for Question 108 would be inappropriate because they would likely have a depressant effect on CNS functions.

109. The answer is c. (*Kandel, pp 282-284. Siegel and Sapru, pp 114-120. Siegel, pp 211-224, 227-247.*) Tyrosine is the amino acid substrate from which dopamine, norepinephrine, and epinephrine are formed. Tyrosine is converted into L-DOPA by tyrosine hydroxylase. L-DOPA is decarboxylated by a decarboxylase into dopamine (and CO_2). Dopamine is converted into norepinephrine by dopamine β-hydroxylase. Norepinephrine is converted into epinephrine by phenylethanolamine-N-methyltransferase. Melatonin is formed from serotonin. 5-hydroxy-indole-O-methyltransferase is part of the final step in the conversion of serotonin into melatonin. Trytophan hydroxylase is the rate-limiting step in the biosynthesis of serotonin.

110. The answer is b. (*Kandel, pp 281-287. Siegel and Sapru, pp 119-120.*) The rate-limiting step or controlling reaction in the biosynthesis of serotonin is tryptophan hydroxylase, which converts tryptophan into 5-hydroxytryptophan. Three of the other enzymes listed as choices—tyrosine hydroxylase, phenylethanolamine-N-methyltransferase, and dopamine β-hydroxylase—are, as noted in the explanation to Question 107, involved in the biosynthetic pathways for norepinephrine and epinephrine. Glutamic acid decarboxylase is utilized in the synthesis of GABA.

111. The answer is d. (*Kandel, pp 1151-1157. Siegel and Sapru, pp 110, 455. Siegel, pp 655-657, 781-787.*) A primary region shown to be affected by Alzheimer disease include the basal nucleus of Meynert (which contains cholinergic neurons that project widely to the forebrain, including the cerebral cortex); although not included in this question, it should be noted that regions also affected include the hippocampal formation and cerebral cortex. The other choices listed in this question included structures that have not been significantly implicated in this disorder.

112. The answer is c. (*Siegel and Sapru, pp 110, 455. Ropper, pp 1022-1023.*) Memantine, an NMDA glutaminergic antagonist has been found to be somewhat effective together with donepezil (Aricept), a reversible acytlycholinesterase inhibitor. Alzheimer brains have been shown to have reduced levels of ACh and cholinergic markers, especially after damage to cholinergic neurons of the basal nucleus of Meynert The other drugs are unrelated to the treatment of Alzheimer disease. Gabapentine and carbamazepine are used for the treatment of epilepsy; haloperidol is a dopaminergic blocker which is used as a sedative; clonidine is a noradrenergic α_2 agonist used for the control of blood pressure; parotxetine and sertraline are serotonin reuptake inhibitors used for the treatment of depression; levodopa is used for the treatment of Parkinson disease, and lithium has been used for treating depression.

113. The answer is c. (*Kandel, pp 1151-1157. Siegel and Sapru, p 455. Siegel, pp 655-657, 781-787.*) One of the clearest neuropathological characteristics of Alzheimer disease is the presence of amyloid deposits and neurofibrillary tangles in the cerebral cortex.

114. The answer is e. (*Kandel, pp 1151-1157. Siegel and Sapru, p 455. Siegel, pp 655-657, 781-787.*) A new and promising strategy that has been applied for the treatment of Alzheimer disease. It involves the attempt to administer small molecules that retard the aggregation of amyloid β peptides that form fibrillar amyloid plaques, which affect the normal functions of neurons.

115. The answer is b. (*Purves, pp 129-131, 169, 280-281, 457. Siegel, pp 268-282.*) The largest numbers of excitatory synapses in the CNS are mediated by glutamate, as it is believed that approximately half of the synapses in the brain release glutamate. For example, functions mediated by fibers that originate from the cerebral cortex and descend to such regions as the neostriatum, thalamus, brainstem, and spinal cord are generally believed to be mediated by glutamate. Many other neuronal systems throughout the brain and spinal cord utilize glutamate as well. Dopaminergic and noradrenergic neurons, while mostly excitatory, can also be inhibitory at some synapses and are less numerous than glutamate. Cholinergic and substance P synapses are also excitatory, but are likewise less numerous than glutamate.

116. The answer is c. *(Purves, p 129. Siegel and Sapru, pp 111-112. Siegel, pp 268-282.)* It has been discovered that one mechanism of neurodegeneration involves prolonged activation of neurons by glutamate. The other choices have not been shown to be related to any process of toxicity.

117. The answer is a. *(Purves, p 129. Siegel and Sapru, pp 111-112. Siegel, pp 268-282.)* It is believed that if glutamate accumulates in the extracellular space and is not removed, the presence of glutamate will effectively stimulate the neuron to death. It has been shown that neurotoxicity is linked to cell death after a stroke, which causes brain ischemia and oxygen deprivation. Glutamate receptors are involved in ischemic cell damage in the following way: glutamate released from the presynaptic terminal would normally activate NMDA and AMPA receptors in the postsynaptic membrane. This results in an increase in the intracellular concentration of Ca^{2+}, which remains long after the initial stimulus is removed, and thus prevents the cell from reestablishing a resting membrane potential (Ca^{2+} activates proteases and DNAses that eat the cell). The net effect here is to produce injury (or death) to the cell.

118. The answer is c. *(Siegel and Sapru, pp 515-518. Siegel, pp 922-923.)* One of the strategies used effectively for the treatment of anxiety disorders is to use classes of drugs that suppress CNS activity. One such class includes benzodiazepine agonists, such as chlordiazepoxide. This drug enhances GABA transmission by binding to the benzodiazepine site on the $GABA_A$-receptor benzodiazepine chloride ionophore complex. The other choices relate to drugs that have opposite effects, namely, ones with excitatory effects on CNS neurons.

119. The answer is c. *(Aminoff, pp 88-89. Siegel and Sapru, pp 515-518. Siegel, pp 922-923.)* As noted in the explanation to Question 118, chlordiazepoxide enhances GABA transmission by binding to the benzodiazepine site on the $GABA_A$-receptor benzodiazepine chloride ionophore complex. In this manner, it acts as a GABA agonist, producing anxiolytic, sedative, and anticonvulsant effects. The other choices would either have little or deleterious effects in the treatment of anxiety disorders.

120. The answer is b. *(Kandel, pp 1214-1222. Siegel and Sapru, p 120. Aminoff, p 259.)* Clonidine has long been used effectively for the treatment of hypertension. Other choices listed are used either as anticonvulsants or for the treatment of headache and are, therefore, inappropriate for the treatment of this patient.

121. The answer is e. (*Brunton, pp 269-271. Cooper, p 201. Kandel, p 1222.*) Prazosin is an adrenergic antagonist whose functions are mediated by its actions upon α_1 receptors. Administration of this drug results in an overall decrease in noradrenergic transmission. Since norepinephrine acts through α_1 receptors in smooth muscle to constrict blood vessels, prazosin is believed to have antihypertensive effects by blocking these noradrenergic receptors in smooth muscles.

122. The answer is b. (*Kandel, pp 480-484. Siegel and Sapru, p 121. Siegel, pp 914-916.*) Research conducted over the past two decades has shown that the actions of morphine are mediated through opioid μ-receptors, while other opioid receptors appear not to play a significant role. Likewise, dopamine receptors are not involved in this process.

123. The answer is c. (*Kandel, pp 480-484. Siegel and Sapru, p 121. Siegel, pp 914-916.*) The region possessing the highest concentration of opioid receptors listed among the structures included in this question is the midbrain periaqueductal gray. This region plays an important role in the modulation of pain and is particularly responsive to opioid activation by morphine as a mechanism in the regulation of pain.

124. The answer is d. (*Siegel and Sapru, pp 111-112. Siegel, pp 287-289.*) As noted above, glutamate has been implicated in ischemia-induced brain damage following brain trauma such as a stroke. It has also been shown that administration of NMDA-receptor antagonists following a stroke is effective by reducing tissue infarction and neuronal cell death. The other choices listed in this question are not known to relate to the reversal of the deleterious effects of stroke.

125. The answer is b. (*Siegel, pp 287-289.*) The NMDA-receptor antagonist is effective in treatment of stroke, in part, by decreasing disruption of the blood-brain barrier. It has been suggested that this becomes manifest by a blockade of the neuronal production of reactive oxygen species that occurs as a result of activation of NMDA receptors. Again, the other choices listed for this question have no known relationship to the process in question.

126. The answer is e. (*Siegel, pp 629-634.*) One of the drugs that have been used effectively for the treatment of epilepsy, especially complex partial seizures involving the temporal lobe, has been gabapentin. The other choices of drugs are ones that enhance convulsive activity either by facilitating excitatory transmitter function or by inhibiting inhibitory transmitter functions. Vigabatrin functions by enhancing GABA-mediated inhibition of neurons, perhaps by the inhibition of GABA-transaminase.

127. The answer is c. (*Siegel, pp 629-635.*) Two current theories underlying drug treatment for the epilepsies are that it is caused either by an excess of excitatory amino acids or by a decrease in GABA levels. As noted in the answer to the previous question, administration of GABAergic compounds are employed that enhance the inhibitory processes characteristic of this inhibitory neurotransmitter. The other choices for this question would have excitatory effects upon neuronal functions and thus would be inappropriate for the treatment of temporal lobe epilepsy.

128. The answer is c. (*Kandel, p 295. Siegel and Sapru, pp 111-112. Purves, pp 121, 149-150. Siegel, pp 568-571.*) Nitric oxide is synthesized from L-arginine when stimulated by nitric oxide synthase. Choline is a precursor of ACh, tyrosine of dopamine and norepinephrine, and tryptophan of serotonin. Glutamate, a neurotransmitter, is synthesized from glutamine and can be converted into GABA by glutamic acid decarboxylase.

129. The answer is a. (*Kandel, p 295. Siegel and Sapru, pp 111-112. Purves, pp 121, 149-150. Siegel, pp 568-571.*) Nitric oxide differs from more classical, or traditional, neurotransmitters, in that, in addition to acting as a neurotransmitter, it is a gas and also acts as a second messenger. After nitric oxide is formed, it diffuses locally and interacts with specific molecules such as the enzyme catalyzing cyclic guanosine 5'-monophosphate (cGMP) synthesis, guanylyl cyclase. A number of different neurotransmitters can have either excitatory or inhibitory effects, depending upon the receptors with which they interact. Since nitric oxide is coupled to a variety of neurotransmitter systems, it is likely that it is also involved in both excitatory and inhibitory processes. Recent studies have shown that nitric oxide is likely involved in a wide variety of processes and is not limited to a single function. Moreover, it is widely distributed throughout both the CNS as well as in the peripheral nervous system. While many transmitters are packaged in synaptic vesicles, nitric oxide differs by diffusing widely without being packaged in synaptic vesicles.

130. The answer is d. *(Kandel, pp 978-980.)* Vasopressin (antidiuretic hormone [ADH]) is produced mainly from the magnocellular neurons of the hypothalamus. The hormone is released into the capillaries of the posterior pituitary. When it is released into the vascular system, it stimulates the kidneys to conserve water. The action of oxytocin is related to functions of the uterus and breasts. This hormone plays a role in the expulsion of the fetus at birth and in the milk ejection reflex following suckling. Substance P, histamine, and somatostatin are not known to relate specifically to this process.

131. The answer is b. *(Siegel, pp 250-252, 261-262, 931-937.)* When an opioid compound, especially a μ-receptor agonist (such as morphine), is administered in response to chronic pain, this causes the release of histamine in neurons. This leads to the activation of histamine H_2 receptors, which play a role in the relief of pain. In fact, there are ongoing attempts now to develop drugs, such as histamine H_3-receptor compounds, which have been shown to mediate antinociception and have anti-inflammatory properties as well. Also note that release of histamine can lead to pruritus (skin infection) after drug administration, which may account for the presence of such infections in drug addicts. The other choices listed in this question are not known to relate to the alleviation of pain, in particular, with respect to morphine administration. In fact, substance P is associated with the elicitation of pain impulses.

132. The answer is a. *(Siegel, 276-279.)* NMDA ion channels are opened by both glutamate and glycine. On the other hand, Mg^{2+} generates a voltage-dependent block of this ion channel. The drug of abuse, PCP, also utilizes a similar mechanism to block NMDA-receptor channels. The other choices do not relate to this mechanism with respect to PCP.

133. The answer is b. *(Siegel, pp 276-289.)* Excitatory amino acids and, in particular, the glutamate family of compounds have long been thought to play an important role in epileptiform activity. Epileptiform activity typically includes AMPA-receptor activation. However, as the seizure becomes more intense, there is increased involvement of NMDA receptors. This is evidenced by the facts that NMDA antagonists can reduce the intensity and length of the seizure activity and that, following removal of human epileptic hippocampal tissue, there is an upregulation of both AMPA and NMDA receptors. Metabotropic glutamate receptors have been shown to be present in the retina but have not yet been demonstrated to be present in regions of the brain that are typically epileptogenic. GABA and glycine are inhibitory transmitters; therefore, seizures would logically block such receptor activation. There has been no substantive evidence concerning the role of cortical nicotinic receptors in epilepsy.

134. The answer is c. (*Purves, pp 143-146. Siegel and Sapru, pp 515-516.*) Cholecystokinin (CCK) agonists have been used to induce panic attacks, and antagonists of CCK receptors have been used to treat anxiety disorders. Cholinergic and noradrenergic agonists would have excitatory effects of behavioral functions and would therefore be contraindicated for the treatment of anxiety disorders. Likewise, antagonists of serotonin 1-A receptors and opioid peptides would likely yield similar excitatory effects upon nervous system functions.

135. The answer is d. (*Kandel, pp 280-286. Purves, pp 119-126, 137-142. Siegel and Sapru, pp 109-121.*) Tryptophan hydroxylase, tyrosine hydroxylase, and choline acetyltransferase are enzymes that are critical for the biosynthesis of serotonin, catecholamines, and ACh, respectively. Dopamine β-hydroxylase converts dopamine to norepinephrine. Catechol-O-methyltransferase and monoamine oxidase are critical for the metabolic degradation of catecholamines.

136. The answer is d. (*Kandel, pp 1213-1216. Siegel and Sapru, p 514.*) Lithium has been used for a number of years as an effective drug for the treatment of bipolar disorders. It has been shown to decrease the length, severity, and recurrence of manic states as well as the depressive components of this disorder. The mechanism of action of lithium in effectively combating bipolar disorder is not absolutely clear, since it has a wide variety of biological effects. In part, these include changes in the expression of some G-proteins and subtypes of adenyl cyclase, alteration of the coupling

of G-proteins to neurotransmitter receptors, alterations of monoamine levels and receptors, and effects upon ion channels. Monoaminergic drugs are
generally used for the treatment of panic disorders and, to some extent, to
treat anxiety. Anxiety attacks are also treated with benzodiazepine drugs.
For schizophrenia, a wide range of drugs have been used; these include
those that affect monoaminergic, cholinergic, and GABAergic systems. See
Question 453 and its answer for further discussion.

137. The answer is c. *(Kandel, pp 280-286. Purves, pp 137-140.)* These
findings can best be explained in terms of a mechanism that involves presynaptic autoreceptors. These receptors modulate the release of a catecholamine by responding to the concentration of this transmitter within
the synapse. It thus represents a specific negative feedback mechanism. For
example, if the concentration of transmitter in the synapse is high, then
release will likely be inhibited. Less inhibition (ie, more transmitter release)
will occur if concentrations are low. Other choices are incorrect. The presence of a GABAergic neuron at the synapse, postsynaptic inhibition, and
collateral inhibition are unrelated, since they refer to events that are associated with the postsynaptic neuron, not the catecholamine (presynaptic)
neuron. As a result of the phasic nature of this phenomenon, destruction of
the catecholamine cell body would produce events that were not phasic;
indeed, there would be permanent loss of the neuron's capacity to release
transmitter.

138. The answer is e. *(Kandel, pp 281-286. Purves, pp 120-135. Siegel and
Sapru, pp 109-111.)* There are three mechanisms by which a transmitter is
removed from the region of the synapse. The most common one is reuptake, in which transporter molecules mediate high-affinity reuptake that is
specific for the transmitter in question. Other mechanisms include diffusion, which removes some components of the transmitter substance, and
enzymatic degradation of the amine achieved by the enzymes monoamine
oxidase and catechol-O-methyltransferase.

The Spinal Cord

Questions

139. A college student received an injury as a result of being tackled in a football game. After the game, the student was treated at a local hospital and was found to be unable to abduct and rotate the left arm at the shoulder, flex the elbow, and extend the wrist of the left side. Further examination revealed depression of the biceps reflex of this limb, but the reflex activity involving the other limbs was normal. Which of the following is the most likely site of the injury?

a. Precentral gyrus
b. Basilar pons
c. Ventral horn cells at C1
d. Nerve roots of C5 to C6
e. Triceps muscle

140. A neurological examination of a 75-year-old male reveals that when the abdominal wall is stroked, the muscles of the abdominal wall of the side of the body stimulated fail to contract. Other neurological tests appear normal. Which of the following is the most likely region of the injury?

a. C1 to C5 spinal segments
b. C6 to T1 spinal segments
c. T2 to T7 spinal segments
d. T8 to T12 spinal segments
e. L1 to L5 spinal segments

141. A 65-year-old female has weakness when attempting to flex her left knee and extend the hip. Neurophysiological analysis of the affected regions reveals a reduced number of motor units firing with fasciculations and slowed conduction velocity. There is no depression of tendon reflexes or muscle wasting. Likewise, plantar and abdominal reflexes are normal, there is little sensory loss, and there are no signs of sphincter disturbances. Which of the following is the best explanation for this disturbance?

a. Peripheral neuropathy of nerves on the left side of the body that exit the spinal cord at L4 to S1
b. Damage to the neuromuscular junctions associated with nerves that exit the left side of the spinal cord between T8 and L3
c. Degeneration of nerve cells in the ventral horn of the left side of the spinal cord between T8 and T12
d. Degeneration of fibers contained in the lateral funiculus of the left side of the thoracic spinal cord
e. Damage to the dorsal horn of the spinal cord of the left side between L1 and L4

142. A 55-year-old man reports pain in the neck and right arm and weakness in extending the fingers of his right hand, with loss of sensation in the right thumb and middle fingers. A neurological examination reveals weakness of the right biceps reflex, but other neurological signs cannot be detected. Which of the following is the most likely diagnosis?

a. Syringomyelia involving the cervical cord
b. A knife wound of the right arm completely severing nerves innervating the biceps muscle
c. Prolapse of a cervical disk
d. Poliomyelitis involving the cervical cord
e. AIDS

143. A 60-year-old woman was hospitalized with a severe respiratory infection for several weeks. Afterward, she displayed symptoms of myalgia and weakness of the lower limbs. In addition, she also showed loss of muscle tone and some flaccidity, with loss of tendon reflexes. Examination also revealed a weakness of facial muscles. This constellation of symptoms progressed for approximately 2 weeks and persisted for more than a year, at which time recovery took place at a slow rate. There was also some demyelination coupled with lymphatic inflammation at the site of the demyelination. Which of the following is the most likely cause of this patient's condition?

a. Myasthenia gravis
b. Muscular dystrophy (MD)
c. Multiple sclerosis (MS)
d. Guillain-Barré syndrome
e. Lumbar disk prolapse

144. Over a period of time, a 46-year-old man found that he developed progressive bilateral weakness of both upper and lower limbs beginning with the muscles of the hands. However, testing revealed that sensory functions appeared normal. Eventually, this individual was found to have wasting of muscles, fasciculations, and evidence of upper motor neuron (UMN) dysfunction, together with an increase in tendon reflexes. After a few additional months, the patient developed facial weakness and an inability to swallow (dysphagia). Further analysis revealed abnormalities in the electromyogram (EMG) of the upper and lower extremities, resulting in denervation atrophy. However, the cerebrospinal fluid (CSF) remained normal. Which of the following is the most likely diagnosis?

a. Multiple sclerosis (MS)
b. Amyotrophic lateral sclerosis (ALS)
c. Poliomyelitis
d. Myasthenia gravis
e. A cerebral cortical stroke

145. A 38-year-old woman is referred to a neurologist because she complained of visual loss and muscle weakness. Subsequent examination reveals impairment of other sensations, which included tingling and burning sensations, weakness of the lower limbs, paralysis of the upper limbs, progressive impairment of gait, signs of UMN involvement (ie, spasticity and increased tendon reflexes), and bladder disturbances. No signs of infection are detected as measured by blood analysis, cultures, and chest x-ray. However, elevations in CSF protein are noted as well as an abnormal immunoglobulin G (IgG) synthesis. Which of the following is the most likely diagnosis?

a. Diffuse cerebellar degeneration
b. ALS
c. MS
d. A peripheral neuropathy
e. A prefrontal cortical brain tumor

146. A 68-year-old male receives a diagnosis of ALS after experiencing weakness in his legs. Over the next year, the disease is progressive and he loses mobility in the use of his arms and legs, as well as some cranial nerve functions. Which region or regions of the spinal cord are primarily affected by this disorder?

a. Dorsal horns of the spinal cord
b. Lateral columns of the spinal cord
c. Ventral horns of the spinal cord
d. Dorsal columns and ventral horns of the spinal cord
e. Ventral horns and lateral columns of the spinal cord

Questions 147 to 155

Match each of the following vignettes with the labeled area of the brain with which it is most closely associated. Each lettered option may be used once, multiple times, or not at all.

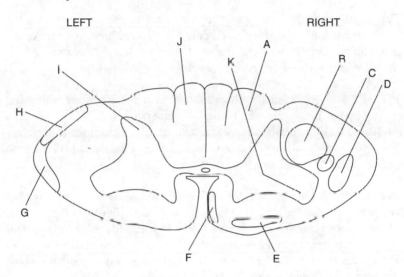

147. An 18-year-old male receives a knife wound in his right arm, partially severing the peripheral nerve. Afterward, he complains about loss of some sensation. A neurological examination indicates a loss of ability to experience vibration sensation, two-point discrimination, and some pain. Which structure that mediates two-point discrimination and vibration sensation is affected by the injury?

148. A 44-year-old woman experienced excruciating pain emanating from her left leg. It was concluded that she was suffering from a disorder of unknown etiology for which drug treatment proved ineffective. A decision was made to surgically cut the pathway mediating pain from the left leg to the brain. Which labeled area was cut by the neurosurgeon?

149. A middle-aged woman is admitted to the hospital after suffering a stroke limited to the motor cortex. The patient presented with a classic UMN paralysis. Which labeled area degenerated as a result of the stroke?

150. An elderly man is brought to the emergency room after fainting in his home. An MRI suggests the presence of a small stroke limited to the medial aspect of the rostral part of the midbrain tegmentum. Which labeled area is most likely affected by the stroke?

151. A 30-year-old man is brought to the emergency room after sustaining a work-related injury that damaged part of his spinal cord. A neurological examination reveals considerable loss of extensor muscle function. Which labeled area was damaged that could account for this defect?

152. A 58-year-old female was admitted to a local hospital following reports by her family that she had recent experiences of falling as well as displaying lack of coordination of movement. Her neurological examination revealed primarily a gait ataxia coupled with some dysarthria and nystagmus. Which labeled area was most likely affected by this lesion?

153. A 30-year-old male was referred to a neurologist after complaining of severe pain in his back. The neurologist provided him with a new drug whose actions have previously been shown to block the release of the neurotransmitter from terminal endings of first-order neurons in the spinal cord which thus prevented transmission of pain impulses to the brain. Which labeled area in the figure did this drug act to reduce pain transmission?

154. A 64-year-old woman suffers from a massive stroke of the motor regions of the cerebral cortex, causing voluntary loss of movement. Among the fiber pathways that are affected by the stroke is a component that passes through the ipsilateral spinal cord. Which labeled area is most likely to be affected by the stroke?

155. An 18-year-old male was involved in a serious football injury which left him temporarily motionless on the ground after he was tackled by two players of the opposing team. A neurological analysis revealed significant compression of the spinal cord, in particular, along its lateral extent. The analysis further revealed clinical signs such as hypotonia, decreased tendon reflexes, and some ataxia. Which labeled area would most likely be involved in compression of the spinal cord?

Questions 156 to 158

Each of the following cases may be caused by a lesion or other damage at a particular site. **Match the location of** the loci of each of the causative lesions listed below. Each lettered option may be used once, multiple times, or not at all.

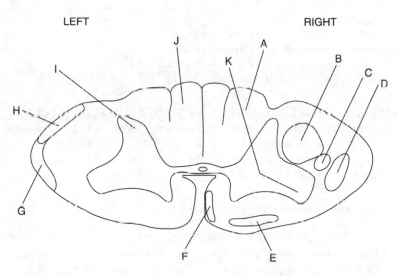

156. A patient suffering from a disease of unknown etiology reports that he cannot move his hands and arms. Neurological analysis revealed a flaccid paralysis of the upper limbs with diminished reflex activity in these limbs.

157. A 76-year-old woman is rushed to an emergency room after she was found unconscious in her apartment. Sometime later, she regains consciousness but cannot move her right arm or hand. Further neurological analysis reveals hyperreflexia and hypertonia in the affected limb.

158. A 25-year-old male is stabbed after having been assaulted and is taken to the emergency room for treatment. A physical examination indicated that the knife wound penetrated the spinal cord and a neurological examination reveals that when he tries to walk, he has difficulty in walking in that he has ataxia of movement. Other aspects of movement appear normal.

159. A 24-year-old man becomes intoxicated and gets into a barfight, during which he is stabbed in the back. He is taken to the emergency room and following a thorough neurological examination, it is determined that the knife wound destroyed the right half of the spinal cord at the level of the lower cervical cord. Which of the following deficits will most likely result from the knife wound?

a. Impaired bladder functions only
b. Impaired movements of the lower limb only
c. Impaired movements of the upper limb only
d. Loss of sensory functions of the lower limb only
e. Loss of sensory and motor functions of upper and lower limbs

160. A 48-year-old male suffers a brain stem stroke that resulted in an upper motor neuron syndrome, which includes loss of voluntary movement of the limbs, hyperreflexia, and hypertonia. With respect to hyperreflexia and hypertonia, which of the following explanations can best explain these symptoms?

a. Abnormal stimulation of unmyelinated C fibers
b. Sequential excitation and inhibition of 1A fibers
c. Abnormal stimulation of gamma motor neurons
d. Sequential excitation and inhibition of alpha motor neurons
e. Abnormal stimulation of general visceral efferent fibers

161. An individual suffers a severe injury that results in the crushing of the peripheral nerves that normally enter the spinal cord at levels C7 to T1, causing both motor and sensory loss. Which of the following regions would most likely be affected by the injury?

a. Back of the head
b. Neck
c. Shoulder
d. Hand
e. Back

162. A 42-year-old female complains about a painful and burning sensation in both hands and arms. Following a neurological examination, it was determined that the patient is suffering from a peripheral neuropathy caused by a virus that selectively attacked sensory fibers in the arms mediating pain and temperature signals. Concerning the distribution and sites of termination of these sensory fibers in the central nervous system (CNS), their sites of termination include which of the following regions?

a. Laminae I and II of the gray matter of the spinal cord ipsilateral to their site of entry into the cord
b. Laminae III and IV of the gray matter of the spinal cord contralateral to their site of entry into the cord
c. Laminae VIII and IX of the gray matter of the spinal cord ipsilateral to their site of entry into the cord
d. Laminae VIII and IX of the gray matter of the spinal cord contralateral to their site of entry into the cord
e. Lower brain stem nuclei ipsilateral to their site of entry into the cord

163. Efforts were made by a pharmaceutical company to develop a drug that reduces or eliminates pain associated with neuropathies. The approach was to utilize a neurotransmitter-receptor blocker against the neurotransmitter released by the first-order pain pathway. The drug under development is an antagonist against which of the following neurotransmitters?

a. Enkephalins
b. Acetylcholine (ACh)
c. Substance P
d. γ-Aminobutyric acid (GABA)
e. Serotonin

164. A 56-year-old female is examined by a neurologist following complaints that she could not recognize any pain sensation in her arms or legs. A detailed neurological examination suggests the presence of a viral disorder that selectively affected sensory fibers that enter the spinal cord and which pass through Lissauer marginal zone. Which of the following statements correctly characterizes the fibers in this region?

a. They mediate unconscious proprioception.
b. This zone is composed of coarse, heavily myelinated fibers.
c. Fibers within Lissauer marginal zone may ascend or descend several segments.
d. These fibers synapse with alpha motor neurons of extensor muscles.
e. Cells in this zone typically project to thalamic nuclei.

165. A 63-year-old male was involved in an automobile accident and sustained a small peripheral nerve injury. The damage involved some of the axons that enter the spinal cord at L1, which affected principally fibers that innervate the nucleus dorsalis of Clarke. Which of the following is the primary dysfunction resulting from this injury?

a. Loss of autonomic functions
b. Loss of unconscious proprioceptive information
c. Loss of pain and temperature sensation
d. UMN paralysis
e. LMN paralysis

166. A patient is diagnosed with a form of motor neuron disease that initially affects neurons situated in the dorsolateral aspect of the ventral horn at L1 to L4. Which of the following arrangements best describes the deficit likely to be present?

a. LMN paralysis involving the hand
b. UMN paralysis of the upper limb
c. LMN paralysis of the back muscles
d. LMN paralysis of the leg
e. UMN paralysis of the leg

167. A small vascular lesion that affected the region of the ventromedial white matter of the cervical cord was discovered in a middle-aged man during a neurological examination. The neurologist came to the conclusion that the lesion affected the descending fibers of the medial longitudinal fasciculus (MLF). Which of the following deficits did the neurologist observe that led him to this conclusion?

a. The patient presented with a UMN paralysis.
b. The patient displayed difficulties in regulating his head position in response to postural changes.
c. The patient displayed an LMN paralysis.
d. The patient displayed ataxia of movement, nystagmus, and diplopia.
e. The patient experienced significant difficulties in regulating blood pressure and bladder functions.

168. A 26-year-old woman complains of loss of some sensation on both sides of her body that seems to be localized around the region of her waist. A neurological examination reveals that the primary sensations lost are pain and temperature, although some bilateral loss of light touch is also noted. Which of the following is the most likely locus of the lesion?

a. Dorsal funiculus on both sides
b. Dorsal root ganglion, bilaterally
c. Region surrounding the central canal
d. Midline region of the lower medulla
e. Region of the ventral horn, bilaterally

169. A 49-year-old male is given a brief neurological examination as part of an overall examination provided by his physician. One such test includes the patellar tendon reflex which is tested during the course of a routine neurological examination. Which of the following statements accurately characterizes this reflex?

a. Inhibited by homonymous alpha motor neuron
b. A monosynaptic reflex
c. A disynaptic reflex
d. Activated by Golgi tendon organ
e. Inhibited by gamma motor neurons

170. An 83-year-old male complains of weakness in his leg muscles. Following a neurological examination, the neurologist concludes that the patient is experiencing loss of muscle spindle receptor function in the affected limbs. Which of the following functions best describes the loss associated with muscle spindles activity in the affected limbs?

a. Loss of capacity to detect the rate of change of muscle length
b. Loss of ability to function as high-threshold receptors
c. Loss of anatomical arrangement in series with the extrafusal muscle fibers
d. Loss of anatomical capacity to project directly to thalamus
e. Loss of capacity to serve as tension detectors

171. An 18-year-old male is shot in the back and is taken to the emergency room. A neurological examination reveals that there was a hemisection of the right half of the spinal cord that extended from T8 to T12. Which of the following deficits will most likely result from this injury?

a. Loss of pain and temperature sensation from the right leg; loss of conscious proprioception from the left leg; UMN paralysis of the left leg
b. Loss of pain and temperature sensation from the left leg; loss of conscious proprioception from the right leg; UMN paralysis of the left leg
c. Loss of pain and temperature sensation from the left arm and leg; loss of conscious proprioception from the right leg and arm; flaccid paralysis of the right leg
d. Loss of pain and temperature sensation from the left leg; loss of conscious proprioception from the right leg; UMN paralysis of the right leg
e. Bilateral loss of pain and temperature sensation and conscious proprioception, both from the lower half of the body; UMN paralysis of the left leg and flaccid paralysis of the right leg

172. A 45-year-old woman is brought to her local hospital's emergency room by her husband because of several days of progressive weakness and numbness in her arms and legs. Her symptoms began with tingling in her toes, which she assumed to be her feet "falling asleep." However, this feeling did not disappear, and she began to feel numb, first in her toes on both feet, then ascending to her calves and knees. Two days later, she began to feel numb in her fingertips and had difficulty lifting her legs. When she finally was unable to climb the stairs of her house because of her leg weakness, had difficulty gripping the banister, and experienced shortness of breath, her husband urged her to go to the emergency room. The neurologist who examines the patient in the emergency room notices that she was short of breath while sitting in bed. He asked the respiratory therapist to measure her vital capacity (the greatest volume of air that can be exhaled from the lungs after a maximal inspiration), and the value for this was far lower than would be expected for her age and weight. Her neurological examination showed that her arms and legs were very weak, so she had difficulty lifting them against gravity. She was unable to feel a pin or a vibrating tuning fork at all on her legs and below her elbows, but was able to feel the pin on her upper chest. The neurologist could not elicit any reflexes from her ankles or knees. He subsequently advises the emergency room staff that the patient needed to have a spinal tap and be admitted to the intensive care unit immediately. Where in the nervous system is the damage most likely to be found?

a. Frontal lobe
b. Temporal lobe
c. Peripheral nerves and nerve roots
d. Spinal cord
e. Parietal lobe

173. In testing for the presence or absence of sensory functions, a neurologist administered a number of tests to a patient. One of them involved a pinprick placed in certain locations on different parts of the body. Which receptor is activated following such stimulation?

a. Merkel tactile disk
b. Ruffini corpuscle
c. Pacinian corpuscle
d. Free nerve endings
e. Meissner corpuscle

174. A 35-year-old male, who had his leg partially crushed in an industrial accident, was examined by a neurologist. The patient reported loss of sensory functions and the neurologist made use of a tuning fork as one of his tools to test sensory functions. If sensory processes were functioning properly, which receptor would be activated by the application of the tuning fork to the surface of different parts of the affected leg?

a. Free nerve endings
b. Muscle spindles
c. Pacinian corpuscle
d. Golgi tendon organ
e. Meissner corpuscle

175. A 55-year-old patient is involved in a severe motor vehicle accident and admitted to the emergency room. The patient complains of abnormal sensations such as burning and tingling in the left arm. A neurological examination further reveals little change in motor or other sensory functions. Which of the following regions was most likely affected by the accident?

a. Dorsal horn of the spinal cord
b. Ventral horn of the spinal cord
c. Ascending pathways in lateral funiculus of the left spinal cord
d. Dorsal columns of spinal cord
e. Nerve roots associated with the cervical cord

176. A 45-year-old male is involved in an industrial accident and develops a complete flaccid paralysis and loss of sensation of the lower limbs. After a week, the patient regains movement of the limbs but at the same time experiences pain in the region of the lower limbs coupled with bladder dysfunction. All of these defects are most likely the result of which of the following?

a. Compression of the dorsal roots at L2
b. Compression of the entire spinal cord at L2
c. Compression of the dorsal columns at L2
d. Compression of the lateral funiculus at L2
e. A lesion transecting the corticospinal tracts at T1

177. A 35-year-old man, who had been in good health, noticed that his right leg was weak. As the day progressed, he found that he was dragging the leg behind him when he walked, and finally asked a friend to drive him home from work because he was unable to lift his right foot up enough to place it on the gas pedal. He also noticed that his left leg felt a little bit numb. Finally, his wife convinced him to go to the emergency room of his local hospital.

In the emergency room, he had a great deal of difficulty walking. He informed the physician that it started slowly several days before but he had ignored the symptoms. His language function, cranial nerves, and motor and sensory examinations of his arms were within normal limits. When the physician examined his right leg, it was markedly weak, with very brisk reflexes in the knee and ankle. Vibration and position sense in the right leg were absent. Pain and temperature testing were normal in the right leg, but these sensations were absent on the left leg and abdomen to the level of his umbilicus. Reflexes in the left leg were normal, but when the physician scratched the lateral portion of the plantar surface on the bottom side of his right foot, the great toe moved up. The remainder of the patient's examination was normal. Which of the following is the primary site of the lesion?

a. Lower brain stem
b. Cervical spinal cord
c. Thoracic spinal cord
d. Lumbar spinal cord
e. Peripheral nerves

178. As a result of a hemisection of the spinal cord, a patient has loss of vibration and position sense in the right leg. Which of the following pathways was affected by the lesion?

a. Right fasciculus cuneatus
b. Right fasciculus gracilis
c. Left fasciculus cuneatus
d. Left fasciculus gracilis
e. Right Lissauer tract

179. Following hemisection of the spinal cord at the level of approximately T3, a patient experiences loss of pain and temperature on the left side of the leg. Which of the following tracts was affected by the hemisection of the cord that could account for this deficit?

a. Right fasciculus cuneatus
b. Right fasciculus gracilis
c. Right spinothalamic tract
d. Left spinothalamic tract
e. Left corticospinal tract

180. After a hemisection of the spinal cord takes place at T3, a patient experiences marked weakness in the right leg. Which of the following best accounts for this weakness?

a. There was muscle damage in the right leg.
b. There was damage in his left frontal lobe.
c. There was damage to the right corticospinal tract.
d. The dorsal root was damaged.
e. There was damage to the right femoral nerve.

181. In testing for motor dysfunctions, a neurologist identifies an upward movement of the patient's toe when the plantar surface of his foot is scratched. This response is indicative of a lesion of a part of the nervous system. Which of the following is linked to this response?

a. UMNs
b. LMNs
c. Peripheral nerves
d. Skeletal muscles
e. Autonomic nerves

The Spinal Cord

Answers

139. The answer is d. *(Siegel and Sapru, pp 140-142. Aminoff, pp 177, 200-218.)* In this case, disruption of the root fibers of C5 to C6 (Erb palsy) involve components of the brachial plexus and affect muscle groups such as the deltoid, supraspinatus, infraspinatus, biceps, and flexor carpi radialis. These muscles govern abduction of the arm, rotation of the arm at the shoulder, and flexion of the elbow and wrist. Reflex activity would also be affected due to disturbance of both alpha and gamma motor neurons serving the biceps muscle. Lesions involving the cerebral cortex or pons, especially the region of the pyramidal tracts, would produce a UMN paralysis, which would include hyperreflexia and hypertonia. An LMN paralysis involving the ventral horn cells at C1 would not affect the brachial plexus and the muscle groups indicated in this question. The triceps muscle is not involved in producing the movements affected by the injury.

140. The answer is d. *(Aminoff, pp 200-218.)* In this case, there is a loss of superficial abdominal reflexes, which require that spinal segments T8 to T12 be intact. The test for these reflexes is to stroke a quadrant of the abdominal wall with an object such as a wooden stick. The normal response is for the muscle of the quadrant stimulated to contract and for movement of the umbilicus in the direction of the stimulus.

141. The answer is a. *(Siegel and Sapru, pp 140-142. Aminoff, pp 200-218.)* The nerves innervating the knee and hip exit the spinal cord between L4 and S1. Typical characteristics of a peripheral neuropathy include muscle weakness directed in a more pronounced manner upon the proximal muscles. Depression of tendon reflexes is generally not seen, and muscle wasting might occur only at a very late stage of the disease. Damage to the neuromuscular junction, such as myasthenia gravis, produces a different constellation of deficits. These include muscle fatigue and weakness that is fluctuating. This disorder also typically affects cranial nerves. In addition, the spinal segments indicated (T8-L3) are not associated with the muscle groups in question. Damage to the ventral horn would produce an LMN (flaccid) paralysis, which is not characteristic of the muscle weakness of this patient. Likewise, damage to the lateral funiculus would produce a UMN (spastic) paralysis, and dorsal horn damage would produce sensory deficits as well as affect muscle tone. In addition, the spinal segments indicated in this last choice (e) do not relate to the muscle groups affected in the patient.

142. The answer is c. (*Aminoff, pp 177, 227, 229.*) The most likely cause of the condition in this patient is a cervical disk prolapse. This disorder would produce pain in the neck and arm, which increases with movement of the head. It would also cause loss of some sensation in the thumb and other fingers, as well as weakness in both finger extension and of the biceps reflex. Syringomyelia would produce bilateral segmental loss of pain and temperature. A knife wound completely severing the nerve would result in a functional loss similar to that experienced with an LMN paralysis. Polio results in loss of LMNs, thus also producing an LMN (flaccid) paralysis. One of the effects of AIDS is that it produces damage to the lateral and dorsal columns, resulting in the appearance of a UMN disorder.

143. The answer is d. (*Siegel and Sapru, pp 70-71, 74. Aminoff, pp 180, 212-213.*) Guillain-Barré syndrome is an acute polyneuropathy whose occurrence classically follows a respiratory or gastrointestinal (GI) infection. It results in a progressive form of ascending paralysis, beginning with myalgia of the lower limbs, loss of muscle tone and tendon reflexes, and some flaccidity, and then extending to the trunk, arms, and bulbar muscles. The disorder can also affect the seventh cranial nerve. The disorder can produce diffuse demyelination of the peripheral nerves with an increase in lymphocytes present at the sites of demyelination. The other disorders listed are generally progressive where eventual recovery without intervention is not known to occur. Myasthenia gravis and lumbar disk prolapse would not show demyelination and lymphocyte increases near the sites of demyelination. MS involves CNS structures; therefore, the constellation of symptoms would be different. MD is progressive, with effects upon both proximal muscles and later in distal muscles.

144. The answer is b. (*Siegel and Sapru, p 156. Aminoff, pp 175-176, 200-208.*) ALS is characterized by a progressive loss of motor functions, first seen as weakness in limb muscles, especially those of the fingers, and later of the other limbs. Sensory functions are not affected. Over time, there is wasting, atrophy, and fasciculations of limb muscles, followed by UMN signs and the patients ultimately die because of respiratory failure or complications of pneumonia. Electromyogram abnormalities can also be observed of the upper and lower extremities. In MS, there is also sensory loss, such as loss or blurring of vision, as well as bladder problems. Poliomyelitis and myasthenia gravis involve LMN symptoms, while a cerebral cortical stroke would result in a UMN disorder without LMN signs.

145. The answer is c. (*Siegel and Sapru, p 156.*) MS is a demyelinating autoimmune disease that affects CNS function. This disorder produces a wide variety of symptoms, including sudden sensory dysfunction and loss, which affect vision and the somatosensory system, causing tingling, pain, and hypesthesia. Broad functional motor disturbances also occur, including weakness of the upper or lower limbs, UMN signs, and gait impairment. There is also bladder dysfunction as well as an increase in CSF protein and IgG synthesis. Diffuse cerebellar degeneration would produce gait ataxia and deficits in the accuracy of intentional movements. As noted earlier, ALS would produce both a UMN and an LMN paralysis, which typically does not extend to sensory functions. Likewise, a peripheral neuropathy would not produce UMN signs, visual deficits, and extensive motor disturbances as described in this case. A tumor of the prefrontal cortex would affect some cognitive and emotional functions, but it would not affect sensory processes such as vision and somatosensation, nor would it produce signs of a UMN disorder or muscle weakness.

146. The answer is e. (*Siegel and Sapru, p 156. Aminoff, pp 200-208.*) In ALS, there is damage initially to ventral horn cells of the spinal cord, producing LMN signs. As the disease progresses, there is involvement of UMNs located in the lateral columns of the spinal cord (ie, corticospinal dysfunction), thereby producing UMN signs such as an increase in tendon reflexes and the presence of an extensor plantar response. Sensory neurons are not involved in this disorder.

147 to 155. The answers are 147-A, 148-D, 149-B, 150-C, 151-E, 152-H, 153-I, 154-F, 155-H. (*Afifi, pp 47-66. Nolte, pp 233-260. Rowland, pp 790-791. Siegel and Sapru, pp 142-155.*) Sensory fibers that terminate in the medulla are located in the dorsal columns. Fibers mediating conscious proprioception from the upper limb are contained in the fasciculus cuneatus (A).

The lateral spinothalamic tract (D) transmits pain and temperature information directly to the thalamus. The lateral corticospinal tract (B) originates in the contralateral cortex and crosses over at the level of the lower medulla. This important pathway mediates control over volitional movements. When these fibers are cut, there is a clear loss of ability to produce volitional movements. The rubrospinal tract (C), situated adjacent to the lateral corticospinal tract, originates from the red nucleus of the midbrain and facilitates the actions of flexor motor neurons. The lateral vestibulospinal tract (E) powerfully facilitates alpha motor neurons of extensor muscles. This tract is located in the ventral funiculus adjacent to the gray matter. The axons of the cells situated in this part of the gray matter (ie, ventral horn) innervate extensor motor neurons. The posterior (or dorsal) spinocerebellar tract (H) transmits information from muscle spindles to the cerebellum via the inferior cerebellar peduncle. This tract is located on the lateral aspect of the lateral funiculus of the cord, just above the anterior (or ventral) spinocerebellar tract. In the genetic disorder, autosomal spinocerebellar ataxia, which may appear during childhood as well as in early or later adulthood, the patient presents with a significant gait ataxia, resulting in loss of balance and coordination as well as nystagmus and dysarthria. These effects have typically been attributed to disruption of the dorsal spinocerebellar pathway (H) and its target neurons in the cerebellum. The dorsal spinocerebellar pathway, located in the lateral aspect of the spinal cord, mediates unconscious proprioception from muscle spindles and Golgi tendon organs to the anterior lobe of cerebellum. Therefore, damage to this pathway will likely result in signs such as hypotonia and decreased tendon reflexes in addition to the above-described characteristic of damage to the anterior cerebellum. First-order pain and temperature fibers from the periphery terminate directly in the region of the dorsal horn, called the *substantia gelatinosa* (I). Blockade of the synaptic endings of the first-order neurons would prevent transmission of pain impulses to the brain. A smaller component of the corticospinal tract, the anterior corticospinal tract (F), originates from the cerebral cortex and passes ipsilaterally to the spinal cord. In its ventromedial position, the fibers are ipsilateral to their cortical origin. Just prior to their termination, many of the fibers are distributed to the contralateral side of the cord. The anterior (or ventral) spinocerebellar tract (G) arises from wide regions of the gray matter of the cord. These fibers pass contralaterally to the lateral aspect of the lateral funiculus to reach a position just below the dorsal spinocerebellar tract.

These fibers then ascend to the cerebellum via the superior cerebellar peduncle, conveying information from Golgi tendon organs located in the lower limbs.

156 to 158. The answers are 156-K, 157-B, 158-J. *(Afifi, pp 47-66. Nolte, pp 233-260. Siegel and Sapru, pp 155-157.)* Ventral horn cells (K) constitute the final common path for descending motor pathways controlling movement, since they directly innervate skeletal muscle. Therefore, they are referred to as LMNs, and lesions involving any component of these neurons result in an LMN deficit. The deficit is characterized by a flaccid paralysis of the muscle groups innervated by these neurons. In contrast, neurons from the cerebral cortex (and elsewhere in the brain) that pass in the lateral funiculus of the cord (B) and innervate ventral horn cells rather than skeletal muscle are referred to as UMNs. Lesions of these fibers produce a UMN syndrome, which is characterized by a spastic paralysis (hyperreflexia and hypertonicity). The fasciculus gracilis (J) conveys, in part, information from joint capsules of the lower limbs to the brain. Disruption of these fibers will block the transmission to the cerebral cortex of these signals that indicate the position of the lower limb following or preceding movement of that limb. Such loss will prevent the necessary feedback signals concerning one's position in space to reach the cortex. As a result, there will be a compensatory motor response characterized by a wide ataxic gait. In contrast, the fasciculus cuneatus mediates similar sensory modalities to the brain, but from the upper limb, and therefore damage to this pathway could not account for ataxia of movement.

159. The answer is e. *(Afifi, pp 47-66. Nolte, pp 233-260. Siegel and Sapru, pp 141-142.)* The section depicted in the diagram is taken from the lower cervical cord. The cervical level of the spinal cord can be distinguished from other levels of the cord by the following characteristics: the presence of a well-defined fasciculus cuneatus, situated immediately lateral to the fasciculus gracilis; the presence of well-defined motor nuclei that are clumped into six different groups, three of which can be distinguished; an absence of an intermediolateral cell column; and relatively extensive quantities of both white and gray matter. Thus, a knife wound that destroyed the right half of the spinal cord results in a Brown-Séquard syndrome. The knife wound would cause loss of sensory and motor functions of both upper and lower limbs. The sensory loss of lower limbs would occur because of the damage to ascending fibers from spinothalamic and the fasciculus gracilis (causing loss of pain and temperature of the contralateral side of the body and conscious proprioception of the ipsilateral side), which would also include some loss of these sensations from the upper limb. At the lesion, there is additional loss of these sensations from the upper limb, which enter the cord at this level of spinal cord. Here, there would also be some bilateral pain and temperature loss at the level of the lesion because of the presence of crossing fibers. Because the lesion occurred at the cervical level, it would result in an LMN paralysis of the upper limb and a UMN paralysis involving the lower limb. Klumpke palsy, a form of brachial plexus palsy, is characterized by weakness of the wrist and finger flexors and of small muscles of the hand, as well as loss of sensation along the medial aspect of the arm.

160. The answer is c. (*Kandel, pp 715-724. Siegel and Sapru, pp 157-159, 259-261.*) Gamma motor neurons innervate the polar regions of the muscle spindle and, when excited, cause resetting of the spindle by stretching it, resulting in a lowering of the threshold for activation of that receptor by an external force. Excessive or abnormal stimulation (activation) of gamma motor neurons will result in significant hyperexcitation of the reflex response (reflected by hyperreflexia and hypertonicity) due to the highly significant reduction of the threshold for activation of the muscle spindle receptor. Unmyelinated C fibers mediate nociceptive sensations from the periphery to the spinal cord and thus do not relate to this question. 1A fibers arise from the nuclear region of the spindle and mediate spindle activity to the spinal cord, and thus form the afferent limb of the monosynaptic stretch reflex. Alpha motor neurons arise in the ventral horn of the spinal cord and innervate extrafusal muscle fibers, causing movement of the limb when excited. It does not innervate the polar regions of the spindle. General visceral afferent fibers exit from the intermediolateral cell columns (at T1-L3 for sympathetics and S2-S4 for parasympathetics) of the spinal cord and innervate postganglionic neurons for these respective autonomic systems. Such fibers, therefore, do not relate to muscle spindles, including their polar regions.

161. The answer is d. (*Nolte, pp 200-224. Afifi, pp 59-89.*) First-order neurons that convey pain and temperature sensations to the spinal cord from C7 to T1 are associated with innervation of the region of the hand.

The back of the head is innervated from fibers that enter the spinal cord at C2, the neck at C3, the shoulder at C3 to C6, and the back at T2 to T12.

162. The answer is a. *(Nolte, pp 237-249. Afifi, pp 56-59.)* First-order neurons that convey pain and temperature sensations to the spinal cord terminate principally in the ipsilateral laminas I and II upon dendrites of cells located in adjacent laminas.

163. The answer is c. *(Afifi, pp 56-62.)* Immunocytochemical studies have demonstrated that the sensory neurons that terminate in laminas I and II of the dorsal horn of the spinal cord stain intensely for substance P. These neurons are believed to mediate pain impulses. Other transmitter substances, while present within the spinal cord, have not been associated directly with first-order sensory afferent fibers.

164. The answer is c. *(Afifi pp 56-62. Nolte, pp 237-247. Siegel and Sapru, pp 139-141.)* Lissauer marginal zone, located on the dorsolateral margin of the dorsal horn of the spinal cord, receives many incoming pain and temperature fibers that are either unmyelinated or finely myelinated. These fibers principally mediate pain and temperature sensations. The fibers contained in this bundle may ascend or descend several segments, serving to integrate different levels of the substantia gelatinosa, which receives these inputs. These fibers are not known to make synaptic contact with motor neurons. Neurons in the substantia gelatinosa do not generally ascend beyond the spinal cord.

165. The answer is b. *(Afifi, pp 47-69. Siegel and Sapru, p 145.)* The nucleus dorsalis of Clarke is situated in the medial aspect of lamina VII of the cord at thoracic and lumbar levels, but does extend up to C8. It receives first-order inputs from fibers that convey muscle spindle and Golgi tendon organ information (ie, unconscious proprioception). Fibers from the nucleus dorsalis of Clarke run laterally to form the dorsal spinocerebellar tract on the ipsilateral side, which terminates mainly in the anterior lobe of the cerebellum.

166. The answer is d. *(Afifi, pp 47-69. Nolte, pp 237-238, 259-262. Siegel and Sapru, pp 155-157.)* The fact that the disorder affected the neuronal cell bodies of the ventral horn indicates that the patient will present with an

LMN paralysis. The affected neurons from L1 to L4 innervate the muscles of the lower limb; therefore, the LMN paralysis would affect the leg normally innervated by these neurons.

167. The answer is b. (*Nolte, p 275. Siegel and Sapru, pp 153-155.*) A principal descending component of the MLF arises from the medial vestibular nucleus, and, accordingly, this bundle is sometimes referred to as the *medial vestibulospinal tract*. The overall function of the MLF is to help coordinate changes in position or balance with the position of the head and eyes. The descending fibers of the MLF provide the anatomic substrate by which the inputs from the vestibular apparatus can influence the manner in which the head will be positioned. It accomplishes this by modulating upper cervical neurons that innervate muscles of the neck that control the position of the head. Since the projection is to the cervical cord, it would not likely have any direct effect upon extensor reflex activity of the lower limbs. Likewise, these descending fibers do not affect any structures that would cause alterations in blood pressure. Only damage to the ascending component of the MLF would result in nystagmus and diplopia. This pathway does not innervate neurons of the spinal cord that supply the upper or lower limbs. Therefore, a UMN paralysis would not be expected. In addition, these fibers do not innervate the cerebellum or mediate conscious proprioception. Only if there were damage to the cerebellum or fibers mediating this form of sensation, would one expect ataxia to occur.

168. The answer is c. (*Afifi, pp 47-69. Siegel and Sapru, pp 147-149.*) Both the lateral and the anterior spinothalamic tracts cross over to the contralateral white matter of the cord relatively close to the central canal. Therefore, a lesion of this region would result in segmental loss of pain and temperature (plus some tactile sensation) because these fibers would be damaged. The dorsal funiculus mediates conscious proprioception; the dorsal root ganglion mediates all sensory processes, which are not limited to pain and temperature sensation; the midline region of the lower medulla contains second-order neurons that mediate conscious proprioception from the body; and the ventral horn contains motor but not sensory neurons. Concerning other pathways in the spinal cord, the anterior corticospinal tract represents approximately 10% of the fibers descending from the cortex as corticospinal fibers. These fibers pass ipsilaterally through the brain stem to the spinal cord, reaching the anterior funiculus of the cord. Near the level at which these fibers terminate, most anterior corticospinal fibers cross over in the commissure of the spinal cord to supply the intermediate gray of the ventral horn. The anterior spinocerebellar tract crosses over to the contralateral side and ascends as a distinct fiber pathway in the far lateral aspect of the white matter immediately below the position occupied by the dorsal spinocerebellar tract. Posterior spinocerebellar fibers, which arise from Clarke nucleus dorsalis, do not cross in the spinal cord. Instead, they pass laterally from their cell of origin and ascend within the dorsal half of the far lateral aspect of the white matter to the cerebellum. Lateral vestibulospinal fibers arise from the lateral vestibular nucleus and descend ipsilaterally within the ventral funiculus to all levels of the spinal cord, where they terminate upon neurons in the ventral horn. Dorsal column fibers are first-order neurons that arise from the periphery and enter the spinal cord at all levels. They ascend ipsilaterally in the fasciculus gracilis and cuneatus to the level of the dorsal column nuclei of the medulla, where they terminate.

169. The answer is b (*Siegel and Sapru, pp 157-159.*) The tendon (stretch) reflex is an example of a monosynaptic reflex. The afferent limb of the reflex arc includes a 1A fiber eminating from the muscle spindle whose axon terminal makes synapse with and excites an alpha motor neuron, which innervates the homonymous extrafusal muscle, thus causing the muscle to contract, resulting in the initiation of the reflex response (ie, extension of the limb). This reflex is facilitated by the action of the gamma efferent fibers, since they activate the polar ends of the intrafusal muscle, thus causing the spindle to be reset and to discharge. The Golgi tendon organ gives rise to 1B fibers, which inhibit the stretch reflex.

170. The answer is a. (*Kandel, pp 715-724. Siegel and Sapru, pp 157-159.*) In contrast to Golgi tendon organs, which detect tension, muscle spindles respond to the rate of change in the length of the muscle and are referred to as velocity detectors. They are low-threshold detectors and are connected in parallel with the extrafusal muscle fibers; stretching the muscle results in an elongation of intrafusal fibers, which stretches the sensory nerve endings in the spindle, producing an increase in the discharge rate. The muscle spindle actually contains three different types of intrafusal fibers—dynamic nuclear bag, static nuclear bag, and nuclear chain fibers—all of which are innervated by a single 1A afferent fiber. Static nuclear bag fibers and nuclear chain fibers are innervated by group II afferent fibers. The various properties of these intrafusal fibers combine in generating the firing patterns of the spindle.

171. The answer is d. *(Afifi, pp 72-73. Siegel and Sapru, p 156.)* Hemisection of the right side of the spinal cord that involves segments T8 to T12 will result in contralateral loss of pain and temperature sensation below the level of the lesion and ipsilateral loss of conscious proprioception below the level of the lesion (called the Brown-Séquard syndrome). Thus, this patient will experience loss of pain and temperature in the left leg and loss of conscious proprioception in the right leg. In addition, there will be damage to the descending corticospinal fibers that normally are essential for activation of the LMNs that control muscles of the right leg (ie, UMN paralysis of the right leg). However, since the lesion is situated below the entry of sensory fibers as well as the origin of anterior horn cells that innervate the upper limbs, no loss of sensation to the upper limbs will ensue, nor will there be an LMN or UMN paralysis of the upper limbs. The pain and temperature fibers ipsilateral to the site of the lesion are unaffected because the second-order neurons decussate at the approximate level of their cell bodies of origin and ascend on the side contralateral to the lesion, leaving this system intact.

172. The answer is c. *(Adams, pp 45-47, 1121-1127. Siegel and Sapru, pp 70, 74.)* This patient does not have a UMN lesion (spinal cord or above) because of the absent reflexes and ascending paralysis bilaterally involving all of the extremities. Lesions in the brain almost always give unilateral findings, and spinal cord lesions provide clues which identify the distinct level of spinal cord involvement. The damage cannot be in the muscle, because the patient has sensory involvement as well. This case is an example of Guillain-Barré syndrome, or an inflammatory disease of the peripheral nerve resulting from demyelination. Inflammatory cells are found within the nerves, as well as segmental demyelination and some degree of Wallerian degeneration. This damage can cause an ascending paralysis and sensory loss, affecting the arms, face, and legs. The CSF often has a high protein level, making a spinal tap a useful test for the diagnosis of Guillain-Barré syndrome. Nerve conduction studies are also helpful in making the diagnosis. Most neurologists believe Guillain-Barré syndrome to be an immunological reaction directed against the peripheral nerve, and some patients have a history of having had some type of infection prior to developing Guillain-Barré syndrome. However, a clear-cut cause is rarely found. Most patients recover from Guillain-Barré syndrome, although the speed of recovery varies. Treatment is currently available (administration of gamma globulin or plasmapheresis), and, if instituted early in the course of the disease, decrease in the length of the illness is possible.

173. The answer is d. *(Kandel, pp 430-440. Siegel and Sapru, p 262.)* Pain is mediated by free nerve endings which give rise to Cδ and Aδ nerve fibers in the skin. (See explanations in response to Question 174.)

174. The answer is c. *(Kandel, pp 430-440. Siegel and Sapru, pp 257-258.)* Pacinian corpuscles are low-threshold, rapidly adapting receptors that effectively respond to high-frequency vibration and thus mediate the (high-frequency vibration) sensation induced by a tuning fork. Free nerve endings mediate pain impulses; muscle spindles are low-threshold receptors that mediate changes in the intrafusal muscle fibers; the Golgi-tendon organ is a high-threshold receptor that responds to muscle tension and the movement of groups of muscles; Meissner corpuscles are low-threshold, rapidly adapting receptors that respond best to tactile stimulation and low-frequency vibration.

175. The answer is e. *(Aminoff, pp 171-182.)* The pain and paresthesia experienced by the patient in the upper left arm is most likely the result of a moderate concussion of the nerve roots associated with the dermatomes in that limb. The concussion was severe enough to generate these abnormal sensations but not sufficiently devastating to cause complete sensory loss in the limb. Damage to the dorsal horn would cause loss of pain and temperature sensation, as well as affecting tactile sensation; likewise, damage to the lateral funiculus would cause loss of pain and temperature sensation associated with the right limbs; the ventral horn mediates motor functions and is thus unrelated to this disorder; the dorsal columns mediate signals associated with conscious proprioception, but not pain.

176. The answer is b. *(Aminoff, pp 172-173.)* Only compression of the entire spinal cord at L2 would produce the initial LMN paralysis, which after spinal shock, would induce bladder dysfunction and pain in the lower limbs. The other choices could not explain the combination of deficits observed in this patient. Compression of the dorsal roots, dorsal columns, or lateral funiculus could not account for the bladder dysfunction; similarly, damage to the corticospinal tracts could not account for the pain that the patient experienced.

177. The answer is c. (*Afifi, pp 72-73. Siegel and Sapru, p 156.*) The patient received a diagnosis of *Brown-Séquard syndrome*, or hemisection of the spinal cord. The lesion is not at the cervical level because motor functions of the upper limbs were considered normal. The examiner can pinpoint the location of the lesion by using the "sensory level," or level at which the loss of pain and temperature begin, by remembering that the lesion affects fibers that have entered the spinal cord one or two levels below it, and then cross to the contralateral side. Therefore, a loss of sensory function at the T10 level indicates a lesion at the T8 or T9 level, a level at which motor deficits may be helpful in diagnosis. In lesions of the thoracic spinal cord, muscles innervated by thoracic nerves are difficult to test. The examiner still expects weakness in the lower extremities, and this helps to make the diagnosis. If the lesion involved the lumbar level, there would be a flaccid paralysis of the lower limb. The disorder could not have been the result of a peripheral nerve injury, because such a possibility could not account for the preservation of pain and temperature in the right leg but with a loss of conscious proprioception associated with that limb. Brown-Séquard syndrome may occur as a result of different types of tumors, infections of the spinal cord, or as a result of a knife or bullet wound.

178. The answer is b. (*Afifi, pp 72-73.*) Because one-half of the spinal cord is damaged, the dorsal columns are damaged, and the patient will have loss of proprioception and vibration ipsilateral to and below the level of the lesion. Since the lower right limb was affected, the loss must be below T6 and ipsilateral because fibers mediating this type of sensation cross above the level of the lesion in the lower medulla. The fasciculus gracilis carries fibers originating from the sacral, lumbar, and lower thoracic levels, and the fasciculus cuneatus carries those from the upper thoracic and cervical levels. Lissauer tract carries pain and temperature fibers via the dorsal root entry zone.

179. The answer is c. (*Afifi, pp 49-73. Siegel and Sapru, pp 147-149.*) The spinothalamic tract carries fibers mediating pain and temperature.

The primary pain fibers enter the spinal cord and pass one or two segments in Lissauer marginal zone before making a synapse with neurons that form the lateral spinothalamic tract. Fibers of the lateral spinothalamic tract then cross to the contralateral side one or two segments above or before, where the primary afferent fibers have entered the cord. Accordingly, pain and temperature are lost below the lesion on the contralateral side. The cuneate and gracile fasciculi mediate proprioception and vibration in association with the same side of the body from which these fibers originate, and the corticospinal tract mediates voluntary motor function.

180. The answer is c. (*Afifi, pp 59-60, 235, 394. Siegel and Sapru, pp 149-152.*) The corticospinal tract mediates voluntary motor function. The fibers cross in the medullary pyramids; thus, lesions below this structure cause ipsilateral weakness. The reflexes are brisk, since in a UMN lesion there is a loss of inhibition to spinal reflexes. Muscle, dorsal root, and femoral nerve damage are all examples of lesions distal to the spinal cord. A frontal lobe lesion would not cause sensory or motor level damage, and would probably cause problems more proximally, including slurred speech.

181. The answer is a. (*Afifi, pp 59-60, 235, 394. Siegel and Sapru, pp 149-152.*) A positive Babinski sign, or dorsiflexion of the great toe when the lateral portion of the plantar surface of the foot is scratched, is a sign of a UMN defect involving the corticospinal tract. Peripheral nerve lesions are a component of LMN lesions, which cause a flaccid paralysis and which do not produce a positive Babinski sign. Damage to the autonomic nervous system does not produce a positive Babinski sign and has little effect upon movement involving the limbs.

The Autonomic Nervous System

Questions

182. A 58-year-old female was suffering from hypertension and the drugs presently available to her seemed to be of little help. Recently, a new drug was approved for distribution and the patient's physician recommended that she try it. The specific feature of this drug is that it selectively blocks synaptic transmission in autonomic ganglia in order to control blood pressure. Which of the following best characterizes this drug?

a. Cholinergic antagonist
b. Noradrenergic antagonist
c. Serotonergic antagonist
d. γ-Aminobutyric acid (GABA)ergic antagonist
e. Peptidergic antagonist

183. A researcher working for a pharmaceutical company is attempting to identify the possible role that peptides may play in regulating autonomic function. From what is presently known, which of the following statements accurately depicts the locus and function of peptides in autonomic function?

a. They are present only at preganglionic axon terminals of the parasympathetic nervous system.
b. They are present only at postganglionic axon terminals of the parasympathetic nervous system.
c. They are present in sympathetic ganglia, where they function primarily as neurotransmitters.
d. They are present in sympathetic ganglia, where they function primarily as neuromodulators.
e. They have not been localized in any of the autonomic ganglia.

184. A patient with elevated heart rate and blood pressure is examined by a battery of physicians and they conclude that his condition is due to a deficiency or loss of the carotid sinus reflex. Which of the following is a component of this reflex?

a. Baroreceptor afferent fibers from cranial nerve XI
b. Glossopharyngeal efferent fibers
c. Interneurons within the nucleus ambiguus of the medulla
d. Efferent fibers contained in the intermediate component of the facial nerve
e. Vagal efferent fibers

185. A patient has a tendency to have elevated blood pressure and heart rate, which can be controlled in part by a calcium channel blocker. Which of the following statements most accurately characterizes the effects of neurotransmitters upon calcium currents in heart muscle cells?

a. They are reduced by norepinephrine acting through β-receptors.
b. They are increased by norepinephrine acting through β-receptors.
c. They are increased by acetylcholine (ACh) acting on muscarinic receptors.
d. They are increased by ACh acting on nicotinic receptors.
e. They are increased by serotonin acting on serotonin 1A receptors.

186. A 78-year-old male presents with loss of voluntary control of bladder functions. Which of the following conditions most likely accounts for the loss of bladder functions?

a. Loss of vagal and sacral efferent fibers only
b. Loss of vagal, sacral, and descending fibers from the cerebral cortex
c. Loss of lumbar and sacral efferent fibers only
d. Loss of lumbar, sacral, and descending fibers from the cerebral cortex
e. Loss of upper thoracic and cervical fibers only

187. After receiving a diagnosis of having elevated blood pressure, an attempt is made to control blood pressure by preventing the synthesis and storage of norepinephrine. Which of the following should be applied to achieve this result?

a. Guanethidine sulfate
b. Reserpine
c. Phenoxybenzamine hydrochloride
d. Hexamethonium chloride
e. Metoprolol

188. A patient is diagnosed with a hypothalamic tumor that results in significant alteration of autonomic functions, including loss of regulation of blood pressure and heart rate. Such effects upon autonomic functions can be understood in terms of the functional connections of the hypothalamus with a brain stem or spinal cord structure. Which of the following structures normally receives such inputs?

a. Ventrolateral nucleus of the thalamus
b. Nucleus accumbens
c. Solitary nucleus
d. Red nucleus
e. Ventral horn cells at the level of C8 to T12 of the spinal cord

The Autonomic Nervous System

Answers

182. The answer is a. *(Kandel, pp 970-974. Siegel and Sapru, pp 399-400.)* The transmitter released from preganglionic endings of both sympathetic and parasympathetic fibers is ACh. The other transmitters listed are not involved at this synapse. Evidence in support of this view is derived, in part, from studies that demonstrated that drugs that block nicotinic receptors (eg, hexamethonium chloride, curare) also block the output of these systems.

183. The answer is d. *(Kandel, pp 970-972.)* Recent studies demonstrate that a wide variety of peptides are found within most sympathetic ganglia. Evidence further suggests that these peptides do not act as transmitters, but instead serve as neuromodulators. In this manner, the action of peptides in autonomic ganglia is to alter the efficiency of neuronal excitability and the effectiveness of cholinergic transmission at autonomic synapses.

184. The answer is e. *(Kandel, pp 879-880.)* The carotid sinus reflex involves several neuronal elements. The afferent side of the reflex begins with stretch receptors in the walls of the carotid sinus. These receptors signal pressure as a result of stretch of the low-capacitance vessel. This causes an afferent volley of action potentials to pass along the glossopharyngeal nerve into the medulla, where the fibers synapse with neurons in the solitary nucleus. These neurons, in turn, synapse upon neurons in the dorsal motor nucleus (and nucleus ambiguus) of the vagus nerve whose axons innervate the heart. Activation of this reflex results in a decrease in heart rate and force of contraction. As a consequence of the decrease in cardiac output, there is an ensuing decrease in blood pressure as well.

185. The answer is b. *(Kandel, pp 964-973.)* The calcium current of heart muscle cells is enhanced by the release of norepinephrine, which acts on β-adrenergic receptors. This effect is additionally mediated by modulation of the potassium current, which serves to keep the action potential of the muscle cells constant. The pacemaker current is also affected by this process since its threshold is decreased as a result of activation of the β-receptors (which further involves the second-messenger system–cAMP-dependent protein kinase). Lowering the threshold of the pacemaker current serves to increase heart rate. Serotonin is not involved in postsynaptic regulation of the heart. ACh has an inhibitory effect upon the heart muscle by acting through different mechanisms.

186. The answer is d. (*Kandel, pp 963-972. Siegel and Sapru, pp 395-396.*) The smooth muscle of the bladder is innervated by postganglionic fibers of the sympathetic nervous system that arise from the inferior mesenteric ganglion. This ganglion, in turn, receives its inputs from T12 to L2 of the intermediolateral cell column of the spinal cord. The smooth muscle of the bladder also receives inputs from postganglionic parasympathetic fibers that are innervated by preganglionic fibers arising from S2 to S4. The external sphincter of the bladder (striated muscle) is innervated by ventral horn cells from the spinal cord. These ventral horn cells, in turn, receive inputs from supraspinal neurons that arise, in part, from the cerebral cortex. It is these neurons that form a part of the substrate for voluntary control over bladder functions (in combination with the parasympathetic and sympathetic fibers from sacral and lumbar levels, respectively).

187. The answer is b. (*Cooper, pp 216-220, 264. Siegel, pp 211-222.*) Noradrenergic activity can be blocked by a number of mechanisms. Reserpine, for example, prevents the synthesis and storage of norepinephrine in sympathetic nerve terminals. Guanethidine sulfate affects noradrenergic transmission by blocking the release of norepinephrine at the sympathetic endings. Competitive α-receptor blockers include phenoxybenzamine hydrochloride and phentolamine, whereas metoprolol blocks β$_1$-receptors. Since ACh is the transmitter at preganglionic synapses of both the parasympathetic and the sympathetic nervous systems, hexamethonium chloride is an effective ganglionic blocker at these synapses.

188. The answer is c. (*Kandel, pp 965-967.*) The solitary nucleus of the medulla plays a significant role in the neural control of autonomic functions because it receives input from several different regions of the brain that regulate such functions. These inputs include fibers that arise from the hypothalamus, central nucleus of the amygdala, midbrain periaqueductal gray, and sensory processes (ie, visceral afferents) of the glossopharyngeal and vagus nerves. The last signal reflects changes in blood pressure and levels of oxygen and carbon dioxide in the blood. The ventrolateral nucleus of the thalamus, red nucleus of the midbrain, and ventral horn cells of the spinal cord are associated with somatomotor rather than autonomic function. The nucleus accumbens is believed to be associated with motivational processes.

The Brainstem and Cranial Nerves

Questions

189. The following test is administered to a patient: a cotton applicator is gently applied to the cornea of the eye as the patient is asked to look upward. The patient does not blink in response to stimulation of the cornea. Which of the following cranial nerves are normally involved in this reflex?

a. Nerves II and III
b. Nerves III and IV
c. Nerves III and V
d. Nerves V and VII
e. Nerves VII and IX

190. A 62-year-old male over a period of weeks begins to experience difficulty in swallowing and hoarseness in speech. A thorough examination reveals the presence of a growing tumor. Which of the following loci best accounts for this deficit?

a. Geniculate ganglion
b. Facial canal
c. Jugular foramen
d. Ventral aspect of pons
e. Dorsal midbrain

191. As a result of an infection, a 56-year-old woman experiences a loss of taste affecting the front of her tongue and the ability to smile. If the sensory loss involves damage of cell bodies, which of the following specific group of neurons would be so affected?

a. Otic ganglion
b. Nodose (inferior) ganglion
c. Pterygopalatine ganglion
d. Geniculate ganglion
e. Trigeminal ganglion

192. A 55-year-old man, who has been suffering from hypertension for the past 8 years, experiences attacks of pain in the regions of the pharynx and ear which are usually preceded by swallowing and coughing spells. These attacks, each of which lasts for an average of 1 minute, occur a number of times; ultimately, this condition showed remission. Although the neurological examination is basically normal, a subsequent magnetic resonance imaging (MRI) is taken and reveals an abnormality at the base of the skull. Which of the following cranial nerves is most likely involved in this disorder?

a. Cranial nerve V
b. Cranial nerve VII
c. Cranial nerve IX
d. Cranial nerve XI
e. Cranial nerve XII

Questions 193 to 197

Match each of the following vignettes with the labeled area of the brain with which it is most closely associated. Each lettered option may be used once, multiple times, or not at all.

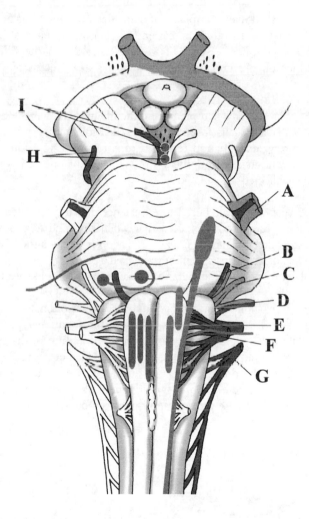

193. A 15-year-old boy was struck in the face by a baseball thrown by the opposing pitcher in a baseball game. The next day, he experienced difficulty smiling and was unable to blink his eye in response to irritation caused by a piece of dirt that came into the eye. On the illustration shown which of the cranial nerves was most likely affected by this accident?

194. A 46-year-old male complains of pain affecting wide areas of his face and jaw. It is determined that the patient is suffering from a viral infection involving the peripheral aspect of a cranial nerve. On the illustration shown, which of the cranial nerves was most likely affected by the viral infection?

195. A 64-year-old male complains of difficulty in swallowing and salivating. The patient also fails to elicit a gag reflex following stroking of the pharynx. Further examination reveals a tumor impinging upon a cranial nerve just beyond its exit from the brain. Which cranial nerve in the figure is most likely affected?

196. A 69-year-old female began to experience difficulty in extending her tongue. After a few days, she noted that when she tried to protrude her tongue, it extended outward to the left. A diagnosis revealed the likely presence of a viral infection that specifically attacked a peripheral branch of one of her cranial nerves. Which cranial nerve in the figure is most likely affected?

197. Three weeks following a complaint by a 58-year-old male concerning hoarseness and disturbances of the stomach, his situation rapidly worsened as indicated by loss of voice and further ulceration of the stomach. After being admitted to a local hospital, he soon died of asphyxia. An autopsy revealed the presence of what appeared to be a rapidly growing tumor that compressed a peripheral component of a cranial nerve. Which cranial nerve in the figure was affected by the tumor?

198. An 80-year-old woman displays marked rigidity of the lower limbs following a stroke. Which of the following brain regions is the most likely location of the stroke?

a. Posterior half of thalamus
b. Anterior hypothalamus
c. Dorsal half of midbrain
d. Dorsal half of pons
e. Ventral horn of spinal cord

199. A 37-year-old male suffers a massive brainstem stroke destroying much if not all of the midbrain and leaving the patient unconscious and unresponsive to sensory stimulation. However, he presents with marked rigidity in his limbs. Which of the following pathways best accounts for the rigidity because its actions are now unopposed?

a. Rubrospinal tract
b. Lateral vestibulospinal tract
c. Corticospinal tract
d. Medial vestibulospinal tract
e. Lateral reticulospinal tract

200. A 43-year-old male was recovering from an infectious disease and experienced a marked instability in his blood pressure, with episodes of spiking of blood pressure. After a series of extensive examinations, it was concluded that this disorder was due to the effects of the infectious agent upon a component of the peripheral nervous system. Which of the following constitute logical sites where an infectious agent could produce such an effect?

a. Superior ganglia of cranial nerves IX and X
b. Geniculate and trigeminal ganglia
c. Otic and superior salivatory ganglia
d. Carotid sinus and aortic arch
e. Carotid and aortic bodies

201. A patient is subjected to a procedure by his cardiologist involving massaging of the neck, which lowered his blood pressure. The procedure involved activation of the carotid sinus receptors. Which of the following receptors or mechanisms associated with the carotid sinus are activated as a result of the procedure that are essential for the initiation of impulses essential for lowering of his blood pressure?

a. Stretch
b. Change in chloride ion concentration
c. Contractions of the gut
d. Decrease in oxygen concentration
e. Increase in carbon dioxide concentration

202. A 55-year-old female is admitted to a local hospital for hypertension and is found to have a localized brainstem stroke resulting in partial barore-flex dysfunction, increased sympathetic activity, and paroxysmal hypertension. Which of the following is the most likely location of the stroke?

a. Trigeminal spinal nucleus
b. Fastigial nucleus
c. Midbrain reticular formation
d. Solitary nucleus
e. Autonomic nuclei of the facial nucleus (cranial nerve VII)

203. An individual has difficulty adjusting his head, especially after he changes his posture. Which of the following is the most likely pathway affected that might cause this deficit?

a. Lateral vestibulospinal tract
b. Medial vestibulospinal tract
c. Medial reticulospinal tract
d. Lateral reticulospinal tract
e. Rubrospinal tract

204. An individual experiences an ipsilateral paralysis of the soft palate and pharynx, producing hoarseness and dysphagia (inability to swallow) and, in addition, displays a loss of the carotid sinus reflex. Which of the following nerve groups is most likely affected?

a. Cranial nerve XII
b. Cranial nerve XI
c. Cranial nerve X
d. Cranial nerve VII
e. Ventral horn cells of the cervical cord

205. In a case involving a patient who experienced hoarseness and dysphagia, it was concluded that the patient suffered from a lesion affecting selective brainstem neurons. Which of the following is most likely to be damaged in this case?

a. Solitary nucleus
b. Deep pontine nuclei
c. Nucleus ambiguus
d. Ventral horn cells of cervical cord
e. Inferior salivatory nuclei

206. Concerning a patient who is unable to salivate nor express a gag or uvular reflex, which of the following best characterizes the neurons associated with loss of these functions?

a. General somatic efferent and special visceral efferent
b. General visceral efferent and special visceral efferent
c. General somatic efferent and general visceral efferent
d. General visceral efferent and general visceral afferent
e. Special visceral efferent and special visceral afferent

207. A patient complains that he cannot move his right eye to the right and that the right side of his face is expressionless. Which of the following is the likely locus of the lesion?

a. Dorsal aspect of the medulla
b. Ventromedial medulla
c. Dorsal pons
d. Ventromedial pons
e. Medial midbrain

208. A 64-year-old woman is admitted to the emergency room after she experienced dizziness. Several days later, a neurological examination reveals that the patient is unable to move her right eye medially. Which of the following is the likely locus of the lesion?

a. Dorsal medulla
b. Ventromedial medulla
c. Dorsal pons
d. Ventromedial pons
e. Medial midbrain

209. A 72-year-old male experiences difficulty in walking downstairs and reports some double vision as well. In this instance, which of the following is the most likely locus of the lesion?

a. Medulla
b. Dorsal pons
c. Ventromedial pons
d. Midbrain
e. Spinal cord

210. An elderly male is admitted to the emergency room after having experienced double vision. Further examination reveals the presence of pressure that is exerted upon the wall of the cavernous sinus. When asked by the neurologist to follow the movement of his fingers when they are directed downward in a medial position, the patient is unable to do so with his right eye. Which of the following cranial nerves is affected in this patient?

a. Cranial nerve VIII
b. Cranial nerve VII
c. Cranial nerve VI
d. Cranial nerve IV
e. Cranial nerve III

211. A patient is admitted to the emergency room after having lost consciousness. Later on, a neurological examination reveals loss of ability to move his right eye laterally when requested to do so. An MRI further reveals the presence of a brainstem infarction. Which of the following is the most likely locus of the infarction?

a. Ventromedial medulla
b. Ventrolateral medulla
c. Dorsolateral pons
d. Dorsomedial pons
e. Dorsomedial midbrain

212. An experiment was conducted to identify the primary groups of neurons in the central nervous system (CNS) which supply the inferior olivary nucleus. The experiment involved the placement of a recording microelectrode in the inferior olivary nucleus and the placement of stimulating electrodes in the neuronal groups that project to the inferior olivary nucleus. In which of the following sites should the investigator place his stimulating electrodes?

a. Hypothalamus and amygdala
b. Caudate nucleus and subthalamic nucleus
c. Solitary nucleus and nucleus of the ventrolateral medulla
d. Red nucleus and spinal cord
e. Deep pontine nuclei and vestibular nuclei

213. An investigator sought to determine the primary neuronal target structure in the brain which receives inputs from the inferior olivary nucleus. In order to complete this study, the investigator microinjected a tracer substance into the inferior olivary nucleus which was then transported from the cell bodies in the inferior olivary nucleus down the axons to their target structures. Which of the following structures would contain the tracer substance indicating that it constitutes a principal projection target of the inferior olivary nucleus?

a. Cerebral cortex
b. Midbrain periaqueductal gray
c. Vestibular nuclei
d. Dorsal column nuclei
e. Cerebellar cortex

214. An elderly female patient complains that she cannot taste the food she eats. A careful neurological examination reveals no evidence of peripheral damage of the taste receptors. The evidence suggests, instead, that there is selective damage to certain regions of the brainstem. Which of the following sites would include damage that could result in the selective loss of taste?

a. Superior olivary nucleus
b. Inferior salivatory nucleus
c. Solitary nucleus
d. Spinal nucleus of the trigeminal nerve
e. Reticular tegmental nucleus of the pons

Questions 215 to 217

Match each of the following vignettes with the labeled area of the brain with which it is most closely associated. Each lettered option may be used once, multiple times, or not at all.

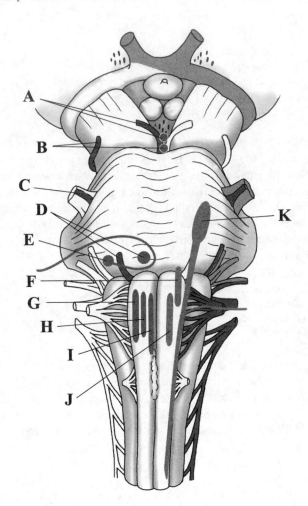

215. A 24-year-old male was hiking in the Rockies on a winter day and became lost. He was discovered a day later and was admitted to a local hospital for a precautionary examination. The patient suffered from overexposure to the cold and, when given a neurological test, had difficulty in closing his eyes, displayed a loss of both the eye-blink reflex and increased sensitivity to sounds, and had difficulty displaying his teeth and chewing food, especially on the side of the mouth. In addition, his speech was somewhat slurred and he was unable to whistle upon request. Which of the cranial nerves shown in the diagram was affected by the cold in this individual?

216. As a result of a brainstem infarction, an elderly woman is unable to move her right eye to the right in following an object moving from left to right across her visual field. Which of the structures shown in the diagram is affected by this infarction?

217. Following a viral infection, a 64-year-old male has a hard time biting down on food and the jaw is noted to deviate to one side. Which of the structures shown in the diagram is being affected by this infarction?

Questions 218 and 219

218. A 68-year-old woman suffered from an infectious disorder for several weeks. Following recovery from this disorder, she experienced some loss of taste and an increase in salivation, together with painful spasms in the region of the pharynx, which extended into the ear. She also experienced some bradycardia and cardiac arrhythmia, as well as deviation of the uvula to the unaffected side. Which of the following cranial nerves was most directly involved in this deficit?

a. Cranial nerve VII
b. Cranial nerve IX
c. Cranial nerve X
d. Cranial nerve XI
e. Cranial nerve XII

219. In the case described in Question 218, which of the following sites is the most likely locus of the lesion affecting this nerve?

a. Upper medulla
b. Lower medulla
c. Lower pons
d. Upper pons
e. Base of the skull

220. A 40-year-old male who suffers from a disorder of unknown origin complains to his physician that he has difficulty producing a smile from the left side of his face. Further analysis shows that the affected muscles are flaccid and the eyelids are open. Where do the cell bodies of origin within the CNS lie whose peripheral innervation of skeletal muscles are affected by this disorder?

a. Upper medulla
b. Lower pons
c. Upper pons
d. Lower midbrain
e. Upper midbrain

221. An elderly female suffering from an infection complains that she cannot salivate and is unable to display lacrimation on the right side of her face. Following a neurological examination, it is determined that a peripheral component of a cranial nerve is affected by this disorder. Which of the following cell bodies of origin form the origin of the affected cranial nerve?

a. Dorsal motor nucleus of the vagus
b. Nucleus ambiguus
c. Inferior salivatory nucleus
d. Superior salivatory nucleus
e. Edinger-Westphal nucleus of cranial nerve III

222. Due to the presence of a tumor, a patient reports that he is unable to experience the sense of taste from the anterior two-thirds of his tongue. Which of the following structures is most likely affected by the tumor?

a. Motor nucleus of the cranial nerve VII
b. Inferior and superior ganglia of cranial nerve IX
c. Cell bodies of the geniculate ganglion of cranial nerve VII
d. Nucleus ambiguus of inferior ganglion of cranial nerve IX
e. Dorsal motor nucleus of the cranial nerve X

Questions 223 to 227

Match each description with the appropriate site shown in the figure. Each lettered option may be used once, multiple times, or not at all.

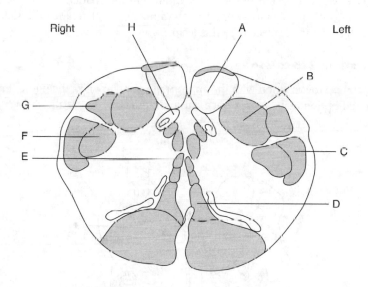

223. A middle-aged woman suffers a vascular occlusion involving part of the brainstem, resulting in selective loss of sensation in her left leg and concomitants ataxia. Which structure is most likely affected?

224. A 65-year-old male is admitted to the emergency room following a brief loss of consciousness. After he regained consciousness, he was examined by a neurologist who discovered that he lost sensation in his left hand. Further analysis revealed that the loss of sensation was due to a vascular lesion. Which structure is associated with the loss of sensation in his hand?

225. A 47-year-old male is brought into the emergency room and is diagnosed with a small brainstem stroke. The patient presents with an inability to display reflex movements of the head in response to vestibular stimulation. Which structure is most likely affected by this lesion?

226. In order to alleviate excruciating pain to the face, a surgical lesion of the fiber bundle mediating pain sensation from the face is made. Which structure is associated with the surgical lesion?

227. A vascular lesion of the lower brainstem in a patient results in the loss of conscious proprioception in the limbs contralateral to the lesion. Which structure is affected by this lesion?

Questions 228 to 236

Match each description with the appropriate site shown in the figure. Each lettered option may be used once, multiple times, or not at all.

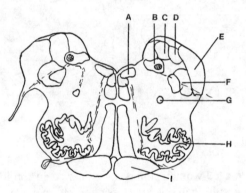

228. A young adult male suffers an injury to the region of the face that affects in part the peripheral nerve innervating the tongue, which results in some loss of ability to identify the taste of foods. Which structure in the brainstem would normally receive these peripheral taste inputs?

229. A stroke involving a part of the lower brainstem resulted in loss of the ability to coordinate movements of the head in response to changes in posture. Which structure is associated with this loss of function?

230. A midbrain stroke results in significant damage to the red nucleus, causing major degeneration of the descending fibers from this nucleus. Which structure present in the lower brainstem is now devoid of this input?

231. A 49-year-old male was admitted to the emergency room after he received a routine physical examination and was shown to have had a sudden increase in blood pressure. Further medical examination indicated that the patient suffered a limited occlusion of the brainstem. Which structure is likely affected, resulting in this change in blood pressure?

232. A patient who suffered a brainstem stroke was examined by a neurologist. He presented with ataxia and lack of coordinated movements. The neurologist concludes that the primary focus of the lesion affected the structure whose neurons contribute the largest number of fibers that are contained in the inferior cerebellar peduncle that supply the cerebellum. Which structure is affected?

233. As a result of a stroke involving the lower brainstem, a 64-year-old man presents with a loss of swallowing and the gag reflex. Which structure is affected?

234. A 75-year-old male is found unconscious in his home and taken to the emergency room of a local hospital. When he recovered consciousness, he was unable to move his right arm or leg and each of these limbs showed spasticity upon testing. Which of the structures shown in the figure was damaged by the stroke?

235. Following a vascular lesion of the lower brainstem, a patient is tested for cranial nerve functions. When asked to stick out his tongue, it deviates to the side. Which structure is affected?

236. A 48-year-old male is suffering from intractable pain of the face for which no drug therapy was effective in alleviating the pain. At the suggestion of the consulting neurosurgeon, the neuronal pathway in the brainstem mediating pain sensation from the face region is surgically interrupted. Identify the structure in question on this figure.

Questions 237 to 242

Match each description with the appropriate site shown in the figure. Each lettered option may be used once, multiple times, or not at all.

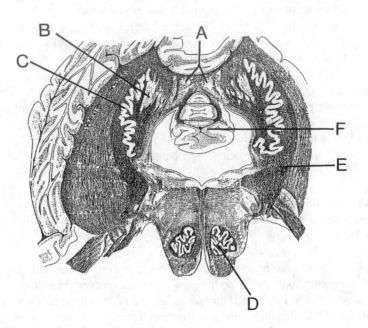

237. A 74-year-old female has been experiencing a loss of balance and, shortly afterward, she is seen by a neurologist. During the neurological examination, the patient presents with a loss of balance, ataxia of movement, and irregularities in blood pressure when taken several times over a period of about 90 minutes. An MRI suggests the presence of a vascular lesion in the region depicted in the diagram shown above. Which structure, if damaged, would most likely result in this group of deficits?

238. An elderly female is seen by a neurologist after complaining about losing her balance. Further examination reveals the presence of ataxia of movement, nystagmus, and some erratic changes in blood pressure. The neurologist concludes that she is suffering from a vascular lesion that was limited to a single structure, and that there is degeneration of axons that normally issue from this structure that supply the vestibular nuclei and reticular formation. Which of the structures shown in this diagram is affected by this lesion?

239. A middle-aged male was admitted to the hospital having suffered a stroke. The patient presented with loss of ability to produce coordinated movements of the upper limbs with little loss of balance. Which is the most likely site of this lesion?

240. A 56-year-old male noticed that when he tried to make purposeful movements, they appeared to lack smoothness and were somewhat inaccurate. This trend tended to become progressively worse over time. After examining the patient, the neurologist concluded that the patient developed a small tumor at a structure whose axons normally supply the red nucleus but which are now disrupted by the tumor. A neurosurgeon was called to remove the tumor. In the diagram shown above, which structure was removed?

241. A 73-year-old male, who displayed a wide, ataxic gait, is seen by a neurologist after being encouraged to do so by his family. The neurologist observed that the patient, in addition to displaying ataxia, also presented with nystagmus. An MRI revealed the presence of a tumor of the vermal region of cerebellar cortex. Which structure shown in the diagram, which normally receives inputs from the vermal region of the cerebellar cortex, is now devoid of such inputs because of the tumor?

242. A 39-year-old male began to have difficulties in coordinating simple movements such as opening a door or reaching for an object that he needed to access. After having seen a neurologist, he was given an MRI which revealed the presence of a large tumor impinging upon the lateral aspect of the cerebellar hemisphere. In the diagram shown above, indicate the structure whose inputs are disrupted by the tumor.

Questions 243 to 249

Match each description with the appropriate site shown in the figure. Each lettered option may be used once, multiple times, or not at all.

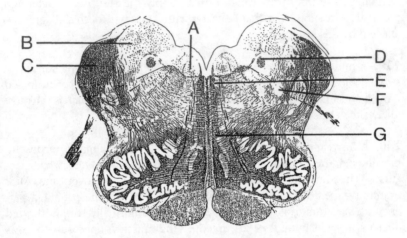

243. A person suffers a facial injury that results in dizziness and some loss of balance. Which structure would lose inputs as a result of the injury?

244. An individual suffers from a discrete brainstem lesion affecting ascending and descending axons. The patient presents with loss of postural adjustment of the head in response to changes in position of the body and some nystagmus. Which structure is most likely affected by the lesion?

245. A patient complains that she lost her sense of taste. A subsequent MRI suggests the presence of a small vascular lesion of the brainstem. Which structure is likely to be affected by this lesion?

246. When a patient attempts to protrude his tongue, it deviates to the side. Damage to which structure would account for this loss?

247. Following a vascular lesion of the lower brainstem, a middle-aged woman is unable to feel the presence of a tuning fork when placed on her leg or arm of one side of her body. On the affected side of her body, she is also unable to sense the position of her leg when asked to move it. Where is the lesion that would result in this deficit?

248. A patient presents with loss of pain sensation from one side of the face. It is discovered that it was probably due to a small brainstem lesion. Where is the likely locus of this lesion?

249. Following a lesion of a portion of the spinal cord, there is damage to the pathway conveying muscle spindle afferents to the cerebellum. Which of the structures shown in this diagram contains the axons that are now damaged as a result of lesion in the spinal cord?

Questions 250 to 254

Match each description with the appropriate site shown in the figure. Each lettered option may be used once, multiple times, or not at all.

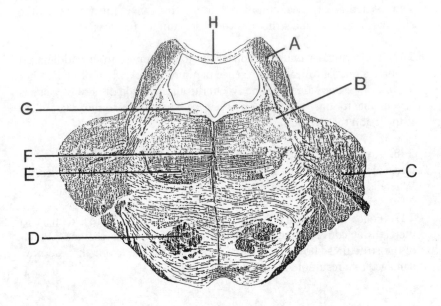

250. An individual suffers from a rare autoimmune disorder that destroyed neuronal cell bodies situated in the basilar aspect of the pons. The patient presents with loss of coordination of movements of the forelimbs when attempting to make a purposeful response. Which fibers degenerated as a result of the autoimmune disorder?

251. A 63-year-old female complains about having difficulties in chewing food and this problem has become progressively worse over time. A neurological examination and subsequent MRI reveals the presence of a discrete brainstem lesion that appears to be responsible for the disruption of the reflex mediating the chewing of food. In the figure shown which is the most likely structure affected by the lesion?

252. An individual is admitted to a hospital after falling unconscious. Later, he presents with a UMN paralysis and is told that he had a stroke involving part of his brainstem. Damage to what structure would account for his deficit?

253. A 49-year-old male complained of loss of sensation along the arm, leg, and trunk of the same side of the body. The patient is given an MRI which detects the presence of a tumor restricted to a single structure at the level of the brainstem shown in the diagram above. Indicate on the diagram above the structure most directly affected by the tumor.

254. A person suffers from a degenerating disease that selectively destroys his deep cerebellar nuclei. The axons of which structure would most likely show significant degeneration as a result of this disorder?

Questions 255 to 259

Match each description with the appropriate site shown in the figure. Each lettered option may be used once, multiple times, or not at all.

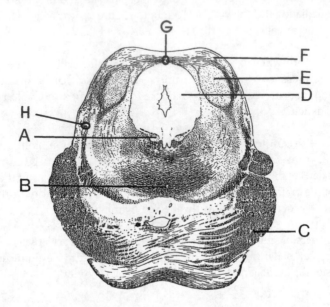

255. An individual suffered a stroke involving part of his midbrain and, when tested by an audiologist, it was revealed that he had lost some ability in auditory discrimination, acuity, and ability to localize sound in space. The loss of which structure could possibly account for these deficits?

256. A person was admitted to a hospital after inhaling a toxic agent, which was later found to produce significant cerebellar damage. The patient subsequently died, an autopsy was performed, and brainstem sections were taken. The pathologist noted significant damage of a structure within the midbrain. Which structure would most likely show such a deficit?

257. A 79-year-old woman was admitted to the emergency room after suffering a stroke. The stroke involved parts of the cerebral cortex, resulting in a contralateral UMN paralysis. Which fibers would be degenerated?

258. A middle-aged man was admitted to the emergency room after falling downstairs. Later, he complained about having double vision and, during a neurological examination, was found to have difficulty moving his eye downward, especially when attempting to look medially. The neurologist concluded that the patient had a small vascular lesion of the brainstem. Which structure was most likely affected by the lesion?

259. An individual was diagnosed with a brainstem tumor and presented with increased sensitivity to pain, a reduction in blood pressure, and a general change and irregularity in emotionality. Which structure was most likely affected by the tumor?

Questions 260 to 264

Match each description with the appropriate site shown in the figure. Each lettered option may be used once, multiple times, or not at all.

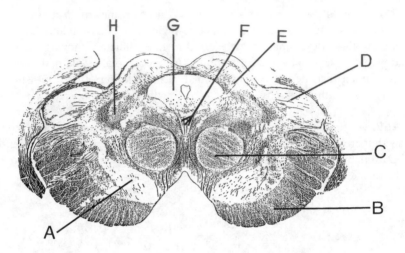

260. A patient was observed to have difficulty moving his eyes up or down as well as following moving objects. Subsequent diagnosis suggested that there was compression of part of the brainstem. Which was the principal structure most likely affected by this compression?

261. A 58-year-old female was examined by an audiologist because she had difficulty in clearly hearing words. The examination revealed a reduction in auditory acuity, discrimination of sounds, and localization of sounds. The patient was referred to a neurologist and was given an MRI. The MRI indicated the presence of a localized tumor in the brainstem at the level indicated in the diagram shown above. In this diagram, identify the structure that could account for this sensory loss?

262. A patient presented with motor dysfunctions characterized by rigidity, tremor, and akinesia. At which site could a lesion produce such a constellation of motor deficits?

263. A person presented with a contralateral limb ataxia, together with a weakness of the medial rectus muscle and a fixed dilated pupil. The neurologist concluded that the patient sustained an infarction of the brainstem. Which structure constituted the principal focus of the infarction?

264. A rare autoimmune disorder that specifically destroys neuronal cell bodies affected a 72-year-old female. As a result, she was unable to direct her eyes medially or vertically, and her pupils did not constrict in response to light. Which structure was damaged by this disorder?

265. A 60-year-old male suffered from excruciating pain on the left side of his face. Since drug therapy was found to be ineffective in alleviating the pain, surgery was indicated. Which of the following structures should be surgically cut or destroyed in order to alleviate the pain?

a. First-order descending sensory fibers contained in the ipsilateral spinal tract of cranial nerve V
b. Neurons in the ventral posterolateral nucleus of the thalamus
c. Cells contained in the main sensory nucleus of the trigeminal nerve
d. Substantia gelatinosa
e. Midbrain periaqueductal gray

266. After eating a meal that contained spoiled food, a 15-year-old boy experiences a rather extensive bout of emesis. Which of the following structures most closely relates to this function?

a. Ventromedial hypothalamus
b. Posterior thalamus
c. Primary motor cortex
d. Dorsolateral pontine tegmentum
e. Area postrema

267. An individual experienced the following constellation of symptoms following a brainstem lesion associated with a stroke of that region: hoarseness, difficulty in swallowing, diminished gastric secretions, and loss of some cardiovascular reflex functions. To which of the following structures can these symptoms be attributed?

a. Cranial nerve VII
b. Cranial nerve IX
c. Cranial nerve X
d. Cranial nerve XI
e. Pontine reticular formation

268. After examining a patient, a neurologist concluded that he suffers a stroke involving the dorsolateral medulla. Which of the following deficits did the neurologist see that allowed him to reach this conclusion?

a. Loss of pain and thermal sensation on the ipsilateral half of the face
b. Loss of pain and temperature sensation on the ipsilateral side of the body
c. Dysphonia
d. Hemiparesis
e. Intention tremor

269. A 7-year-old male was having difficulty in understanding speech sounds, especially in the presence of background noise. Further neurological examination revealed damage, due to a viral infection, to the brainstem that appeared to affect the olivocochlear bundle. Which of the following statements concerning the olivocochlear bundle correctly describes its principal function?

a. It arises from the inferior olivary nucleus and projects to the cochlea.
b. Stimulation of it inhibits acoustic fiber responses to auditory stimuli.
c. It communicates directly with the medial lemniscus.
d. It can be seen easily in brainstem sections taken from the upper pons.
e. It is part of the ascending auditory pathway to the dorsal cochlea nucleus.

270. An elderly woman is brought to see an audiologist after complaining about hearing difficulties. The audiologist notes that she is suffering from unilateral deafness and refers her to a neurologist for further examination. On the basis of his examination, damage to which of the following structures most likely accounts for her present condition?

a. The auditory cortex of one side
b. The lateral lemniscus of one side
c. Cranial nerve VIII on one side
d. The medial geniculate
e. The medial lemniscus

271. A 68-year-old male suffered a brainstem stroke that affected his ability to experience a certain reflex response associated with the head region. What was unusual about the damage caused by the brainstem lesion is that it affected the cell bodies of first-order sensory neurons associated with this reflex which is located within the CNS. Which of the following cell bodies of first-order sensory neurons most likely was affected by the brainstem stroke?

a. Geniculate ganglion
b. Spiral ganglion
c. Mesencephalic nucleus of cranial nerve V
d. Solitary nucleus
e. Scarpa ganglia

272. A middle-aged person is referred to a neurologist after experiencing certain visual deficits. Through the use of an MRI and other diagnostic procedures, it is concluded that there is some damage to a part of his nervous system. The patient presented with a lateral gaze paralysis, in which both eyes were conjugatively directed to the side opposite the lesion. In this condition, which of the following is the locus of the lesion?

a. Root fibers of cranial nerve III
b. Nucleus of cranial nerve III
c. Root fibers of cranial nerve VI
d. Nucleus of cranial nerve VI
e. Nucleus and root fibers of cranial nerve IV

273. An individual is referred to a neurologist because he is having difficulty moving his eyes horizontally to one side. The neurologist concludes that the individual has a vascular lesion. Which of the following structures was most likely affected by this lesion?

a. Paramedian pontine reticular formation
b. Ventrolateral medulla
c. Cranial nerve IV
d. Primary motor cortex
e. Ventral posterolateral nucleus of thalamus

274. A patient displays an ipsilateral paralysis of lateral gaze coupled with a contralateral hemiplegia. Which of the following is the most likely site of the lesion?

a. Ventromedial medulla
b. Dorsomedial medulla
c. Ventrocaudal pons
d. Dorsorostral pons
e. Ventromedial midbrain

275. A 15-year-old male was examined by a neurologist because of a complaint that he had a difficult time in appreciating the taste of food. Upon further analysis, it was discovered that he suffered from a rare genetic disorder that affects receptors that respond to changes in the chemical milieu of the environment. Which of the following sets of cranial nerves contain the special property of responding to changes in the chemical milieu?

a. Cranial nerves V, VII, and IX
b. Cranial nerves III, VII, and XII
c. Cranial nerves IX, X, and XI
d. Cranial nerves II, VII, and VIII
e. Cranial nerves I, VII, and IX

276. A patient displays the following constellation of symptoms: UMN paralysis of the left leg, paralysis of the lower half of the left side of the face, and a left homonymous hemianopsia. Which of the following regions most likely contains the lesion?

a. Medulla
b. Basilar pons
c. Pontine tegmentum
d. Midbrain
e. Forebrain

277. When a patient is asked to follow an object placed in the right side of his visual field, he is unable to move his right eye either up or down. Which of the following regions would most likely contain the lesion?

a. Medulla
b. Basilar aspect of the pons
c. Pontine tegmentum
d. Midbrain
e. Cerebellum

278. A patient is capable of displaying pupillary constriction during an accommodation reaction but not in response to a direct-light stimulus. Which of the following is the most likely site of the lesion?

a. Optic nerve
b. Ventral cell column of cranial nerve III
c. Pretectal area
d. Visual cortex
e. Edinger-Westphal nucleus of cranial nerve III

279. A person complains that he has a hard time sensing the taste of foods. A subsequent neurological examination reveals that he had a significantly diminished sense of taste. Which of the following groups of structures are the most logical sites where a lesion would lead to impaired sensation of taste?

a. Geniculate ganglion, chorda tympani, and medial lemniscus
b. Solitary nucleus, parabrachial nucleus, and ventral posteromedial nucleus
c. Solitary nucleus, ventral posterolateral nucleus, and postcentral gyrus
d. Solitary nucleus, ventral posteromedial nucleus, and superior parietal lobule
e. Geniculate ganglion and ventral posterolateral nucleus

Questions 280 and 281

280. A 79-year-old woman was found unconscious in her apartment and taken to the emergency room of a local hospital. Upon regaining consciousness, the patient was examined by a neurologist and she presented with loss of sensation on one side of her face, some difficulty in chewing, loss of pain and temperature on one side of the body, signs of a Horner syndrome on one side of her face, some difficulty in hearing and localizing sound, and tremors and poor coordination in movement of one of her arms. An MRI indicated the presence of a brainstem stroke. An occlusion of which of the following arteries would result in the lesion at part A in the diagram shown here?

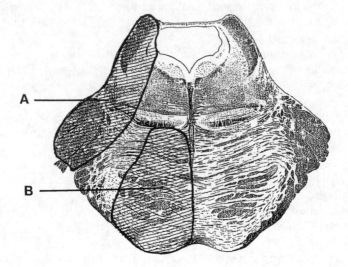

a. Basilar artery
b. Superior cerebellar artery
c. Anterior spinal artery
d. Vertebral artery
e. Posterior inferior cerebellar artery

281. An 84-year-old female fainted while attending a family party and was immediately taken to the emergency room of a local hospital. When she regained consciousness, she presented with an upper motor neuron paralysis on one side of her body and weakness of muscles on the other side of her face. An occlusion of which of the following arteries would result in the lesion at B in the diagram shown in the previous question?

a. Paramedian branch of the basilar artery
b. Circumferential branch of the basilar artery
c. Superior cerebellar artery
d. Anterior inferior cerebellar artery
e. Anterior spinal artery

282. A 72-year-old male is seen by a neurologist after he complained of weakness in his facial muscle and hands, clumsiness, problems in articulating his speech, and difficulty in swallowing. An MRI revealed the presence of a vascular lesion in the brain. Which of the following regions most likely includes the site of the lesion?

a. Dorsomedial medulla
b. Ventromedial medulla
c. Basilar pons
d. Pontine tegmentum
e. Midbrain tegmentum

283. A 59-year-old female presents with difficulty in chewing and ipsilateral sensory loss of much of her face. In addition, she also presents with a contralateral upper motor neuron hemiplegia. Further analysis revealed the presence of a vascular occlusion. Which of the following regions most likely includes the site of the lesion?

a. Rostral aspect of dorsomedial medulla
b. Ventral aspect of caudal medulla
c. Caudal aspect of basilar pons
d. Rostral aspect of basilar pons
e. Basilar aspect of caudal midbrain

Questions 284 to 286

284. A 34-year-old male is seen by an ophthalmologist after complaining about not being able to follow objects such as the movement of cars along a road. He is referred to a neurologist and a subsequent MRI reveals an arterial occlusion in the region shown at A in the figure above. Identify the artery that supplies the region shown at A whose occlusion could account for this visual deficit.

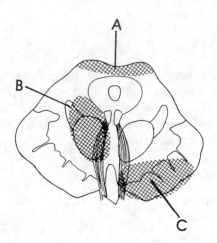

a. Posterior cerebral artery
b. Anterior spinal artery
c. Anterior cerebellar artery
d. Basilar artery
e. Posterior inferior cerebellar artery

285. A patient presents with loss of tactile sensation, pressure, and conscious proprioception as well as tremor and some loss of coordination in the limb on the same side of the body where sensory loss is reported. A subsequent MRI reveals that there is a localized tumor present in the region indicated by B in the figure in the previous question. Which of the following structures are likely affected by this tumor that could account for these deficits?

a. Red nucleus and medial lemniscus
b. Red nucleus and raphe nucleus
c. Superior cerebellar peduncle and substantia nigra
d. Reticular formation and oculomotor nerve
e. Lateral lemniscus and trochlear nerve

286. A patient presents with an ipsilateral paralysis involving an inability to move his eye vertically, and the affected eye is also abducted. The patient also presents with an upper motor neuron paralysis that includes part of the face. The lesion, determined from an MRI, is depicted at C in the diagram in Question 284 shown on the previous page. Which of the following structures are affected by this lesion?

a. Substantia nigra and crus cerebri
b. Red nucleus and crus cerebri
c. Crus cerebri and cranial nerve III
d. Red nucleus and substantia nigra
e. Substantia nigra and cranial nerve III

287. A newborn suffers from an inborn error in development in which the neurons in the ventral aspect of the midbrain, which included the substantia nigra and ventral tegmental area, failed to form. The consequence of this developmental abnormality impact significantly upon the neurochemistry and functions that relate to other regions of the brain. Which of the following statements best describes the results of such an error in development?

a. There was extensive loss of noradrenergic input limited to limbic system, basal ganglia, and cerebral cortex.
b. There was loss of peptidergic input limited to the limbic system and hypothalamus.
c. There was loss of serotonergic input limited to the basal ganglia and hypothalamus.
d. There was extensive loss of GABAergic input to limbic system, basal ganglia, and cerebral cortex.
e. There was extensive loss of dopaminergic input to basal ganglia, limbic system, and cerebral cortex.

288. A 60-year-old male suffers an upper pontine stroke that selectively damages neuronal pathways mediating auditory signals from the lower brainstem to other relay neurons in higher levels of the brainstem. Which of the following is the principal ascending auditory pathway of the brainstem affected by the stroke?

a. Medial lemniscus
b. Lateral lemniscus
c. Trapezoid body
d. Trigeminal lemniscus
e. Brachium of the superior colliculus

Questions 289 and 290

289. A 64-year-old woman who has had heart disease for many years. While carrying chemicals down the stairs of the dry-cleaning shop where she works, she suddenly lost control of her right leg and arm. She fell down the stairs and was able to stand up with some assistance from a coworker. When attempting to walk on her own, she had a very unsteady gait, with a tendency to fall to the right side. Her supervisor asked her if she was all right, and noticed that her speech was very slurred when she tried to answer. He called an ambulance to take her to the nearest hospital. Upon admission, her face appears symmetric, but when asked to protrude her tongue, it deviates toward the left. She is unable to tell if her right toe is moved up or down by the physician when she closes her eyes, and she can not feel the buzz of a tuning fork on her right arm and leg. In addition, her right arm and leg are markedly weak. The physician can find no other abnormalities in the remainder of the patient's general medical examination. Where in the nervous system did the damage occur?

a. Right lateral medulla
b. Occipital lobe
c. Left lateral medulla
d. Right cervical spinal cord
e. Left medial medulla

290. In the patient in Question 289, where in the nervous system could a lesion occur that would cause her arm and leg weakness but spare her face?

a. Right corticospinal tract in the cervical spinal cord
b. Left inferior frontal lobe
c. Right medullary pyramids
d. Occipital lobe
e. Right side of basilar pons

291. A 65-year-old male with a history of heart disease is admitted to the emergency room after having been found unconscious in his home. When the patient regains consciousness and is examined by a neurologist, it was discovered that he cannot identify the presence of a tuning fork, pencil, or pressure applied to his left leg. In addition, the patient is unable to move his left leg or arm. Other clinical signs are not apparent. Which of the following regions most likely accounts for the deficits described?

a. Ventromedial aspect of medulla-spinal cord border
b. Rostral aspect of the ventromedial medulla
c. Dorsolateral aspect of the caudal aspect of medulla
d. Dorsomedial aspect of the pontine tegmentum
e. Dorsomedial aspect of the midbrain tegmentum

292. A patient displays a deviation of the tongue to the left and a hemiparesis on the right side. The lesion is located in which of the following regions?

a. Right hypoglossal nucleus
b. Left hypoglossal nucleus
c. Right inferior frontal lobe
d. Right ventromedial medulla
e. Left ventromedial medulla

293. A patient is suffering from a speech deficit coupled with an ipsilateral loss of pain and temperature from the left side of the face and contralateral loss of pain and temperature from the body, as well as some autonomic dysfunctions. With reference to speech, the physician who was called to see the patient in the emergency room noted that his speech was slurred as if he were intoxicated, but the grammar and meaning were intact. Which of the following types of speech deficit did the patient encounter?

a. Broca aphasia
b. Wernicke aphasia
c. Mixed aphasia
d. Dysarthria
e. Agnosia

Questions 294 and 295

294. A 29 year old female office worker with diabetes awoke one morning with the inability to close her left eye and a left facial droop. Her left eye felt a bit dry as well. She had run out of sick days and, hoping that the problem would go away, went to work. After several coworkers noticed that her face was drooping and that she was especially sensitive to loud noises on her left side, they convinced her to go to the nearest emergency room to make sure she had not had a stroke. She was examined immediately because of her age. The doctor noted right away that her mouth drooped on the left side. Her left eye was slightly closed. He tested her speech and mental status, which were normal, other than some slight slurring of her speech. Her vision and eye movements were also normal. Sensation and jaw movement were also normal, but when she was asked to wiggle her eyebrows, only the right side of her forehead moved. When asked to close her eyes tightly and not allow her to open her eyes, her right eye would not open, but her left eye could not oppose the force. She was not able to hold air in her cheeks when asked to hold her breath, and when asked to smile, only the right side of her mouth elevated. She could not sense an object that had a sweet taste when placed along the anterior aspect of the tongue. She was very sensitive to noise on her left side. A nurse asked if a head CT should be ordered in order to look for a stroke or tumor, but the doctor said that it was not necessary. He told the patient that he would draw some blood and give her a medication to take for a while. Assuming that this was not a stroke, where in the nervous system did the damage occur?

a. Buccinator muscle
b. Trigeminal nerve
c. Facial nerve
d. Glossopharyngeal nerve
e. Hypoglossal nerve

295. In the previous vignette the patient's facial weakness is characteristic of which of the following?

a. A muscle lesion
b. A lesion of the internal capsule
c. A superior brainstem lesion
d. An UMN seventh-nerve lesion
e. A lower motor neuron (LMN) seventh-nerve lesion

296. An 18-year-old male is hit on the side of his head, including the face region, as a result of being tackled in a football game. The next day, he has trouble displaying expression on the right side of his face. He is seen by a neurologist. During the examination, he is asked to protrude his tongue and it does not deviate to either side, but if he closes his eyes and sugar water is placed on the right side of the anterior portion of his tongue, he cannot identify it. Where was the damage that most likely produced the defect in taste in the anterior two-thirds of his tongue?

a. Trigeminal ganglion
b. Proximal aspect of glossopharyngeal nerve
c. Distal aspect of lingual nerve
d. Solitary nucleus
e. Proximal aspect of the chorda tympani nerve

297. An individual had no prior problems with his hearing but was subsequently struck in the face by an object, causing him to become extremely sensitive to noise. Assuming that there was no prior damage to the cochlear nerve or with his ears, damage to the nerve supply of which of the following muscles could cause the sensitivity to or distortion of noises?

a. Digastric
b. Platysma
c. Buccinator
d. Geniohyoid
e. Stapedius

298. A 68-year-old female was admitted to the emergency room following an inability to move her left eye to the left, as well as a failure to show a smile on the left side of her face. However, she experienced no loss of taste from any part of her tongue. Damage to which of the following structures would most likely account for these deficits?

a. The trigeminal and abducens nerves
b. The facial and trigeminal nerves, distal to their exit from the brainstem
c. The facial and abducens nerve nuclei within the pons
d. The facial nerve, distal to the chorda tympani nerve
e. The facial nerve, distal to the geniculate ganglion

Questions 299 to 300

299. A second-year medical student was asked to see a nursing home patient as a requirement for a physical diagnosis course. The patient was a 79-year-old man who was apparently in a coma. The student was not certain how to approach this case, so he asked the patient's wife, who was sitting at the bedside, why this patient was in a coma. The wife replied, "Oh, he isn't in a coma. But he did have a stroke." Slightly confused, the student leaned over and asked the patient to open his eyes. He opened his eyes immediately. However, when asked to lift his arm or speak, the patient did nothing. The student then asked the patient's wife whether she was certain that his eye opening was not simply a coincidence and whether he really was in a coma, since he was unable to follow any commands. The wife explained that he was unable to move or speak as a result of his stroke. However, she knew that he was awake because he could communicate with her by blinking his eyes. The student appeared rather skeptical, so the patient's wife asked her husband to blink once for "yes" and twice for "no." She then asked him if he was at home, and he blinked twice. When asked if he was in a nursing home, he blinked once. The student then asked him to move his eyes, and he was able to look in his direction. However, when the student asked him if he could move his arms or legs, he blinked twice. He also blinked twice when asked if he could smile. He did the same when asked if he could feel someone moving his arm. The student thanked the patient and his wife for their time, made notes of his findings, and returned to class. In the case described above, where in the nervous system could a lesion occur that can cause paralysis of the extremities bilaterally, as well as in the face, but not of the eyes?

a. High cervical spinal cord bilaterally
b. Bilateral thalamus
c. Bilateral basal ganglia
d. Bilateral basilar pons
e. Bilateral frontal lobe

300. In the previous vignette which of the following arteries could have been subjected to an infarct that would account for the lesion described in this case?

a. Anterior spinal artery
b. Vertebral artery
c. Basilar artery
d. Middle cerebral artery
e. Posterior cerebral artery

301. A patient experiences paralysis in both arms and legs, but is able to control his gaze in a vertical direction and to blink his eyes. Which of the following pathways would be damaged as a result of an infarct of a blood vessel in the brain to account for paralysis of the limbs?

a. Corticospinal and corticobulbar tracts
b. Spinothalamic tract
c. Solitary tract
d. Superior cerebellar peduncle
e. Inferior cerebellar peduncle

302. A patient is admitted to the emergency room following what appeared to be a stroke. He presents with an ipsilateral paralysis of lateral gaze, a facial paralysis, and Horner syndrome. Which of the following regions of the CNS could have damaged that would best account for the constellation of dysfunctions described in this case?

a. Rostral aspect of the lateral medulla
b. Caudal aspect of the lateral medulla
c. Caudal aspect of the lateral pons
d. Rostral aspect of the lateral pons
e. Caudal aspect of the lateral midbrain

303. An individual was admitted to the emergency room following loss of consciousness. After the patient regained consciousness, he was examined by a neurologist and presented with a right side hemiplegia, loss of sensation on the left side of the face, and his ability to chew. Which of the following arteries was most likely subjected to an infarct that could account for the deficits described in this individual?

a. Posterior inferior cerebellar artery
b. Anterior inferior cerebellar artery
c. Circumferential branches of basilar artery
d. Paramedian branches of basilar artery
e. Anterior spinal artery

Questions 304 and 305

304. A 62-year-old man who smoked two packs of cigarettes per day for 35 years was suffering from a chronic cough that was attributed to his smoking habit by his physician. One day the patient noticed that his right eyelid drooped slightly and that his right pupil was smaller than the left. He also noticed that the inner side of his right hand was numb and that he had begun to drop things from his right hand. He had no other symptoms. He consulted his physician, who directed him to a neurologist. The neurologist noted that although the right pupil was smaller than the left, it was still reactive to light. Although the patient's right eyelid drooped slightly, he could close his eyes tightly when asked to do so. The neurologist noted that he did not sweat on the right side of his face, was unable to feel a pinprick on the inner surface of his right hand, and his right triceps and hand muscles were weak.

With respect to the patient described above, assuming for the moment that the damage included a part of the CNS, which of the following structures could have been damaged that would account for his disorder?

a. Left oculomotor nerve
b. Right oculomotor nerve
c. Edinger-Westphal nucleus
d. Descending hypothalamic sympathetic fibers
e. Parasympathetic fibers coursing from the Edinger-Westphal nucleus

305. Concerning the case in the previous vignette the patient's small pupil was due to which of the following?

a. Unopposed action of the muscles with parasympathetic innervation
b. Unopposed action of the muscles with sympathetic innervation
c. Both sympathetic and parasympathetic damage
d. A lesion in the nucleus of the third nerve
e. A lesion in distal branches of the trochlear nerve

Questions 306 and 307

306. A 59-year-old male is admitted to the emergency room following a brief loss of consciousness. Upon awakening, he is examined by a neurologist who notes a left side oculomotor nerve paralysis as well as a tremor the limbs on the right side coupled with some somatosensory loss on the right side of the body. Which of the following is the most likely locus of the lesion described in this case?

a. Lateral aspect of the caudal forebrain
b. Lateral caudal midbrain tegmentum
c. Medial rostral midbrain tegmentum
d. Medial rostral pontine tegmentum
e. Lateral caudal pontine tegmentum

307. In the patient in Question 306, it is determined that the patient's condition is the result of an occlusion of an artery. Which of the following arteries is most likely occluded?

a. Posterior cerebral artery
b. Middle cerebral artery
c. Superior cerebellar artery
d. Cirumferential branches of basilar artery
e. Paramedian branches of basilar artery

308. A patient from Question 306 presents with a dilated pupil and double vision and receives a diagnosis of an oculomotor paralysis. It is determined that there is a defect in the neurotransmitter mechanism associated with the postganglionic neuron supplying the smooth muscle of the eye. Which of the following neurotransmitters is most likely affected in this case?

a. Acetylcholine
b. Norepinephrine
c. GABA
d. Dopamine
e. Serotonin

Questions 309 and 310

309. A 35-year-old man who had optic neuritis (an inflammation of the optic nerve causing blurred vision) for several years was told that he had a 50% chance of eventually developing multiple sclerosis (MS), a degenerative disease of the CNS white matter. One day he noticed that he had double vision and felt weak on his right side. Although he noted that the symptoms were becoming steadily worse throughout the day, he attributed this to stress from his job as a stockbroker, and in order to relax he decided to take a drive in his car. While he was driving, his vision became steadily worse. As he was about to pull over to the side of the road, he saw two trees on the right side of the road. Uncertain which was the actual image, he attempted to place his right foot on the brake pedal. He suddenly realized that he was unable to lift his right leg, and his car collided with the tree. A pedestrian on the side of the road called the emergency medical service (EMS), and the man was brought to a nearby emergency room.

A neurologist is called to see the patient because the emergency room physicians thought he might have had a stroke, despite his young age. The neurologist speaks to him, then examines him. He finds that his left eye was deviated to the left and down. When the patient attempts to look to his right, his right eye moves normally, but his left eye is unable to move farther to the right than the midline. His left pupil is dilated and does not contract to light from a penlight. His left eyelid droops, and he has difficulty raising it. In addition, the right side of his mouth remains motionless when he attempts to smile, but his forehead is symmetric when he raises his eyebrows. His right arm and leg are markedly weak. The neurologist tells the patient that he is not certain that this was necessarily a stroke, but admits him to the hospital for observation and tests. A lesion in which of the following nerves most likely caused the patient's double vision?

a. Optic nerve
b. Oculomotor nerve
c. Cervical sympathetic fibers
d. Trochlear nerve
e. Abducens nerve

310. In the patient in Question 309, which of the following muscles are affected by nerve damage, causing his left eye to be deviated toward the left side and down?

a. Superior rectus, superior oblique, inferior rectus, inferior oblique
b. Superior rectus, inferior rectus, inferior oblique, lateral rectus
c. Superior rectus, inferior rectus, inferior oblique, medial rectus
d. Lateral rectus, superior oblique, medial rectus, inferior rectus
e. Lateral rectus, superior oblique, inferior oblique, medial rectus

Questions 311 and 312

311. A 62-year-old male is found unconscious by his wife in their home. He is admitted to the emergency room of a local hospital and, when he regains consciousness, is examined by an emergency room physician and then by a neurologist. The patient presented with a left side UMN paralysis of the arm and leg. In addition, his right eye was dilated, the pupil of that eye was unresponsive to light, the eyelid was drooping, and the eye deviated downward. Which of the following is the likely locus of the lesion?

a. Dorsomedial pons of right side
b. Right frontal eye field of cerebral cortex
c. Ventromedial midbrain of right side
d. Dorsolateral pons of right side
e. Dorsomedial midbrain of right side

312. In the patient in Question 311, which combination of structures described below was most likely damaged by the lesion?

a. Red nucleus and superior cerebellar peduncle
b. Internal capsule and optic tract
c. Substantia nigra and cerebral peduncle
d. Third nerve and cerebral peduncle
e. MLF and pontine tegmentum

313. A patient presents with an inability to gaze upward, some nystagmus upon attempting to gaze downward, a large pupil with an abnormal elevation of the upper lid, and paralysis of accommodation. An MRI reveals the presence of a cascular lesion. Which of the following is the most likely locus of this lesion?

a. Pretectal area and postereior commissure
b. MLF and dorsal pontine tegmentum
c. Cerebral peduncle and red nucleus
d. Trochlear nerve and inferior colliculus
e. Superior colliculus and periaqueductal gray

Questions 314 and 315

314. A 17-year-old high school football player is sent to a neurology clinic because his mother thinks he may have acquired neck problems during a game. A month before, he sustained a concussion from a blow to his head from another player. Shortly after, she noted that he intermittently tilted his head to the side. When asked what was the matter, he simply said that sometimes he had double vision and that the images were situated on top of each other vertically, making it difficult to go downstairs. When he is examined, there is no neck pain or limitation of motion. He tends to keep his head tilted to the right side. When asked to follow the doctor's finger with his head in a straight position, his left eye does not move downward when his eyes are turned to the right, and they tend to remain slightly deviated toward the left. At this point, he states that he has double vision and feels better if his head is tilted to the right. The remainder of his eye movements, as well as the remainder of his examination, are normal. Where did the damage most likely occur?

a. The oculomotor nerve
b. The abducens nerve
c. The trochlear nerve
d. The trigeminal nerve
e. The facial nerve

315. In the patient in Question 314, which of the following muscles was most likely weakened?

a. Superior rectus
b. Inferior rectus
c. Lateral rectus
d. Superior oblique
e. Inferior oblique

316. A 70-year-old female suffered a stroke affecting parts of the left frontal lobe of the cerebral cortex. Upon testing, the patient was later unable to move her eyes to the right when requested to do so. Which of the following pathways if disrupted, could best account for this deficit?

a. Frontal lobe projections to the ipsilateral superior colliculus
b. Frontal lobe projections to the contralateral occipital cortex
c. Frontal lobe projections to the ipsilateral trochlear nucleus
d. Frontal lobe projections to the contralateral oculomotor complex
e. Frontal lobe projections to the contralateral pontine gaze center

317. A patient's eyes are seen to be deviated to the left and he is unable to move his eyes to the right. An MRI reveals a brain infarction. Which of the following regions or structures is most likely affected to account for this deficit?

a. Right frontal lobe
b. Left frontal lobe
c. Right vestibular nuclei
d. Right oculomotor nucleus
e. Left abducens nucleus

318. A 67-year-old female who complained of headaches was given an MRI and found to have a small tumor situated on the dorsolateral roof of the midbrain. Which of the following deficits is most likely to occur as a result of this tumor?

a. Inability to move the eyes in a horizontal direction
b. Inability to move the eyes upward
c. Loss of the accommodation reflex
d. Double vision upon attempt at downward gaze
e. Nystagmus upon attempt at moving the eyes horizontally

The Brainstem and Cranial Nerves

Answers

189. The answer is d. (*Aminoff, p 362. Afifi, p 118. Siegel and Sapru, pp 235-240.*) The reflex described in this question is the corneal reflex. It involves the reflex activation of the ophthalmic division of the sensory component of cranial nerve V in response to touching of the cornea and the motor division of the facial nerve (cranial nerve VII), which produces the motor component (ie, the blinking response).

190. The answer is c. (*Siegel and Sapru, pp 229-233.*) The vagus nerve exits through the jugular foramen. A tumor formed in this region would put pressure on the peripheral components of the vagus nerve, including those portions that innervate the larynx and pharynx. Damage to these muscles would cause deficits in vocalization such as hoarseness as well as difficulty in swallowing. The other choices listed in this question do not relate in any way to the vagus nerve.

191. The answer is d. (*Afifi, pp 307-309.*) Taste associated with the anterior two-thirds of the tongue is mediated by the facial nerve (cranial nerve VII). The geniculate ganglion contains the cell bodies associated with the sensory (gustatory) component of the seventh nerve. The somatic motor component of the seventh nerve mediates the muscles of facial expression. Thus, the sensory and motor components of the seventh nerve affected in this individual can be characterized as special visceral afferent (because this afferent contains chemoreceptors) and special visceral efferent (because the motor component innervates skeletal muscle and is derived from a branchial arch), respectively.

192. The answer is c. (*Afifi, pp 91-92, 99. Siegel and Sapru, pp 233-235.*) Cranial nerve IX, the glossopharyngeal nerve, innervates the skeletal muscles of the pharynx. The motor component involved arises from the nucleus ambiguus of the medulla. This cranial nerve also contains afferents, a component of which arises from the superior ganglion. These sensory neurons convey somatosensory sensation, including pain afferents that ultimately synapse in the spinal trigeminal nucleus. The motor component of the glossopharyngeal nerve mediating swallowing and coughing constitutes a special visceral efferent (because it is derived from a visceral arch), and the sensory component conveying pain is referred to as a general somatic afferent fiber.

193. The answer is c. (*Afifi, pp 131-132. Siegel and Sapru, pp 255-257.*) As noted in the answer to Question 191, the muscles governing facial expression, which includes the ability to smile, display teeth, and close an eye are governed by peripheral branches of cranial nerve VII which innervate the affected muscles.

194. The answer is a. (*Siegel and Sapru, p 225.*) The cranial nerve affected by the assault of the baseball is cranial nerve V, which would account for the pain experienced along the face. It exits the brain laterally in the middle of the pons.

195. The answer is d. (*Siegel and Sapru, pp 225, 233-235.*) The cranial nerve in question is the glossopharyngeal nerve (cranial nerve IX). As noted in answer to the previous question, the special visceral efferent component supplies the muscles of the pharynx and the general visceral efferent component supplies the parotid gland. Therefore, damage to this nerve would affect swallowing and gag reflex as well as one's ability to salivate. This nerve exits the brain at the level of the upper medulla in a lateral position (superior to the inferior olivary nucleus) and just caudal to cranial nerve VIII.

196. The answer is f. (*Siegel and Sapru, pp 225-228.*) The affected nerve was the hypoglossal nerve (cranial nerve XII). Damage to this causes the tongue to be deviated to the side of the lesion upon attempts at protrusion. The hypoglossal nerve exits the brain between the pyramid and the olive. No other cranial nerve exits the brain at this position.

197. The answer is E. (*Siegel and Sapru, pp 225, 229-233.*) As noted in the answer to Question 190, damage to the peripheral branches of the vagus nerve (cranial nerve X) could affect both the special visceral efferent component (ie, nerve fibers that innervate the pharynx and larynx) and general visceral efferent component (ie, preganglionic parasympathetic fibers that innervate wide areas of the body viscera, including the stomach). Consequently, damage to this cranial nerve could produce difficulty in swallowing, aphonia, and ulceration of the stomach. This nerve exits the brain in a lateral position at approximately the same level of the medulla as the hypoglossal nerve and just rostral to the position of exit of the glossopharyngeal nerve.

198. The answer is d. (*Afifi, p 224. Kandel, pp 668-669, 817.*) Rigidity can occur by experimentally producing a decerebrate preparation (ie, severing the brainstem at the level of the pons), and it appears clinically as well. In both experimental and clinical situations, there is extensive destruction of brain tissue below the midbrain in the region of the pons, but the medulla is spared. Damage above the pons would likely produce other kinds of syndromes. Damage to the posterior thalamus would produce sensory deficits; damage to the hypothalamus would produce autonomic deficits affecting the visceral nervous system; and damage to the dorsal midbrain would affect sensory functions such as control of eye movements, ability to follow movements of objects in the visual field, disruption in the regulation of pain, and disruptions in the regulation of autonomic functions, including the development of Horner syndrome. Damage to the ventral part of the spinal cord would produce a flaccid or an LMN paralysis.

199. The answer is b. (*Afifi, p 224. Kandel, pp 668-669, 817.*) The massive stroke basically leaves the patient in a decerebrate condition, not unlike those demonstrated in experimental preparations, thus resulting in marked extensor rigidity presented by this patient. This phenomenon is due to the fact that pathways (from the cerebral cortex) that normally inhibit or suppress extensor motor tone are cut by virtue of the surgery and thus their influences upon motor functions are eliminated. However, the lateral vestibulospinal tract, which does not receive significant input from the cerebral cortex, remains essentially intact. This pathway powerfully facilitates extensor motor neurons and extensor reflexes, thus contributing significantly to the expression of decerebrate rigidity, in particular when the descending inhibitory pathways, which arise from more rostral levels, are disrupted by the experimental procedure or stroke. The rubrospinal tract facilitates flexor motor neurons; the lateral reticulospinal tract suppresses extensor motor tone; the medial vestibulospinal tract integrates movement and positioning of the head in response to vestibular stimulation; and the corticospinal tracts, which govern voluntary movements of the limbs, are associated with a UMN paralysis involving spasticity but not rigidity.

200. The answer is d. (*Afifi, pp 89-90. Kandel, pp 972-975. Siegel and Sapru, pp 225, 229-235.*) Specialized peripheral receptors, which specifically respond to changes in blood pressure, include the carotid sinus (associated with cranial nerve IX) and the aortic arch (associated with cranial nerve X). If these receptors (or the cell bodies associated with these receptors) are damaged, then one of the fundamental regulatory mechanisms for the control of blood pressure would be disrupted. The results of such a disruption would likely lead to increases and instability in blood pressure, with evidence of spiking of blood pressure.

201. The answer is a. (*Afifi, pp 89-90. Kandel, pp 972-975.*) Because these sensory receptors in these structures respond to increases in blood pressure, they are, in effect, stretch receptors and are consequently referred to as baroreceptors. In this case, massaging of the neck causes activation of the baroreceptors in the carotid sinus, thus effecting a reduction in blood pressure.

202. The answer is d. (*Afifi, pp 89-90. Kandel, pp 972-975.*) The baroreflex involves primarily projections from the baroreceptors in the carotid sinus to the solitary nucleus of the medulla, which in turn projects to parasympathetic nuclei such as the dorsal motor nucleus of the vagus nerve, which, when activated, leads to a vagal slowing of the heart (ie, the baroreflex pathway). Therefore, damage to the solitary nucleus would disrupt the baroreflex. Other choices are not related to the regulation of the baroreflex mechanism. The trigeminal nuclei are unrelated to autonomic functions. The fastigial nucleus has been shown to facilitate sympathetic activity and vestibular functions. Likewise, descending fibers from the midbrain reticular formation are mainly sympathetic. The autonomic nuclei of the facial nucleus are parasympathetic and regulate salivation, not blood pressure.

203. The answer is b. (*Afifi, p 61. Siegel and Sapru, pp 152-154.*) The medial vestibulospinal tract arises from the medial vestibular nucleus and descends in the MLF to cervical levels, where it controls lower motor neurons (LMNs), which innervate (flexor) muscles controlling the position of the head. The lateral vestibulospinal tract facilitates extensor motor neurons of the limbs, the rubrospinal tract facilitates flexor motor neurons of the limbs, and the reticulospinal tracts modulate muscle tone of the limbs.

204. The answer is c. (*Martin, pp 42-44. Afifi, pp 91-92. Siegel and Sapru, pp 229-233.*) This individual, who suffers a paralysis of the soft palate and pharynx, as well as loss of the carotid sinus reflex, sustains damage that includes cranial nerve X. It should be noted that several of these symptoms could have resulted from damage to cranial nerve IX as well. However, in this question, cranial nerve IX was not listed as a choice. Damage to the fibers of cranial nerve X would frequently cause dysphagia, hoarseness, and paralysis of the soft palate. In addition, damage to the dorsal motor nucleus of the vagus constitutes an efferent limb for expression of the carotid sinus reflex. Thus, damage to these two groups of axons would produce the constellation of deficits described for this case.

205. The answer is c. (*Afifi, pp 91-92. Martin, pp 42-44. Siegel and Sapru, pp 233-235.*) The axons of the nucleus ambiguus of cranial nerve X innervate the soft palate and pharynx. As noted in Question 204, damage to these neurons would frequently cause dysphagia, hoarseness, and paralysis of the soft palate. The solitary nucleus is associated with the transmission of taste information to the thalamus and for the regulation of blood pressure. Deep pontine nuclei mediate signals from the cerebral cortex to the cerebellar cortex. The axons of ventral horn cells innervate skeletal muscles of the body, and axons of inferior salivatory nuclei associated with cranial nerve IX contact postganglionic neurons that innervate the parotid gland.

206. The answer is b. (*Afifi, pp 89-92. Martin, pp 42-44. Siegel and Sapru, pp 233-235.*) The nucleus ambiguus (component of cranial nerve IX) is classified as a special visceral efferent fiber because it innervates skeletal muscle and it is derived from a visceral arch, while the inferior salivatory nucleus innervates the parotid gland (through a postganglionic parasympathetic neuron) and is therefore classified as a general visceral efferent fiber.

207. The answer is c. (*Afifi, pp 115-119. Martin, pp 42-49. Siegel and Sapru, p 190.*) The combined deficit in which the patient loses ability to (use his lateral rectus muscle to) abduct his right eye and display facial expression on the right side of the face means that the lesion is located in the dorsal pons at the site where the facial nerve curves around (just above) the motor nucleus of cranial nerve VI (forming the facial colliculus). Thus, a lesion at this site will affect both cranial nerves, causing the combined deficits described in this case.

208. The answer is e. (*Afifi, pp 140-143. Siegel and Sapru, pp 243-244.*) The cranial nerve involved in adduction of the eye is cranial nerve III, in which the act of moving the eye medially is governed by the medial rectus muscle. Cranial nerve III is located near the midline of the rostral half of the midbrain just below the midbrain periaqueductal gray.

209. The answer is d. (*Afifi, pp 133-134. Martin, pp 260-261, 285-286. Siegel, p 240.*) The locus of the lesion is the posterior half of the medial midbrain, which includes the trochlear nerve (cranial nerve IV). To walk downstairs, one has to have the ability to move the eyes down when they are in the medial position. This involves the use of cranial nerve IV, which innervates the superior oblique muscle (whose action is to pull the eye downward when in the medial position). If there is damage to this nerve on one side, the eyes will not be able to focus on the same visual field, thus producing double vision. Cranial nerve IV is classified as a general somatic efferent fiber because it innervates skeletal muscle and it is derived from somites.

210. The answer is d. (*Martin, pp 260-261, 285-286. Afifi, pp 133-143. Siegel and Sapru, pp 240-242.*) As noted in the answer to Question 209, the trochlear nerve controls downward movement of the eyes when it is situated in a medial position. After exiting the brain, this cranial nerve enters the cavernous sinus (along with cranial nerves III, V, and VI) and enters the orbit through the superior orbital fissure. Therefore, pressure exerted on the cavernous sinus could easily affect the function of this nerve.

211. The answer is d. (*Siegel and Sapru, pp 240-242.*) The patient was suffering from a lateral gaze paralysis resulting from an infarction of the dorsomedial pons, thus affecting the abducens nerve (cranial nerve VI), whose nucleus is located in the region of the infarction. The fibers of the abducens nerve pass ventrally, exiting the brain in a relatively medial position at the level of the lower pons.

212. The answer is d. (*Afifi, pp 85-86.*) Two of the principal afferent fiber systems that project to the inferior olivary nucleus include the red nucleus and the spinal cord. These inputs serve important functions of enabling the inferior olivary nucleus to transmit information related to both sensory (spinal cord) and motor (red nucleus) processes to the cerebellar cortex. The other structures indicated in this question do not have known projections to the inferior olivary nucleus.

213. The answer is e. (*Afifi, pp 85-86. Siegel and Sapru, p 361.*) The primary projection pathway of the inferior olivary nucleus exits this nucleus, enters the inferior cerebellar peduncle of the contralateral side of the brain, and passes into the cerebellar cortex, terminating on apical dendrites of Purkinje cells throughout the cerebellar cortex in a somatotopic manner. As indicated in the explanation of the previous question, this pathway represents an important source of input to the cerebellum from significant regions mediating sensory and motor information (via the inferior olivary nucleus). Other suggested answers do not include known projection targets of the inferior olivary nucleus.

214. The answer c. (*Afifi, pp 307-309. Siegel and Sapru, pp 316-320.*) The central pathways mediating taste include the following: primary afferent taste fibers associated with taste receptors of cranial nerves VII, IX, and X synapse in the solitary nucleus. Many fibers from the solitary nucleus project to the ventral posteromedial nucleus of the thalamus, which in turn project to the ventrolateral aspect of the postcentral gyrus.

215. The answer is e. (*Siegel and Sapru, pp 225, 235-237.*) The cranial nerve affected by the cold was the facial nerve (cranial nerve VII). Damage to the facial nerve will produce manifestations of facial paralysis, such as failure to close an eye, loss of the eye-blink reflex, inability to whistle, and difficulty in exposure of the teeth. In this diagram, the facial nerve passes around the dorsal aspect of cranial nerve VI and exits in a lateral position at the level of the lower pons.

216. The answer is d. (*Siegel and Sapru, pp 225, 240-243.*) The inability to move the right eye to the right (ie, in a lateral direction) is the result of damage to the right abducens nerve (cranial nerve VI). Normally, activation of the right abducens nerve causes the right eye to be moved laterally to the right. This cranial nerve exits the brain at the level of the lower pons just above the medulla at a position medial to the exit of the facial nerve. The cell bodies of origin of this nerve lie in the caudal aspect of the dorsomedial pons at a position just below where the facial nerve arches over and around cranial nerve VI before it exits the brainstem.

217. The answer is C. *(Siegel and Sapru, pp 225, 237-240.)* The motor branch of the trigeminal nerve (cranial nerve V) innervates the muscles of mastication. Damage to this nerve will affect the ability for jaw closing. Since a branch of the trigeminal nerve innervates the pterygoid muscle, there will also be a deviation of the jaw to the affected side when the patient is asked to open his mouth. The trigeminal nerve exits the brainstem laterally at the level of the middle of the pons. It consists of a very large sensory component and a smaller motor component.

218. The answer is b. *(Afifi, pp 91-92, 99. Siegel and Sapru, pp 233-235. Aminoff, pp 70, 72, 84, 283, 363.)* The cranial nerve that was directly affected was the glossopharyngeal nerve (cranial nerve IX). This is a mixed and complex nerve containing (1) special visceral efferents from the nucleus ambiguus that supply the stylopharyngeus muscle (for elevation of pharynx in speech); (2) special visceral afferent fibers that transmit taste impulses from the posterior third of the tongue and general visceral afferent fibers associated with the inferior ganglion whose receptors lie in the carotid sinus that regulates cardiovascular functions; (3) general somatic afferents whose cell bodies lie in the superior ganglion of cranial nerve IX and which mediate somatosensory information, including pain from the pharynx; and (4) general visceral efferent fibers that originate in the inferior salivatory nucleus, which are preganglionic and synapse in the otic ganglion. The postganglionic fiber from the otic ganglion innervates the parotid gland and mediates, in part, salivation. Thus, when this nerve is affected by an infectious agent, it results in the constellation of symptoms presented in this case.

219. The answer is e. *(Afifi, pp 91-92, 99. Siegel and Sapru, pp 233-235. Aminoff, pp 70, 72, 84, 283, 363.)* When the glossopharyngeal nerve is affected by an infectious agent, it results in the constellation of symptoms presented in Question 216. Since the cell bodies of motor (or visceral motor) fibers (mediating motor and visceral effects) as well as the terminals of sensory afferents (mediating pain from the pharynx) lie in different regions of the medulla, it is very unlikely that such an effect could be the result of damage within the brainstem. A much more likely occurrence is that the infectious agent produced disruption of the glossopharyngeal nerve peripherally, such as at the base of the skull or jugular foramen, where all the components run together and can be more easily affected.

220. The answer is b. (*Afifi, pp 112-114, 124. Siegel and Sapru, pp 235-237. Aminoff, pp 26, 70-74, 83-85, 182, 229, 363.*) The nerve affected by this disorder is cranial nerve VII (facial nerve). The cell bodies of origin, which innervate the muscles of facial expression (special visceral efferents), arise from the facial nucleus, which are located in the ventrolateral aspect of the lower pons.

221. The answer is d. (*Afifi, pp 112-114. Siegel and Sapru, pp 235-237. Simon, pp 347-348.*) The preganglionic parasympathetic neurons associated with lacrimation and which contribute to salivation arise from the superior salivatory nucleus of the lower pons. These preganglionic neurons synapse with postganglionic neurons in the submandibular and pterygopalatine ganglia. Since the disorder affected parts of the facial nerve, other choices are clearly incorrect since they relate to other cranial nerves. The inferior salivatory nucleus governs salivation associated with the parotid gland but has no relationship to lacrimation.

222. The answer is c. (*Siegel and Sapru, pp 235-237.*) The geniculate ganglion contains the cell bodies of special visceral afferents of cranial nerve VII, mediating taste impulses from the anterior two-thirds of the tongue to the CNS. The other choices are not appropriate. Sensory components of cranial nerve IX are not involved because they mediate taste from the posterior third of the tongue. Neither are the motor nucleus of cranial nerve VII, nucleus ambiguus, or dorsal motor nucleus because they are either somatomotor or autonomic neurons and do not mediate information associate with taste.

223 to 227. The answers are 223-A, 224-B, 225-E, 226-C, 227-D. (*Afifi, pp 81-84. Siegel and Sapru, pp 142-149, 237-239.*) The nucleus gracilis (A) contains cells that respond to movement of the lower limb as a result of joint capsule activation. Damage to this region will result in loss of conscious proprioception associated with the ipsilateral (ie, left) leg, and, additionally, the loss of conscious proprioception will result in ataxia because this input is essential for normal ambulation to occur. The nucleus cuneatus (B) contains cells that respond to a variety of stimuli applied to the upper limb, including vibratory stimuli. Damage to this nucleus causes loss of sensation in the ipsilateral arm and hand (ie, left hand and arm). One component of the descending MLF (E) contains fibers that arise from the medial vestibular nucleus that project to cervical levels and contribute to reflex activity associated with the position of the head. The descending track of the trigeminal nerve (C) contains first-order fibers mediating pain and temperature information from the head region. Because of its lateral position in the brainstem, a surgical procedure is sometimes carried out to cut these fibers as a means of alleviating excruciating pain. Fibers of the medial lemniscus (D) arise from the contralateral dorsal column nuclei and ascend to the ventral posterolateral nucleus of the thalamus. These fibers transmit the same information noted earlier for the dorsal column nuclei, which includes two-point discrimination and conscious proprioception from the opposite side of the body.

228 to 236. The answers are 228-B, 229-C, 230-H, 231-B, 232-H, 233-G, 234-I, 235-A, 236-F. *(Afifi, pp 91-101. Nolte, pp 252-254. Siegel and Sapru, pp 227-235, 302-306, 316-320, 361.)* Different groups of neurons of the solitary complex (B) respond to taste stimuli and to inputs that signal sudden changes in blood pressure. A lesion of the solitary nucleus would most likely result in alterations in blood pressure such as sudden hypertension. The medial vestibular nucleus (C) receives direct vestibular inputs from the otolith organ and semicircular canals. Axons of medial vestibular neurons descend to the spinal cord in the MLF and serve to regulate reflexes associated with the head. Also note that the inferior vestibular nucleus (D) also receives vestibular inputs, but does not project its axons to the spinal cord. The inferior olivary nucleus (H) receives inputs from the red nucleus and spinal cord, and it projects its axons through the inferior cerebellar peduncle (where it constitutes its largest component) to the contralateral cerebellar cortex, where they synapse with the dendrites of Purkinje cells. Fibers contained in the inferior cerebellar peduncle (E) comprise the largest single-most input into the cerebellum (approximately 40% of afferents) and these fibers arise from cells located in both the spinal cord and the brainstem. A lesion of the inferior olivary nucleus would likely affect several of the feedback mechanisms essential for the expression of normal purposeful movements of the limbs and may induce ataxia as well. The nucleus ambiguus (G) is a special visceral efferent nucleus that is situated in a position ventrolateral to that of the hypoglossal nucleus. Its axons innervate the muscles of the larynx and pharynx and, therefore, are essential for the occurrence of such responses as the gag reflex. The pyramids (I), located on the ventromedial aspect of the brainstem, contain fibers that arise from the sensorimotor cortex. These neurons serve as essential UMNs that mediate voluntary control of motor functions. A brainstem lesion would produce an upper motor neuron paralysis of the contralateral limbs. The hypoglossal nucleus (A), a general somatic efferent nucleus, is located in the dorsomedial aspect of the medulla. Its axons innervate the muscles of the tongue and cause extrusion of the tongue toward the opposite side, but when this structure is damaged, the tongue protrudes to the side of the lesion when extended. Descending first-order fibers mediating pain and temperature from the face are contained in the lateral aspect of the lower brainstem (F) and are thus accessible to surgical intervention. In cases of very severe pain, these fibers are sometimes cut surgically in order to eliminate or reduce facial pain.

237 to 242. The answers are 237-A, 238-A, 239-C, 240-B, 241-A, 242-C. (*Afifi, pp 200-220. Nolte, pp 505-516 Siegel and Sapru, pp 371-374.*) The efferent projections of the cerebellum arise from three distinct groups of nuclei called deep cerebellar nuclei. The nucleus located in the most medial position is the fastigial nucleus (A). It gives rise to at least two important projections: one that is distributed to the reticular formation and another that is distributed to the vestibular nuclei. In this manner, the fastigial nucleus contributes to the regulation of balance and ambulation via its connections with the vestibular system and to the regulation of blood pressure (as well as muscle tone) via its connections with reticular formation. The nucleus situated most laterally is the dentate nucleus (C). It projects through the superior cerebellar peduncle and its axons innervate principally the ventrolateral nucleus of the thalamus, which in turn projects to the motor cortex. In this way, the dentate nucleus contributes to the regulation of coordinated movements of the distal musculature. Damage to any component of this circuit would seriously affect the capacity to produce coordinated movements of the arms and hands.

Neurons of the emboliform (B) and globose (not labeled) nuclei lie in an intermediate position between the fastigial and dentate nuclei and therefore are often referred to as the interposed nuclei. Their axons project through the superior cerebellar peduncle principally to the red nucleus. Therefore, in order to obtain orthodromic recordings of monosynaptic action potentials in the red nucleus, stimulation has to be applied at a primary afferent source of the red nucleus, namely, the interposed nuclei. The projections from the cerebellar cortex to the deep cerebellar nuclei are topographically organized. Cells located in the far medial aspect of the cerebellar cortex, the vermal region, project (via Purkinje cell axons) to the fastigial nucleus (A). Damage to this region of cerebellar cortex or its projections to the fastigial nucleus would result in ataxia and nystagmus. In contrast, the lateral aspects of the cerebellar hemispheres project to the dentate nucleus (C), which is the most lateral of the deep cerebellar nuclei. Damage to any of the components of this pathway would result in intentional tremors and loss of coordination of movements.

243 to 249. The answers are 243-B, 244-E, 245-D, 246-A, 247-G, 248-F, 249-C. *(Afifi, 200-220. Nolte, pp 267-293, 255-274, 284-307. Siegel and Sapru, pp 174-175, 227-228, 304-306, 316-320, 361-364.)* The inferior vestibular nucleus (B) lies immediately medial to the inferior cerebellar peduncle (shown at C) and receives direct inputs from first-order vestibular fibers that arise from the vestibular apparatus. The MLF (E) contains second-order vestibular fibers, the majority of which ascend in the brainstem to innervate cranial nerve nuclei III, IV, and VI. A small component of this bundle also descends to cervical levels of the spinal cord from the medial vestibular nucleus. As noted previously, the descending component of the MLF integrates vestibular signals, which help to regulate the position of the head with changes in position of the body. Damage to this structure will also affect the ascending fibers, which innervate the neurons controlling the extraocular eye muscles. Such damage would result in nystagmus. The solitary nucleus (D) receives inputs from first-order taste fibers and is thus a special visceral afferent nucleus that transmits taste signals to the ventral posteromedial nucleus of the thalamus. The solitary nucleus also receives cardiovascular inputs from cranial nerve IX and, for this reason, has properties of a general visceral afferent nucleus as well. The hypoglossal nucleus (A) innervates the muscles of the tongue, causing it to protrude outward and to the opposite side. Thus, when this nerve is damaged, the opposite (normal) nerve causes the tongue to deviate to the side of the lesion when the patient attempts to stick out his tongue.

The medial lemniscus (G) ascends to the thalamus and transmits information associated with conscious proprioception from the contralateral side of the body as a result of the decussating fibers of the medial lemniscus. This bundle constitutes a second-order neuron that arises from the dorsal column nuclei of the lower medulla. The dorsal column nuclei receive first-order signals that mediate conscious proprioception from fibers contained within the dorsal columns of the spinal cord. Damage to the medial lemniscus would result in loss of vibration and conscious proprioception on the side of the body opposite the lesion. The spinal nucleus of cranial nerve V (F) receives pain and temperature fibers from first-order trigeminal neurons that arise from the head. Damage to this region would result in loss of pain sensation from the ipsilateral side of the face. The inferior cerebellar peduncle (C) is one of two principal cerebellar afferent pathways. One major fiber group contained within the inferior cerebellar peduncle arises from brainstem structures such as the contralateral inferior olivary nucleus and reticular formation. The other groups of fibers contained within this bundle arise from the spinal cord. Of the fibers that ascend in this bundle from the spinal cord, many constitute second-order muscle spindle afferents that arise from the nucleus dorsalis of Clarke.

250 to 254. The answers are 250-C, 251-B, 252-D, 253-E, 254-A. *(Afifi, pp 200-220, 303-320. Nolte, pp 256-259, 267-293, 470-478. Siegel and Sapru, pp 364-365.)* The middle cerebellar peduncle (C) serves as a relay nucleus for the transmission of information from the cerebral cortex to the cerebellum. Fibers in this peduncle arise from the contralateral deep pontine nucleus, which receives its principal afferents from the cerebral cortex. As noted previously, damage to this pathway would affect the cerebral cortex-cerebellar circuit, resulting in movements of the distal musculature that would lack coordination. The motor nucleus of cranial nerve V (B) is an LMN (special visceral efferent) because it innervates the muscles of mastication and controls, in particular, jaw-closing responses. Damage to the sensory or motor nuclei of cranial nerve V would disrupt the reflex mediating chewing responses which includes the masseter reflex and its jaw-closing component of this reflex. Corticobulbar and corticospinal fibers (D) are situated in the ventral aspect of the basilar pons. Damage at any level of the corticospinal system would result in a contralateral UMN paralysis. The medial lemniscus (E) is a somatotopically organized pathway that arises from the dorsal column nuclei and projects to the ventral posterolateral nucleus of the thalamus. Fibers of this pathway that arise from the nucleus gracilis (associated with the leg) project to more dorsolateral aspects of the ventral posterolateral nucleus. Fibers arising from the nucleus cuneatus (associated with the arm) project to more ventromedial aspects of the ventral posterolateral nucleus. Thus, damage to this pathway would result in loss of conscious proprioception and some tactile sensation on the contralateral side of the body. Fibers of the superior cerebellar peduncle (A) arise from the dentate and interposed nuclei of cerebellum and project to both the red nucleus and the ventrolateral nucleus of the thalamus. Therefore, if these cerebellar nuclei were destroyed, then the fibers contained in the superior cerebellar peduncle would show extensive degeneration.

255 to 259. The answers are 255-E, 256-B, 257-C, 258-A, 259-D. *(Afifi, pp 107-109. Nolte, pp 267-293. Siegel and Sapru, pp 194-199.)* The inferior colliculus (E) is situated in the caudal aspect of the tectum and is an important relay nucleus for the transmission of auditory information to the cortex from lower levels of the brainstem. Damage to the inferior colliculus would likely result in some loss of auditory discrimination, acuity, and ability to localize sound in space. The decussation of the superior cerebellar peduncle (B) is also present at caudal levels of the midbrain and is usually seen together with the inferior colliculus. These crossing fibers arise from the dentate and interposed nuclei and terminate in the contralateral red nucleus and ventrolateral nucleus of the thalamus. Damage to the cerebellum would likely result in degeneration of the fibers contained within the superior cerebellar peduncle. The crus cerebri (C) contains fibers that arise from all regions of the cortex and project to all the levels of the brainstem and the spinal cord. As noted previously, damage to the corticospinal tract at any level would result in a UMN paralysis. The trochlear nucleus (cranial nerve IV) (A), which is situated just below the periaqueductal gray at the level of the inferior colliculus, receives direct inputs from ascending fibers of the MLF that arise from vestibular nuclei. The trochlear nucleus governs the downward movements of the eyes, in particular, when they are in a medial position. A fourth nerve paralysis is particularly seen when the patient is attempting to walk down a flight of stairs and cannot move his eyes downward. The midbrain periaqueductal gray (D) contains dense quantities of enkephalin-positive cells and nerve terminals. The transmitter (or neuromodulator) enkephalin plays an important role in the regulation of pain, cardiovascular functions, and emotional behavior.

260 to 264. The answers are 260-E, 261-D, 262-A, 263-C, 264-F.
(*Afifi, pp 129-147. Nolte, pp 278-290. Siegel and Sapru, pp 198-200, 206.*) The
superior colliculus (E), situated at a more rostral level of the tectum, plays
an important role in tracking or pursuit of moving stimuli as well as movements of the eyes up and down. Damage to this region would clearly affect
the ability to produce these movements. The medial geniculate nucleus
(D), which is part of the forebrain, actually sits over the lateral aspect of the
midbrain and can be seen at rostral levels of the midbrain. It is part of an
auditory relay system and receives its inputs from the inferior colliculus via
fibers of the brachium of the inferior colliculus. Damage to this relay
nucleus would affect auditory acuity and one's ability to localize and discriminate sound. The pars compacta is situated in the medial aspect of the
substantia nigra (A) and contains dopamine neurons whose axons innervate the striatum. Damage to these dopamine neurons produces Parkinson
disease, which is characterized by rigidity, tremor, and akinesia. The red
nucleus (C), a structure associated with motor functions, receives direct
inputs from both the cerebral cortex and the cerebellum. The contralateral
limb ataxia could be accounted for by the loss of inputs from the red
nucleus to the cerebellum via the inferior olivary nucleus. The loss of
pupillary constriction and ability to move the eye medially could be
accounted for by the fact that the fibers of the oculomotor nerve pass ventrally in proximity to the red nucleus. Thus, damage to the red nucleus
would also affect the oculomotor nerve. The oculomotor nerve (cranial
nerve III) (F), located at the level of the superior colliculus, contains general somatic efferent components that innervate extraocular eye muscles
and general visceral efferent components whose postganglionic fibers
innervate smooth muscles associated with pupillary constriction and
bulging of the lens. As just noted, damage to the oculomotor nerve would
produce impairment of vertical and medial movements of the eyes as well
as loss of the pupillary light reflex.

265. The answer is a. (*Afifi, pp 117-119. Nolte, pp 270-274, 307-314. Siegel
and Sapru, pp 237-240.*) The spinal trigeminal nucleus receives its sensory
inputs from first-order neurons contained in the ipsilateral descending tract of
cranial nerve V. A central property of the spinal trigeminal nucleus is that it is
uniquely associated with pain inputs (to the exclusion of the main sensory
nucleus and mesencephalic nucleus). Fibers from this nucleus mainly project
contralaterally to the ventral posteromedial nucleus of the thalamus. Surgical

interruption of these descending first-order pain fibers is a practical approach and one that has been carried out by neurosurgeons. Destruction of the ventral posterolateral nucleus would not necessarily destroy the major pain inputs to the cerebral cortex and would additionally be a more difficult structure to destroy surgically. The main sensory nucleus of the trigeminal nerve is not known to convey pain inputs to thalamus and cortex. The substantia gelatinosa conveys pain and temperature sensation from the body and not the head. The midbrain periaqueductal gray constitutes part of a pain-inhibitory system, not one that transmits pain sensations to the cerebral cortex.

266. The answer is e. *(Kandel, pp 1292-1294. Nolte, pp 141, 594.)* The area postrema is of interest because it is a circumventricular organ associated with emetic functions. As a circumventricular organ, the area postrema constitutes a part of the ependymal lining of the brain's ventricular system (in this case, the fourth ventricle). It also contains both fenestrated and nonfenestrated capillaries that allow for enhanced transport, which possibly accounts for the fact that it lies outside the blood-brain barrier. Axons and dendrites from neighboring structures (but not from the forebrain) innervate this structure, which is composed of astroblast-like cells, arterioles, sinusoids, and some neurons. Various peptides (but not monoamine-containing neurons) have also been shown to be present in this structure. Experimental evidence has strongly implicated the area postrema as a chemoreceptor trigger zone for emesis. It responds to digitalis glycosides and apomorphine.

267. The answer is c. *(Afifi, pp 89-91. Siegel and Sapru, pp 229-233.)* Cranial nerve X is a highly complex nerve. Special visceral efferent fibers innervate the constrictor muscles of the pharynx and the intrinsic muscles of the larynx. Damage to this division results in hoarseness and difficulty in swallowing. General visceral efferent fibers constitute part of the cranial aspect of the parasympathetic nervous system; thus, they are preganglionic parasympathetic fibers that innervate the heart, lungs, esophagus, and stomach. Damage to the descending vagus would reduce gastric secretions and disrupt cardiovascular reflex activity. Special visceral afferents include fibers from chemoreceptors for taste associated with the epiglottis and chemoreceptors in the aortic bodies that sense changes in O_2-CO_2 levels in the blood. General visceral afferent fibers arise from the trachea, pharynx, larynx, and esophagus and signal changes in blood pressure to the brainstem. Cranial nerve IX shares a number of similarities with cranial nerve X.

However, damage to cranial nerve IX would not affect gastric secretions. Cranial nerve VII does not relate to functions such as swallowing, speech, and gastric secretions. Cranial nerve XI is a purely motor nerve. The reticular formation of the pons does not regulate gastric secretions, swallowing, or speech.

268. The answer is a. *(Afifi, pp 98-99. Nolte, pp 306-314. Siegel and Sapru, p 176.)* A primary characteristic of a lesion of the dorsolateral medulla is loss of pain and temperature sensation on the contralateral side of the body and ipsilateral half of the face. Damage to the descending tract of the trigeminal nerve and to the spinal nucleus of cranial nerve V will produce loss of sensation on the ipsilateral side of the face. There also will be damage to the lateral spinothalamic tract, which has already crossed at the level of the spinal cord and which conveys pain and temperature sensation from the contralateral side of the body. Hemiparesis would not result from this lesion since the pyramidal tract would remain intact. The cerebellum would also be spared, and intention tremor associated with cerebellar damage would not occur.

269. The answer is b. *(Martin, pp 198. Nolte, pp 361-363.)* The olivocochlear bundle is a most interesting pathway because it arises from the region immediately dorsal to the superior olivary nucleus and projects contralaterally back to the hair cells of the cochlea. Stimulation of this bundle results in inhibition or reduction of responses to auditory signals by auditory nerve fibers. The main function of the olivocochlear bundle is to regulate the function of hair cells and thus affect auditory sensitivity. Damage to this pathway is believed to result in difficulty in discriminating sounds and therefore understanding speech. There is no evidence that the olivocochlear bundle bears any anatomic or functional relationship to the medial lemniscus. Since the pathway arises from the superior olivary nucleus, which is present at the level of the lower pons, it would not be visible in a section taken from the upper pons.

270. The answer is c. *(Afifi, pp 107-109. Nolte, pp 358-363. Siegel and Sapru, pp 299-301.)* Since the auditory relay system is a highly complex pathway in which auditory signals are bilaterally represented at all levels beyond the receptor level, lesions at these levels would not produce a solely unilateral deafness. Such a loss could only result when the lesion involves either the receptor or the first-order neurons of the nerve (ie, cranial nerve VIII itself). The medial lemniscus is not related to the auditory system.

271. The answer is c. *(Afifi, pp 117-118. Nolte, pp 305-307. Siegel and Sapru, pp 237-239.)* In general, first-order sensory neurons form ganglia outside the CNS. There is one exception: the mesencephalic nucleus of cranial nerve V, which transmits unconscious proprioception (ie, muscle spindle activity) from jaw muscles. These inputs serve as the first-order neurons for a disynaptic pathway to the cerebellum, as well as for a monosynaptic pathway with the motor nucleus of cranial nerve V mediating the jaw-closing reflex.

272. The answer is d. *(Afifi, pp 115-116. Nolte, pp 524, 529-534. Siegel and Sapru, p 240.)* Conjugate lateral gaze requires the simultaneous contractions of the lateral rectus muscle of one eye and the medial rectus of the other eye. Recent studies have indicated that there is a region that integrates and coordinates such movements and that the site is part of the nucleus of cranial nerve VI. It is likely that it accomplishes this phenomenon, in part because ascending axons from the abducens nucleus pass through the MLF to the contralateral nuclei of cranial nerve III. Thus, the abducens nucleus serves not only to innervate the lateral rectus muscle but also to integrate signals necessary for conjugate deviation of the eyes. The abducens nucleus appears to be the only cranial nerve structure where lesions of the root fibers and nucleus fail to display identical effects.

273. The answer is a. *(Afifi, pp 115-116. Nolte, pp 280-286, 351-355, 359-373. Siegel and Sapru, pp 244-247.)* The paramedian pontine reticular formation, located in or adjacent to cranial nerve VI (see explanation to Question 272), is an important integrating structure controlling the position of the eyes. It receives inputs from the cerebral cortex (presumably the region of the frontal eye fields) and fibers from the cerebellum, spinal cord, and vestibular complex. Its efferent fibers project to the cerebellum, vestibular complex, pretectal region, interstitial nucleus of Cajal, and nucleus of Darkschewitsch of the rostral midbrain. These are all nuclei concerned with the regulation of eye position and movements. It is not related to any other known motor or auditory functions, nor has it been shown to contain ascending noradrenergic neurons.

274. The answer is c. *(Afifi, pp 124-127. Nolte, pp 302-304, 290-294. Siegel and Sapru, p 190.)* For a lesion to produce both an ipsilateral gaze paralysis and contralateral hemiplegia, it must be situated in a location where fibers regulating both lateral gaze and movements of the contralateral limbs lie close to each other. The only such location is the ventrocaudal aspect of the pons, where fibers of cranial nerve VI descend toward the ventral surface of the brainstem and where corticospinal fibers are descending toward the spinal cord. The other regions listed in the question do not meet this condition.

275. The answer is e. *(Purves, pp 393-392. Siegel and Sapru, p 226.)* The group called special visceral afferent fibers is limited to those cranial nerves that convey impulses to the brain associated with olfaction (I) and taste (VII, IX, and X). Since olfaction and taste involve chemical senses, some authors also include cranial nerves IX and X in the group because these nerves contain components involved in signaling changes in O_2 and CO_2 levels in the blood.

276. The answer is e. *(Purves, pp 294-297. Nolte, pp 442-446.)* Because the deficit includes a homonymous hemianopsia, the lesion has to be located somewhere in the forebrain, such as in the region that includes the optic tract and internal capsule on the right side of the brain. The motor neurons of cranial nerve VII, as well as spinal cord motor neurons, receive cortical fibers that are crossed, which accounts for the fact that motor dysfunctions of the lower face and body involve lesions on the same side.

277. The answer is d. *(Afifi, pp 140-145. Siegel and Sapru, pp 242-244.)* Inability to move the eyes up or down when they are displaced laterally would result from a lesion of the midbrain involving cranial nerve III. Because the somatomotor neurons of cranial nerve III supply, in part, the superior and inferior recti muscles as well as the inferior oblique muscle, cranial nerve III is responsible for up-and-down movements of the eye when they are positioned laterally. Recall that when the eye is positioned medially, it is the superior oblique that is innervated by cranial nerve IV that pulls the eye downward.

278. The answer is c. *(Afifi, p 144. Nolte, p 455. Siegel and Sapru, pp 243-244.)* This disorder is referred to as the Argyll Robertson pupil and occurs with CNS syphilis (tertiary). Although the precise site of the lesion has never been fully established, it is believed to be in the pretectal area. The reasoning is that in the pupillary light reflex, many optic fibers terminate in the pretectal area and superior colliculus region and are then relayed to the autonomic nuclei of cranial nerve III. Impulses from this component of cranial nerve III then synapse with postganglionic parasympathetics that innervate the pupillary constrictor muscles, thus producing pupillary constriction. In the case of the accommodation reflex, retinal impulses first reach the cortex and are then relayed through corticofugal fibers to the brainstem. Some of these fibers are then relayed directly or indirectly to both motor and autonomic components of cranial nerve III, thus activating the muscles required for the accommodation reaction to occur, which includes pupillary constriction.

279. The answer is b. (*Kandel, pp 642-644. Nolte, pp 324-330, 313-316. Siegel and Sapru, pp 316-320.*) The solitary nucleus receives first-order neurons from the taste system and thus serves as a critical relay nucleus for the taste pathway. Axons arising from the solitary nucleus project to the ventral posteromedial nucleus of the thalamus and may also synapse in the parabrachial nuclei of the upper pons. Structures such as the ventral posterolateral nucleus, medial lemniscus, and superior parietal lobule are not associated with the taste pathway.

280. The answer is b. (*Kandel, pp 1309-1313. Nolte, pp 277-292. Siegel and Sapru, pp 47-52, 500-504.*) The superior cerebellar artery supplies the dorsolateral aspect of the upper pons. The basilar artery supplies the medial aspect of the pons. The other arteries (vertebral, anterior spinal, and posterior inferior cerebellar) supply different parts of the medulla. The lateral aspect of the upper pons contains the superior cerebellar artery that supplies spinothalamic fibers, the lateral lemniscus, and the locus ceruleus (situated just dorsal to the motor nucleus of cranial nerve V, which is also affected by the lesion). This lateral pontine lesion produces a syndrome that includes (1) loss of pain and temperature sensation from the contralateral side of the body (damage to the lateral spinothalamic tract), (2) ipsilateral loss of masticatory reflexes (damage to the motor nucleus of cranial nerve V), (3) diminution of hearing (disruption of secondary auditory pathways), and (4) Horner syndrome (disruption of descending fibers from the hypothalamus and midbrain that mediate autonomic functions).

281. The answer is a. (*Kandel, pp 1309-1313. Siegel and Sapru, pp 500-503.*) The paramedian branch of the basilar artery supplies the ventromedial pons (ie, medial basilar pons). The circumferential branch supplies more lateral regions of the pons, as does the superior cerebellar artery. The anterior spinal and anterior inferior cerebellar arteries supply different parts of the medulla. Occlusion of this artery would result in a contralateral upper motor neuron paralysis of the body and weakness of muscles related to the face.

282. The answer is c. (*Afifi, pp 123-125. Kandel, pp 1309-1313. Siegel and Sapru, pp 190-191.*) The lesion described in this case is an example of a basal pontine syndrome involving the basilar pons. It is the result of a vascular lesion affecting corticobulbar and corticospinal fibers. Such damage would account for the weakness in facial nerves, dysarthria, and dysphagia. A lesion placed at the other regions of the brainstem indicated by the other choices does not affect the structures that could account for the syndrome described in this case.

283. The answer is d. (*Afifi, pp 123-125. Kandel, pp 1309-1313. Siegel and Sapru, pp 190-191.*) A lesion of the rostral aspect of the basilar pons would affect the sensory and motor fibers of the trigeminal nerve that exit the brainstem at this level. A lesion of the basilar pons would also affect corticospinal fibers, thus resulting in a contralateral upper motor neuron paralysis. Other choices in the question include regions that do not involve the upper pons where the trigeminal fibers exit the brain.

284. The answer is a. (*Afifi, pp 145-146. Kandel, pp 1312-1314. Siegel and Sapru, pp 199-200.*) The lesion involves the superior colliculus. This structure receives inputs from the cerebral cortex and optic tract, and its neurons respond to moving objects in the visual field. This region is supplied by the posterior cerebral artery. The cerebellar and anterior spinal arteries supply more caudal aspects of the brainstem and the basilar artery supplies more ventral aspects of the pons and midbrain.

285. The answer is a. (*Afifi, pp 145-146. Kandel, pp 1312-1314.*) The lesion will disrupt fibers of the medial lemniscus (lateral aspect of the lesion) and thus produce contralateral loss of conscious proprioception. It will also disrupt fibers passing from the cerebellum to the red nucleus and ventrolateral nucleus of the thalamus, which could account for a tremor of the contralateral limb. Note that there would be no ipsilateral motor loss because functions associated with the red nucleus are expressed on the contralateral side. None of the other structures mentioned in the other choices could account for the deficits presented in this patient.

286. The answer is c. (*Afifi, pp 150-151. Kandel, pp 1312-1314.*) The primary structures damaged by this lesion include the crus cerebri, which results in a UMN paralysis of the contralateral limbs, as well as a paresis of the lower facial and tongue muscles. The other outstanding syndrome present from this lesion is a paralysis that results from damage to cranial nerve III. The disorder described in this case is referred to as a Weber syndrome. Other structures may be marginally affected and cannot account for the disturbances described in this case.

287. The answer is e. (*Siegel, pp 251-252. Afifi, pp 135-136.*) The pars compacta of the substantia nigra contains dopamine neurons whose axons project to the neostriatum. The dopaminergic neurons of the ventral tegmental area project to other areas of the forebrain, such as the hypothalamus, limbic system, and cerebral cortex. Therefore, loss of neurons in these two regions of the ventral midbrain will cause loss of dopaminergic inputs to the basal ganglia, limbic system, and cerebral cortex. While the substantia nigra contains GABA neurons, their projections are directed mainly to the thalamus. These regions of the ventral midbrain are not known to contain either noradrenergic or serotonergic neurons.

288. The answer is b. (*Afifi, pp 107-109. Nolte, pp 271, 358-360. Siegel and Sapru, pp 184-186.*) The principal ascending pathway of the auditory system listed in this question (that was affected by the stroke) is the lateral lemniscus. It transmits information from the cochlear nuclei to the inferior colliculus. The trapezoid body is a commissure that contains some of the fibers of the lateral lemniscus that cross from the cochlear nuclei of one side of the brainstem en route to the inferior colliculus of the other side. The trapezoid body is present at the level of the caudal pons. The brachium of the superior colliculus, trigeminal lemniscus, and medial lemniscus do not transmit auditory sensory information.

289 and 290. The answers are 289-e, 290-a. (*Adams, p 678. Afifi, pp 98-100, 141-143. Siegel and Sapru, pp 501-504.*) The patient had a stroke resulting from occlusion of medial branches of the left vertebral artery, presumably secondary to atherosclerosis (ie, cholesterol deposits within the artery, which eventually occlude it). The resulting syndrome is called the medial medullary syndrome, because the affected structures are located in the medial portion of the medulla. These structures include the pyramids, the medial lemniscus, the medial longitudinal fasciculus, and the nucleus of the hypoglossal nerve and its outflow tract. The patient's symptoms resulted from damage to the aforementioned structures and may have been caused by the same process (atherosclerosis) that resulted in her heart disease. The weakness of her right side was caused by damage to the medullary pyramid (at the level of the hypoglossal nerve) on the left side. Her face was spared because fibers supplying the face exited above the level of the infarct. However, a lesion in the corticospinal tract of the cervical spinal cord above C5 could cause arm and leg weakness and spare the face, because facial fibers exit at the pontine-medulla border. A lesion in the inferior portion of the precentral gyrus of the left frontal lobe would cause right-sided weakness, but would include the face, because this area is represented more inferiorly than are the extremities. Her unsteady gait was a result of the weakness of her right side, but may also have been the result of the loss of position and vibration sense on that side from damage to the medial lemniscus (as demonstrated by the inability to identify the position of her toe with her eyes closed, and the inability to feel the vibrations of a tuning fork). Without position sense, walking becomes unsteady because it is necessary to feel the position of one's feet on the floor during normal gait. Damage to both the medial lemniscus and pyramids at this level causes problems on the contralateral side because this lesion is located rostral to the level where both of these fiber bundles cross to the opposite side of the brain. Damage to the descending component of the MLF could only affect head and neck reflexes, but not gait. Gait is also unaffected by pain inputs. Deviation of the tongue occurs because fibers from the hypoglossal nucleus innervate the genioglossus muscle on the ipsilateral side of the tongue. This muscle normally protrudes the tongue toward the contralateral side. Therefore, if one side is weak, the tongue will deviate toward the side ipsilateral to the lesion when protruded.

291. The answer is b. (*Afifi, pp 99-101. Nolte, pp 272-274, 319-320. Siegel and Sapru, p 176.*) There are similarities between this case and the previous one described in Questions 289 and 290. However, in this case, there were no dysfunctions reported concerning his ability to move his tongue and there were no speech deficits. This indicates that the lesion could not have been at the level of the caudal ventromedial medulla, (especially since the medial lemniscus is not present at this level and the dorsal columns are located in a dorsal position), but rather at a somewhat more rostral level of the ventromedial medulla, which includes the pyramidal tract and medial lemniscus, but not the hypoglossal nucleus and nerve. The other choices do not include pyramids or medial lemniscus.

292. The answer is e. *(Afifi, pp 87-88, 99-101, 319-320. Nolte, p 319. Siegel and Sapru, p 176.)* A lesion of the left ventromedial medulla would produce a disorder referred to as "alternating hypoglossal hemiplegia" in which there is damage to the hypoglossal nerve as it is about to exit the brainstem and to the pyramidal tract. Damage to the hypoglossal nerve causes a deviation of the tongue to the side of the lesion when it is protruded and a contralateral UMN paralysis of the limbs because these descending corticospinal fibers cross at the medulla-spinal cord border. The other choices do not include structures that were affected in this case. The choice involving the right ventromedial medulla is incorrect because the tongue deviated to the left, not the right side and the paralysis was on the right side of the body, not the left.

293. The answer is d. *(Afifi, pp 98-101. Nolte, pp 298-300, 317-318. Siegel and Sapru, p 176.)* The patient's speech was dysarthric (slurred) because the lesion affected the nucleus ambiguus that gives rise to the somatomotor components of cranial nerves IX and X, which innervate the laryngeal and pharyngeal muscles essential for speech. Since this deficit is purely a motor problem, rather than an effect that is manifested by a lesion of higher regions in the cortex (which mediate the structure and function of speech), the grammar, content, and meaning of his speech remained intact.

294 and 295. The answers are 294-c and 295-e. *(Adams, pp 240, 1181-1182. Afifi, pp 114-115. Siegel and Sapru, pp 235-237.)* This is an example of Bell palsy, or damage to the facial nerve lesion distal to its nucleus in the pons. The motor weakness is an LMN because of the involvement of the upper one-third of the face (this has bilateral innervation within the CNS). The loss of taste on the anterior two-thirds of the tongue and the hyperacusis (sensitivity to noise) point to damage that is distal to the brainstem because these are functions whose nerves join the facial nerve distal to its exit from the pons. This type of palsy may be caused by a virus and is more common among people with diabetes. This type of facial paralysis, involving the upper one-third of the facial muscles, is characteristic of an LMN facial nerve lesion. Since there is bilateral innervation within the CNS, from the precentral gyrus, bilaterally, until they synapse at the facial nerve nucleus, all UMN facial weakness spares the forehead. Since there is motor weakness of the face and since the chorda tympani nerve (which subserves taste) joins the facial nerve, it is likely that the lesion exists proximal to where the chorda tympani joins the facial nerve.

296. The answer is e. *(Adams, pp 240, 1181-1182. Afifi, pp 114-115. Siegel and Sapru, pp 235-237.)* As noted in the explanation to the previous questions (Questions 294-295), taste impulses from the anterior two-thirds of the tongue is transmitted over the chorda tympani nerve. The lesion must have involved the proximal aspect of this nerve. If the lesion occurred distal to the chorda tympani nerve, taste would have been spared. The glossopharyngeal nerve mediates, in part, taste from the posterior third of the tongue. The trigeminal ganglion mediates somatosensory sensation from the face, but does not mediate taste impulses. A lesion in the lingual nerve (a branch of the trigeminal) would result in a loss of taste as well, but would also result in a loss of sensation to the face, not motor weakness. A lesion of the solitary nucleus would have produced only loss of taste but no loss of motor functions, which was present in this case.

297. The answer is e. *(Adams, pp 240, 1181-1182. Afifi, pp 114-115. Siegel and Sapru, pp 235-237.)* The assault on the face caused damage to the facial nerve, which contains a branch that supplies the stapedius muscle. Contraction of this muscle normally serves as a mechanism for dampening the motion of the ossicles, thus reducing amount of stimulation reaching the organ of Corti. If this muscle is paralyzed, hyperacusis or increased acuity as well as hypersensitivity to low tones will occur.

298. The answer is c. *(Adams, pp 240, 1181-1182. Afifi, pp 114-116. Siegel and Sapru, pp 235-237.)* The lesion in this case had to be within the brainstem, namely affected the cranial nerves VI and VII. The most likely locus of such a lesion is the region of the nucleus of cranial nerve VI and surrounding region, which includes the fibers of cranial nerve VII, which is just dorsal to the nucleus before it descends in a ventrolateral trajectory prior to its exit from the brainstem. Other choices involving peripheral damage to cranial nerve VII would also affect sensory components of cranial nerve VII, which indeed was not present in this case. Cranial nerve V was not involved in this case.

299 and 300. The answers are 299-d and 300-c. *(Adams, pp 305-306. Afifi, pp 152-153. Siegel and Sapru, p 190.)* This is an example of the locked-in syndrome, or pseudocoma, caused by an infarction of the basilar pons. Because the tracts mediating movement of the limbs and face run through this region, the patient is unable to move the face, as well as both arms and legs. Consciousness and eye movements are preserved. The pontine basilar pons is supplied mainly by the basilar artery. Complete occlusion of this artery causes deficits on both sides, since this artery supplies both sides of the pons. Sensory loss, including loss of proprioception (feeling the movement of a limb), also occurs as a result of damage to the medial lemniscus bilaterally. This tract contains fibers from the dorsal columns and also runs through the pontine tegmentum. Patients with the locked-in syndrome are often mistaken for comatose patients due to their inability to move or speak. If the lesion spares the reticular formation, an area mediating consciousness in the pons, the patient will remain alert.

301. The answer is a. *(Adams, pp 305-306. Afifi, pp 152-153. Siegel and Sapru, p 190.)* Basilar artery occlusion causes damage to the basilar pons, where the corticospinal and corticobulbar tracts run. These tracts contain motor fibers mediating movement of the limb and face, respectively. This results in complete paralysis to both sides of the body and the face. None of the tracts in the other choices mediate conscious movement.

302. The answer is c. *(Siegel and Sapru, p 390.)* The case described in this question is referred to as a caudal tegmental pontine syndrome since it affects structures located in the caudal aspect of the pontine tegmentum. The key structures affected in this syndrome include the nucleus of cranial nerve VI (regulating lateral gaze), fibers of cranial nerve VII (regulating facial expression), and descending hypothalamic fibers (regulating sympathetic functions). Other choices are clearly incorrect since lesions of the medulla, rostral pons, or midbrain would not affect lateral gaze or facial expression.

303. The answer is d. *(Siegel and Sapru, pp 190, 502-503.)* Damage to the paramedian branches of the basilar artery would affect the corticospinal tracts on one side of the brainstem, thus causing paralysis of the contralateral limbs. The distribution of this artery is such that it would also affect both sensory and motor components of cranial nerve V, thus causing loss of ipsilateral facial sensation and the ability to chew. The other choices include arteries that would either not affect the corticospinal tracts (cerebellar arteries) or would not affect the trigeminal fibers (anterior spinal artery).

304 and 305. The answers are 304-d and 305-a. *(Adams, p 188, 242, 313, 464-465. Afifi, pp 62, 71, 151, 100. Kandel, pp 962-974. Siegel and Sapru, pp 199-200, 242-243, 287.)* The patient's drooping eyelid, small pupil, and lack of sweating on the right side are examples of Horner syndrome. This is caused by the interruption of sympathetic fibers anywhere along their course from the hypothalamus and brainstem to the intermediolateral cell column in the upper thoracic levels of the spinal cord, where neurons, supplying sympathetic innervation to the pupil, the levator palpebrae superioris muscle of the eyelid, and sweat glands of the face, are located. Interruption of this sympathetic innervation will result in the drooping of the upper eyelid (ptosis), pupillary constriction (miosis; due to unopposed action of the parasympathetic innervation of the circular muscles of the iris), and lack of sweating on the face. Parasympathetic or oculomotor damage causes pupillary dilation, rather than constriction. The patient could close his eyes tightly because this function is mediated by the seventh nerve, which is not damaged by this lesion. Preganglionic sympathetic neurons are predominantly cholinergic, and postganglionic sympathetic neurons are predominantly noradrenergic. Horner syndrome may be caused by either a preganglionic or a postganglionic lesion. The location may be determined by the use of eyedrops specifically targeted at a particular neurotransmitter. One cause of interruption of the sympathetic fibers is a tumor of the apex (top portion) of the lung, called a Pancoast tumor. Because the apex of the lung is in close proximity to the spine, a Pancoast tumor may compress the upper thoracic spinal cord where the sympathetic fibers exit from it. Compression of the adjacent spinal nerves between C8 and T2, entering the brachial plexus, also interrupts the nerve supply to the hand and triceps muscle, causing numbness and weakness in these areas. Pancoast tumors do not often cause respiratory symptoms early in their course because they are located far from the mainstem bronchi. Because these tumors have this unique location, the neurological abnormalities often predate the respiratory problems. The neurologist suspected that the patient may have a Pancoast tumor in the lung because of his long history of smoking.

306. The answer is c. *(Siegel and Sapru, pp 190, 500-502.)* The case described in this question was an illustration of Benedikt syndrome.

It involves damage to the medial aspect of the midbrain at the level of the superior colliculus. Thus, the neuronal cell groups and axons damaged include the oculomotor complex, causing an ipsilateral oculomotor paralysis, the red nucleus, and fibers of the superior cerebellar peduncle (which pass to the thalamus), causing the contralateral tremor, and parts of the medial lemniscus, causing some loss of somatosensory functions on the contralateral side of the body.

307. The answer is a. *(Siegel and Sapru, pp 190, 500-502.)* The medial aspect of the rostral half of the midbrain tegmentum is supplied by the posterior cerebral artery. The structures supplied include, in part, the oculomotor complex, red nucleus, axons of the superior cerebellar peduncle, and medial lemniscus. These structures were the ones affected in the case described in this question and damage to this region produces Benedikt syndrome. The middle cerebral artery supplies the forebrain, including the lateral aspect of the hemispheres; the superior cerebellar and basilar arteries supply different aspect of the pons, regions which do not include the structures affected in this case.

308. The answer is a. *(Siegel and Sapru, pp 398-399.)* The neurotransmitter released at endings of preganglionic neurons is acetylcholine. The neurotransmitter released at most postganglionic sympathetic synapses is norepinephrine and at all parasympathetic neurons is acetylcholine. The oculomotor nerve is parasympathetic.

309 and 310. The answers are 309-b and 310-c. *(Afifi, pp 62, 71, 151, 100, 126-127, 132-134, 140-145. Siegel and Sapru, pp 242-244.)* The third cranial nerve (oculomotor) controls four of the six extraocular muscles that move the eye. When this nerve fails to function, the eye remains deviated laterally due to the unopposed action of the other two extraocular muscles. When the eyes no longer move together, patients have double vision because the visual cortex now receives two different images. In addition, fibers originating in the third nerve nucleus innervate the levator palpebrae superioris, a muscle that helps to lift the eyelid. Damage to the optic nerve causes loss of vision, blurred vision, and a central scotoma (blind spot in the center of the visual field). Damage to the cervical sympathetic fibers causes Horner syndrome, consisting of ptosis (drooping of the eyelid), miosis (constriction of the pupil), and anhydrosis (loss of sweating), not eye movement abnormalities. The actions of the superior oblique, the muscle innervated by the trochlear nerve, include intorsion, depression, and abduction. The abducens nerve mediates the lateral rectus muscle, which abducts the eye. The eye is depressed and abducted due to the unopposed actions of the superior oblique and lateral rectus muscles, which together move the eye downward and abduct it (see earlier discussion for the actions of these muscles). The other four muscles are innervated by the oculomotor nerve, which presumably has been damaged. This is an example of Weber syndrome, or a lesion involving the third cranial nerve outflow tract and the corticospinal and corticobulbar tracts in the cerebral peduncles of the midbrain. Weber syndrome may occur as a result of an occlusion of the interpeduncular branches of the posterior cerebral artery (which supply this portion of the midbrain), a tumor pressing on this area, an aneurysm (circumscribed dilation of an artery) of the posterior communicating artery, or a plaque (lesion) related to multiple sclerosis.

311. The answer is c. (*Siegel and Sapru, pp 200, 500-501.*) As described in the explanation to Question 310, the patient presented with a disorder known as Weber syndrome. It involves damage to the oculomotor nerve and cerebral peduncle on one side of the brain stem. In order for these structures to be affected, the lesion has to be located in the ventromedial aspect of the rostral aspect of the midbrain at a level where the oculomotor nerve is about to exit from the brainstem. The damage to the oculomotor nerve produces an oculomotor paralysis with loss of function of both somatomotor and parasympathetic components of the oculomotor complex as well as a contralateral UMN paralysis of the limbs because of damage to the corticospinal tracts.

312. The answer is d. (*Siegel and Sapru, pp 200, 500-501.*) As noted above in the explanation to Question 311, the structures involved in producing Weber syndrome include the oculomotor nerve and cerebral peduncle.

313. The answer is a. (*Siegel and Sapru, pp 200, 500-501.*) This condition is known as a gaze palsy or Parinaud syndrome. It results from damage to the region including the pretectal area and posterior commissure. The large pupil relates to the presumed loss of input from the pretectal area into the Edinger-Westphal component of the oculomotor complex, and the upward gaze paralysis results from loss of input into the somatomotor components of the oculomotor complex from the posterior commissure. The posterior commissure normally plays an important role in integrating vertical gaze, in part, because of its inputs into what is believed to be a vertical gaze center proximal to the oculomotor complex.

314 and 315. The answers are 314-c and 315-d. *(Adams, 230, 233-234. Afifi, pp 132-134. Siegel and Sapru, pp 240-242.)* Damage to the trochlear nerve causes weakness of the superior oblique muscle, resulting in the inability of the orbit to deviate downward when the eye is intorted. To compensate for the vertical double vision, the patient tends to tilt his head to the contralateral side, causing the contralateral eye to intort. The trochlear nerve supplies the superior oblique muscle. The trochlear nerve is the only nerve to decussate peripherally, and also to emerge from the dorsal aspect of the brainstem. In this case, the damaged nerve emerged from the right (contralateral) dorsal midbrain. The action of the superior oblique muscle is to rotate the orbit medially and downward. Because the trochlear nerve is not only the smallest cranial nerve but also has the longest course of any cranial nerve, it is especially vulnerable to trauma. One of the most common causes of trochlear nerve palsy is trauma.

316. The answer is e. *(Siegel and Sapru, pp 244-249.)* A region of the frontal called the frontal eye fields (area 8) projects to the contralateral horizontal gaze center of the pons and thus controls "voluntary" horizontal movement of the eyes. Damage to area 8 or to its output pathway to the horizontal gaze center would prevent one's ability to move the eyes horizontally or to the right (in this case). The other choices are incorrect. The superior colliculus does regulate voluntary control over eye movements although this region does play a role in tracking movements of objects. The occipital cortex plays a role in involuntary movements, not voluntary movements of the eyes. Any cortical projections to the trochlear nucleus would only move the eye downward, not horizontally. Projections to the oculomotor complex would move the eye inward.

317. The answer is c. *(Siegel and Sapru, pp 244-249.)* The right vestibular nuclei project to the right pontine gaze center (and right abducens nucleus) as well as to the left oculomotor nucleus. When such inputs are damaged, the eyes become deviated to the left because cranial nerve outputs to the right lateral rectus and left medial rectus muscles are lost. Thus, the unopposed actions of the right medial rectus and left lateral rectus muscles will cause the eyes to become deviated to the left. The other choices are incorrect. Frontal cortical inputs govern voluntary movement of the eyes, not involuntary movements. As noted above, loss of inputs to the left abducens or right oculomotor complex will cause the eyes to be deviated to the right, not the left, which was the situation in this case.

318. The answer is d. (*Siegel and Sapru, pp 240-249.*) Because the tumor was situated on the dorsal aspect of the midbrain, it affected the trochlear nerve, which is the only nerve to exit from the dorsal aspect of the brainstem. All other cranial nerves exit from the lateral or ventral aspects of the brainstem. As indicated in answer to Questions 314 and 315, the trochlear nerve acts to move downward when it is in a medial position. When this nerve is damaged, the two eyes cannot focus upon the same object upon attempts at downward gaze (such as walking downstairs) and thus the patient experiences double vision. The patient typically attempts to compensate for this deficit by turning his head at an angle to the side so as to avoid the double vision. Horizontal movements are governed by cranial nerves III and VI; accommodation and upward movements of the eye are associated with cranial nerve III. Nystagmus is associated with lesions of the MLF and parts of the cerebellum.

Sensory Systems

Questions

319. A 48-year-old woman receives an ophthalmological examination after complaining about blurred vision. Further examination revealed partial degeneration of the optic tract resulting from an unknown etiology. As a result of this disorder, there was presumed retrograde degeneration of the cell bodies of origin which give rise to the optic tract. Which of the following cells is most likely to show degeneration from this disorder?

a. Bipolar cells
b. Horizontal cells
c. Rods
d. Cones
e. Ganglion cells

320. A 5-year-old boy, who was blind by birth, is administered an extensive series of genetic testing. Following this testing, it is concluded that the boy suffers from a rare genetic disorder in which the receptor directly linking the rod and cone cells with ganglion cells is lacking, causing blindness in this boy. Which of the following cell types is absent in this boy?

a. Bipolar cell
b. Horizontal cell
c. Golgi cell
d. Amacrine cell
e. Optic nerve cell

321. Which of the following best characterizes how cones differ from rods?

a. Cones have a higher sensitivity to light than rods.
b. Cones have more photopigment than rods.
c. Cones have pigments that are sensitive to different parts of the light spectrum while rods lack this pigment.
d. Cones have a lower temporal resolution with a long integration time and slow response relative to rods.
e. Cones have lower acuity and are present in fewer numbers in the fovea than rods.

322. An individual is diagnosed with retinitis pigmentosa. Which of the following is the most likely cause of this disease?

a. Degeneration of area 17 of the cerebral cortex
b. Degeneration of bipolar cells of the retina
c. Degeneration of amacrine cells
d. Degeneration of retinal ganglion cells
e. Degeneration of photoreceptors

323. A 21-year-old male, who previously had normal vision, suddenly becomes blind. A detailed examination and analysis of the patient indicates that he was infected by a virus that selectively attacked and destroyed the same retinal cells that are attacked in felines as determined from experimental studies. In such studies, the cells attacked by the virus are ones that produce action potentials in response to changes in position of selective objects presented to the visual field of a cat. Which of the following retinal cells were destroyed by this virus?

a. Amacrine cells
b. Rods
c. Cones
d. Ganglion cells
e. Horizontal cells

Questions 324 and 325

324. A patient is diagnosed by an optometrist as being nearsighted. To correct this person's defect, which of the following lenses should the doctor recommend be put into his eyeglasses?

a. Cylindrical
b. Concave
c. Convex
d. Neutral
e. Rectangular

325. In the previous question, the corrective lens is applied because of which of the following conditions?

a. Retinal damage.
b. The eyeball is too long.
c. The eyeball is too short.
d. The eyeball is oblong.
e. The lens resists change.

Questions 326 and 327

326. A patient is diagnosed by the same optometrist as being farsighted. To correct this person's defect, which of the following lenses should the doctor recommend be put into his eyeglasses?

a. Cylindrical
b. Concave
c. Convex
d. Neutral
e. Spherical

327. In the previous vignette, the corrective lens is applied because of which of the following conditions?

a. Corneal damage.
b. The eyeball is too long.
c. The eyeball is too short.
d. The eyeball is oblong.
e. The lens resists change.

328. A patient is told that he has astigmatism. To correct this defect, the optometrist prescribes which of the following lenses and for which reason?

a. Cylindrical lens because the cornea or lens is oblong.
b. Concave lens because the eyeball is too long.
c. Convex lens because the lens is too short.
d. Neutral lens because the eyeball is normal but the cornea is too thin.
e. Concave lens because the cornea is opaque.

329. A patient complains of having constant headaches involving the frontal region. Further examination reveals increased intraocular pressure, but at the time of examination there is little evidence of visual deficits. Which of the following is the likely diagnosis?

a. Cataracts
b. A tumor of the visual cortex or lateral geniculate nucleus
c. A tumor at the base of the brain impinging upon the optic chiasm
d. Glaucoma
e. Color blindness

330. A routine eye examination reveals the presence of inflammation limited to the left optic disk, probably due to neuritis of this region. Which of the following is the likely visual deficit resulting from this disorder?

a. Total blindness of the left eye
b. Left homonymous hemianopsia
c. Left heteronymous hemianopsia
d. Left enlargement of the blind spot
e. Left upper quadrantanopia

331. As a result of calcification of the internal carotid artery, which impinges upon the lateral half of the right optic nerve prior to its entrance to the brain, a 68-year-old woman experiences certain visual deficits. Which of the following is the most likely visual deficit?

a. Total blindness of the right eye
b. Right nasal hemianopsia
c. Right homonymous hemianopsia
d. Right bitemporal hemianopsia
e. Right upper homonymous quadrantanopia

332. It was discovered that a 29-year-old male had a tumor pressing on the base of the brain, where it impinged upon the optic chiasm. His field of vision was seriously affected. Which of the following defects was present in this individual?

a. Total blindness of both eyes
b. Bitemporal hemianopsia
c. Right homonymous hemianopsia
d. Binasal hemianopsia
e. Right lower homonymous quadrantanopia

333. A routine magnetic resonance imaging (MRI) revealed the presence of a tumor situated in the left optic tract proximal to the lateral geniculate nucleus. The patient complained of having a reduction in his field of vision. Which of the following best characterizes the likely visual deficit?

a. Total blindness of the left eye
b. Bitemporal hemianopsia
c. Right homonymous hemianopsia
d. Left homonymous hemianopsia
e. Left homonymous quadrantanopia

334. A 70-year-old male was admitted to the emergency room and a subsequent MRI revealed the presence of a tumor involving parts of the left temporal lobe. In addition to certain short-term memory deficits, visual deficits were noted as well. Which of the following visual deficits would most likely result from this tumor?

a. Left homonymous hemianopsia
b. Right homonymous hemianopsia
c. Left upper quadrantanopia
d. Right upper quadrantanopia
e. Left lower quadrantanopia

335. A 55-year-old woman complained of headaches and was subsequently diagnosed as having a tumor localized to the left parietal lobe. In addition to a variety of sensory deficits, further examination also revealed a reduction in her visual fields. Which of the following visual deficits would most likely result from this tumor?

a. Left homonymous hemianopsia
b. Right homonymous hemianopsia
c. Left upper quadrantanopia
d. Right upper quadrantanopia
e. Right lower quadrantanopia

336. A 14-year-old boy is involved in a serious sledding accident which affects sensation in his legs. As a result of the accident, he is unable to identify and recognize the position of his legs when he attempts to walk and thus displays an ataxic gait. Which of the following receptors are ineffective in providing the conscious proprioception?

a. Meissner corpuscles
b. Free nerve endings
c. Merkel receptors
d. Joint capsules
e. Pacinian corpuscles

337. A 49-year-old female complains about loss of accuracy in identifying and localizing sensation, in particular, conscious proprioception, tactile sensation, and pressure, from the appropriate sites along her right hand and leg. An MRI indicated the presence of a tumor in the region of the right dorsal columns at the level of the spinal cord-medulla border. The presence of the tumor could account for both loss of sensation and for loss of accuracy in identifying the sites on the limbs associated with the respective sensation because of a general property of inhibition associated with dorsal column functions. Which one or more of the following types of inhibition have been identified within the dorsal column nuclei that are disrupted by the tumor?

a. Feed-forward inhibition utilizing local interneurons only
b. Feedback inhibition utilizing local interneurons only
c. Descending inhibition from fibers arising in the cerebral cortex only
d. Feed-forward, feedback, and descending inhibition
e. Feed-forward and descending inhibition only

338. A 57-year-old male was referred to a neurologist after he complained about difficulties in determining the directionality and orientation of movement of stimuli along his right arm. An MRI was taken of the patient and a CNS tumor was noted. Where in the regions listed below is the tumor most likely to be present?

a. Left spinal cord
b. Medial half of thalamus
c. Ventral pons
d. Internal capsule
e. Cerebral cortex

339. A patient had been seeing a physician for almost a year because she complained of pain in her shoulder. After extensive analysis, the physician determined that the pain in her shoulder reflected referred pain that arose from another source. In this case, which of the following best explains the basis for the referred pain?

a. Inhibitory fibers that block transmission of pain impulses along a given pathway and then transfer the impulses to a different pathway associated with a different part of the body
b. A massive discharge along a given pathway that results in the activation of a separate pathway because of the principle of divergence
c. A convergence of primary afferent fibers from a given region onto second-order neurons that normally receive primary afferents from a different body part
d. The disruption of lateral spinothalamic fibers
e. The blockade of substance P from primary afferent terminals

340. A car door was accidentally closed on the hand of a teenage boy. As a result, he experienced significant pain that persisted for a while. In terms of the neurochemical events that took place at the afferent terminals of the first-order pathway that conveyed the pain sensation to the spinal cord, which of the following transmitters would be released onto dorsal horn neurons of the spinal cord from these primary afferent fibers?

a. Enkephalins alone
b. Glutamate alone
c. Substance P alone
d. Glutamate and substance P
e. Enkephalins, substance P, and glutamate

341. A patient is experiencing severe pain. If it were possible to place an electrode into the gray matter around the cerebral aqueduct of the midbrain and stimulate the cells in this region, it would induce an analgesic response. Which of the following best explains such an effect?

a. Activation of a pathway that ascends directly to the cortex and mediates analgesia
b. A descending pathway that blocks nociceptive inputs at the level of the dorsal horn
c. Activation of local interneurons that block ascending nociceptive signals at the level of the midbrain
d. Activation of an ascending inhibitory pathway that projects to the ventral posterolateral nucleus of the thalamus
e. Activation of cholinergic neurons in the basal forebrain

342. Concerning the analgesic effects mediated by stimulation of the periaqueductal gray indicated in the patient above, which of the following provides the best explanation of the neural substrate(s) underlying this phenomenon?

a. Fibers from the periaqueductal gray that synapse directly on dorsal horn cells
b. Fibers from the periaqueductal gray that synapse on neurons of the nucleus raphe magnus that then synapse on dorsal horn cells
c. Fibers from the periaqueductal gray that synapse on inferior olivary neurons that then synapse on dorsal horn cells
d. Hypothalamic fibers that synapse on neurons of the nucleus solitarius that then synapse on neurons of the dorsal horn
e. Hypothalamic fibers that synapse directly on dorsal horn neurons

343. A neuron that responds with an *on-center* and *off-surround* to generate contrast within the receptive field can be identified in which of the following cells?

a. Retina (ganglion cell)
b. Lateral geniculate nucleus
c. Retina (ganglion cell) and lateral geniculate nucleus
d. Layer IV of the primary visual cortex (area 17)
e. Retina (ganglion cell), lateral geniculate nucleus, and area 18

344. A 34-year-old female began to experience vision difficulties and received an ophthalmological examination. The patient was later seen by a neurologist and was diagnosed with demyelinating disease affecting the optic nerve and optic tracts. As a result of the demyelinating disease, there was degeneration of the optic tracts. Which of the following structures were devoid of inputs from the optic tracts?

a. The lateral geniculate nucleus only
b. The lateral geniculate nucleus and the pretectal area
c. The lateral geniculate nucleus, the pretectal area, and the superior colliculus
d. The lateral geniculate nucleus, the pretectal area, the superior colliculus, and the suprachiasmatic nucleus
e. The lateral geniculate nucleus, the pretectal area, the superior colliculus, the suprachiasmatic nucleus, and the nuclei of cranial nerves III and IV

345. An 18-year-old male is admitted to the emergency room after experiencing extreme pain following ingestion of a "homemade" drug of abuse. It is determined that this drug of abuse blocked the neurotransmitter functions in the dorsal horn of the spinal cord that normally inhibit pain transmission. Which of the following best characterizes the anatomical substrate and neurochemical mechanism underlying this inhibitory mechanism?

a. Opioidergic, and only contact dendrites of postsynaptic neurons that contain opiate receptors
b. Opioidergic, and only contact opiate receptors located presynaptically on nociceptive terminals
c. Opioidergic, and contact both dendrites of postsynaptic neurons and presynaptic terminals, both of which contain opiate receptors
d. Serotonergic, and only contact dendrites of postsynaptic neurons that contain 5-HT
e. Cholinergic, and contact dendrites of both postsynaptic neurons and presynaptic terminals, both of which contain muscarinic receptors

346. An individual lost his sense of smell. After receiving a medical examination, it was determined that the reason for his loss of sensation was due to degeneration of primary afferent fibers that enter the olfactory glomerulus. In a healthy individual, upon which of the following structures do these primary afferent fibers terminate?

a. Granule cell dendrites forming axodendritic synapses
b. Granule cell axon terminals forming axoaxonic synapses
c. Mitral cell dendrites forming axodendritic synapses
d. Mitral cell axon terminals forming axoaxonic synapses
e. Axon terminals of fibers arising from the olfactory tubercle, forming axoaxonic synapses

347. When a cone is hyperpolarized by light, which of the following occurs?

a. The on-center bipolar cell is excited and the off-center bipolar cell is inhibited.
b. The on center bipolar cell will inhibit the ganglion cell with which it makes synaptic contact.
c. The ganglion cell that receives its input from an off-center bipolar cell will discharge because the bipolar cell is excited during the presence of the stimulus.
d. An on-center bipolar cell excites a neighboring ganglion cell that receives its input from an off-center bipolar cell.
e. A transmitter released from a cone cell has the same effect upon all processes with which it synapses.

348. A middle-aged male is involved in an automobile accident that causes brain damage affecting a region of the cerebral cortex, resulting in loss of the conscious perception of smell. Which of the following regions of the cortex is most likely affected?

a. Temporal neocortex
b. Posterior parietal lobule
c. Cingulate gyrus
d. Prefrontal cortex
e. Precentral gyrus

349. An 8-year-old girl was seen by an ophthalmologist and later by a neurologist because she had difficulty in seeing objects clearly. Much of what she sees appears quite blurred. The neurological examination was not particularly revealing but a genetic test indicated that she is suffering from a rare (genetic) disorder in which one of the retinal cell types essential for clarity of vision is missing. A clue to her disorder was revealed after a genetic strain of an animal was developed which was also lacking this cell type. It was further discovered that this cell type is responsible for the presence of lateral inhibition within the retina, and a similar visual deficit was noted in this animal. Which of the following cell types is likely lacking in this patient?

a. Rod cells
b. Cone cells
c. Bipolar cells
d. Ganglion cells
e. Horizontal cells

350. An experiment was performed by a physiologist who was interested in identifying a specific kind of neuron within the visual cortex. The type of neuron sought by the investigator was one that responds to an image in a specific position, has discrete excitatory and inhibitory zones, and is associated with a specific axis of orientation. Which of the following cells would respond to such an image?

a. M cells of the lateral geniculate nucleus
b. P cells of the lateral geniculate nucleus
c. Simple cells of the visual cortex
d. Complex cells of the visual cortex
e. Hypercomplex cells of the visual cortex

351. A 45-year-old female who has difficulty in sensing different odors is examined by her primary physician and then by a neurologist. An MRI scan is negative and the neurologist concludes that the loss of the sense of smell is due to damage to the olfactory receptor mechanism which initially responds to an olfactory stimulus. Which part of the olfactory receptor mechanism that normally responds to an olfactory stimulus is presently unresponsive to such a stimulus?

a. Mitral cell
b. Granule cell
c. Sustentacular cell
d. Basal cell
e. Olfactory cilia

352. A 47-year-old male who had been working in a factory for many years where a strong chemical odor was present finds it now difficult to discriminate different types of odorants. Following a neurological examination, it is concluded that the neural basis of olfactory discrimination is significantly impaired. Which of the following neural properties underlying the patient's ability to discriminate odorants is now disrupted?

a. Specific activation of different cell groups within the amygdala
b. Specific activation of different groups of olfactory glomeruli that are spatially organized and segregated within the olfactory bulb
c. Specific activation of different groups of cells within the olfactory tubercle
d. Temporal summation of olfactory signals in the anterior olfactory nucleus
e. Temporal summation of olfactory signals in the mediodorsal thalamic nucleus

353. A 47-year-old male accidentally inhales a toxic substance which causes him to lose his sense of smell and produces selective damage to his olfactory bulb. Assuming that the toxic substance caused neuronal damage to the principal efferent pathway of the olfactory bulb, which of the following cell types that gives rise to this pathway was damaged?

a. Granule cells
b. Golgi cells
c. Receptor cells
d. Mitral cells
e. Periglomerular cells

354. A patient suffers damage to the olfactory bulb and its output pathways, resulting in the loss of smell. Which of the following combinations of structures listed below is deprived of this direct (monosynaptic) olfactory input?

a. Hypothalamus and prefrontal cortex
b. Amygdala and pyriform cortex
c. Hippocampus and amygdala
d. Prefrontal cortex and medial thalamus
e. Septal area and prefrontal cortex

355. A person is examined by a neurologist after complaining that he keeps having a sensation of smell that he could not clearly define. A subsequent MRI reveals the presence of a brain tumor and that the patient is experiencing uncinate hallucinations. The tumor is most likely situated in which of the following regions?

a. Anterior temporal lobe
b. Medial dorsal thalamic nucleus
c. Parietal cortex
d. Hypothalamus
e. Midbrain periaqueductal gray

356. A 53-year-old male was diagnosed with a tumor localized to the thalamus that disrupted most but not all types of sensations. Which of the sensations listed below would still function despite of the presence of the tumor?

a. Conscious proprioception
b. Taste
c. Olfaction
d. Vision
e. Audition

Sensory Systems

Answers

319. The answer is e. (*Kandel, pp 516-520. Siegel and Sapru, pp 272-278.*) The output of the retina is mediated by the ganglion cells. Ganglion cells receive inputs from photoreceptor and bipolar cells. In turn, ganglion cells give rise to optic nerve fibers, which project through the optic chiasm and optic tracts to the lateral geniculate nucleus of the thalamus. Other cells mentioned in this question only produce local connections within the retina.

320. The answer is a. (*Kandel, pp 514-520. Siegel and Sapru, pp 272-278.*) The bipolar cell receives inputs from the receptor cells (ie, rods and cones). The response of the bipolar cell to the receptor cell input is then mediated to the ganglion cell. (See the discussion that follows for further consideration of the physiology of the retina.) Horizontal and amacrine cells connect neighboring receptor or bipolar cells, Golgi cells are not present in the retina, and optic nerve cells project out of the retina as indicated earlier.

321. The answer is c. (*Kandel, pp 508-515. Siegel and Sapru, pp 272-274.*) Cones differ from rods in that cone cells contain pigments that are sensitive to different parts of the light spectrum, while rod cells are achromatic. The other choices are incorrect: rods have a greater sensitivity to light than cones and have more photopigment than cones. Cones also have a higher temporal resolution with a shorter integration time and more rapid response than rods. Cones also have greater acuity and are present in greater quantities in the fovea than rods.

322. The answer is e. (*Adams, pp 211, 950. Purves, p 265.*) In one form of retinitis pigmentosa, there is a genetic defect with respect to rhodopsin. The result of this defect is the production of defective opsin. As a consequence, rod cells are affected, leading to a reduced response to light. Consequently, there is degeneration of photoreceptors which die by apoptosis. At a later time, cone cells also appear to degenerate. Other components of the retina, such as retina/ganglion cells, and central nervous system (CNS) neurons, such as those located in area 17, are not directly affected and vision is not totally lost.

323. The answer is d. (*Kandel, pp 512-521. Siegel and Sapru, pp 272-278.*) The only cell in the retina that is capable of producing an action potential is the ganglion cell. As indicated earlier, the ganglion cell gives rise to optic nerve fibers, which terminate as optic tract fibers in the lateral geniculate nucleus. As a result of action potentials generated in the ganglion cells, volleys of impulses are transmitted over these fibers, resulting in the appropriate responses in the neurons of the lateral geniculate nucleus. Therefore, the patient became blind of damage to the ganglion cells whose axons form the optic nerve and optic tract, thus depriving the lateral geniculate nucleus and visual cortex from receiving visual inputs.

324 and 325. The answers are 324-b, 325-b. (*Purves, pp 254-257. Siegel and Sapru, pp 285-286.*) To correct for myopia, a person is prescribed a concave (or flat) lens, because objects focus in front of the retina. The concave lens helps to refocus the object onto the retina. The reason that the focus of the object is in front of the retina is that the eyeball is too long.

326 and 327. The answers are 326-c, 327-c. (*Kingsley, pp 436-439. Purves, pp 254-257. Siegel and Sapru, pp 285-286.*) To correct for farsightedness, a person is prescribed a convex lens, because objects focus behind the retina. The convex lens helps to refocus the object onto the retina. The reason that the focus of the object is behind the retina is because the eyeball is too short.

328. The answer is a. (*Kingsley, pp 436-439. Purves, pp 254-257. Siegel and Sapru, p 286.*) In astigmatism, the shapes of the cornea and possibly the lens become oblong, resulting in differences in the curvature of the lens along the long and short axes. Thus, astigmatism is corrected with a cylindrical lens.

329. The answer is d. (*Ropper, pp 226-228.*) Glaucoma is a condition of elevated intraocular pressure caused (perhaps by infection) when debris accumulates in the spaces that lead to Schlemm canal and is occasionally preceded by pupillary dilatation. If not treated, it can rapidly lead to blindness because the pressure can block conduction along the optic nerve. In addition, glaucoma can also be associated with frontal headaches; the diagnosis can be identified by determining the intraocular pressure.

330. The answer is d. (*Aminoff, pp 131-138, 144-147.*) A neuritis involving the optic disk would affect the size of the visual field loss around the optic disk, which corresponds to the blind spot. In general, this kind of neuritis would expand somewhat the size of the blind spot but would cause no further visual loss.

331. The answer is b. (*Aminoff, pp 131-138, 144-147.*) Calcification of the internal carotid artery could serve to disrupt nerve fibers proximal to it. One such group of fibers includes parts of the optic nerve. In this case, the component of the right optic nerve affected includes the lateral aspect, or those fibers that mediate vision associated with the nasal visual field of the right eye. If the damage were more extensive and if it involved the entire nerve, then total blindness of the right eye would have occurred.

332. The answer is b. (*Siegel and Sapru, p 288. Aminoff, pp 131-138, 144-147.*) A tumor pressing on the optic chiasm will disrupt the optic nerve (and tract) fibers that cross to the opposite side. These fibers mediate vision associated with fibers arising from the nasal retina of each eye. Since the nasal retina of each eye is associated with the temporal visual field for each eye, the visual loss is referred to as a *bitemporal hemianopsia*.

333. The answer is c. (*Siegel and Sapru, p 288. Aminoff, pp 131-138, 144-147.*) Disruption of optic tract fibers destined for the lateral geniculate nucleus will cause a homonymous hemianopsia because it affects fibers arising from the temporal retina of the ipsilateral side and from the nasal retina of the contralateral side. Since the damage occurred in the left optic tract, the loss of vision is reflected on the right visual field (ie, the left temporal retina is associated with the nasal [or right] visual field of the left eye, and the right nasal retina is associated with the temporal [or right] visual field of the right eye). Therefore, such a lesion would result in a right homonymous hemianopsia.

334. The answer is d. (*Siegel and Sapru, pp 288-289. Aminoff, pp 131-138, 144-147.*) From the lateral geniculate nucleus, there are two trajectories that the fiber pathways take en route to the visual cortex. One pathway passes dorsally through the parietal lobe and terminates in the upper bank of the calcarine fissure in the ipsilateral primary visual cortex. The second pathway takes a more circuitous (ventral) route—called the *Meyer-Archambault loop*—through the temporal lobe and terminates in the lower bank of the calcarine fissure in the ipsilateral primary visual cortex. The lower bank of the calcarine fissure is associated with the upper visual quadrants of the contralateral visual fields for both eyes, while the upper bank of the calcarine fissure is associated with the lower quadrants of the contralateral visual fields for both eyes. Thus, if there is a lesion of the left temporal lobe affecting the Meyer-Archambault loop, then the right upper quadrant for each eye will be affected. This deficit is referred to as a *right upper quadrantanopia*.

335. The answer is e. (*Siegel and Sapru, pp 288-289. Aminoff, pp 131-138, 144-147.*) The reasoning underlying the answer to this question is exactly as presented in the explanation of the answer to Question 334. In brief, fibers from the left lateral geniculate destined for the upper bank of the calcarine fissure will mediate visual impulses associated with lower quadrants of the right visual fields for both eyes. This deficit is referred to as a *right lower quadrantanopia*.

336. The answer is d. (*Nolte, pp 206-224. Siegel and Sapru, pp 257-258.*) Meissner corpuscles, Merkel receptors, and pacinian corpuscles respond to tactile, pressure, or possibly vibratory stimuli, while free nerve endings are associated with nociceptive stimuli. Joint capsules respond to movement of the limb, and the axons of these receptors contribute to the dorsal column–medial lemniscal system mediating the conscious perception of movement.

337. The answer is d. (*Kandel, pp 433-440, 451-457.*) To generate an excitatory focus with an inhibitory surround, three types of inhibition are present in the dorsal column nuclei. First-order neurons ascending in the dorsal columns make synaptic contact with different cells in the dorsal column nuclei and excite those cells. One such cell may be an inhibitory interneuron that makes synaptic contact with a neighboring dorsal column nuclear cell, thus inhibiting that cell (ie, feed-forward inhibition). In addition, the dorsal column cell that is excited by the first-order neuron may make synaptic contact with another inhibitory interneuron (in addition to its classical ascending projection to the ventral posterolateral nucleus of the thalamus). This inhibitory interneuron makes synaptic contact with an adjacent dorsal column cell and inhibits that cell (ie, feedback inhibition). Finally, a descending fiber from the postcentral gyrus can make synaptic contact with inhibitory interneurons that inhibit dorsal column cells (descending inhibition). The figure illustrates feedback, feed-forward, and descending inhibition. Inhibitory neurons are depicted in black. These types of inhibition are all disrupted by the presence of a tumor.

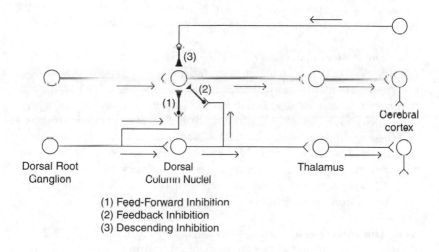

(1) **Feed-Forward Inhibition**
(2) **Feedback Inhibition**
(3) **Descending Inhibition**

338. The answer is e. (*Kandel, pp 456-468.*) As a general rule, neurons that are situated in the cortex in association with any of the sensory systems take on a much higher level of complexity than neurons that are situated at lower levels of the relay network. In the case of the somatosensory system, direction-sensitive cells in the somatosensory cortex will respond to one direction of movement of a stimulus along the receptive field and not to another direction. Orientation-sensitive neurons respond best to movement along one axis of the receptive field. This is not true of neurons that are situated in lower levels of the somatosensory pathway. Thus, a tumor or lesion of this region of cortex is likely to disrupt the neuronal process essential for such discriminations to be made.

339. The answer is c. (*Kandel, pp 472-485. Siegel and Sapru, p 265.*) Referred pain is a phenomenon in which pain impulses, arising from primary afferent fibers from one part of the body (such as from deep visceral structures), terminate on dorsal horn projection neurons that normally receive cutaneous afferents from a different part of the body (such as the arm). In this situation, a person who is suffering a heart attack experiences pain that appears to be coming from the arm. It is the convergence of these distinctly different inputs onto the same projection neurons that provides the basis for this phenomenon. None of the other possible mechanisms listed in this question have an anatomic or physiological basis.

340. The answer is d. (*Kandel, pp 472-485. Siegel and Sapru, pp 263-264.*) Primary nociceptive afferent fibers would have to release an excitatory transmitter in order for normal transmission to take place. Two excitatory transmitters have been identified in association with different classes of primary nociceptive afferents: (1) substance P and (2) excitatory amino acids. The best candidate as an excitatory amino acid is glutamate. Since enkephalins have been shown to be inhibitory transmitters in the pain system, they are not likely to be released from the primary afferents. Instead, other CNS neurons impinge upon the primary afferents, and enkephalins are released from those neurons.

341. The answer is b. (*Kandel, pp 472-485. Siegel and Sapru, pp 262-264.*) Perhaps one of the most important discoveries in pain research made over the past 25 years is that of a descending pathway that originates in the midbrain periaqueductal gray and makes synaptic contacts in the medulla. From the medulla, this pathway descends to the dorsal horn, where these fibers provide the anatomic substrate for suppression of pain inputs that enter the spinal cord from the periphery. There are no known inputs to the cortex that directly produce analgesia. The mechanism governing analgesia appears to operate at lower brain stem and spinal cord levels. The ascending fibers for transmission of pain impulses reach thalamic nuclei directly, and, thus, local interneurons within the midbrain would not be able to interfere with such transmission. The pathway to the ventral posterolateral nucleus of the thalamus is an excitatory one and is not known to have any inhibitory properties. Cholinergic neurons in the basal forebrain have been implicated in memory functions and are not known to have any role in the regulation of pain sensation.

342. The answer is b. (*Kandel, pp 485-487. Siegel and Sapru, pp 262-264.*) The descending pathway for central inhibition of nociception involves the following: fibers that originate in the midbrain periaqueductal gray matter project caudally to the level of the nucleus raphe magnus, upon whose neurons they synapse. Fibers from the nucleus raphe magnus then project further caudally, where they synapse in the dorsal horn of the spinal cord.

343. The answer is c. (*Kandel, pp 512-533. Siegel and Sapru, pp 274-278.*) Both retina ganglion cells and lateral geniculate neurons exhibit an on-center and off-surround with respect to objects in the receptive field. Cells in area 18 of the visual cortex are not known to possess these characteristics. Cells in layer IV of the primary visual cortex do not have circular receptive fields. Instead, these cells respond to such stimuli as lines and bars.

344. The answer is d. (*Afifi, pp 309-315. Siegel and Sapru, pp 281-284.*) Fibers of the optic tract synapse in a number of regions associated with the processing of visual information or visual reflex activity. These include the lateral geniculate nuclei (part of the classical visual pathway for relaying visual information to the visual cortex), the pretectal area (for elicitation of the pupillary light reflex and reflex movements of the eyes), the superior colliculus (for bilateral control of rapid eye movements), and the suprachiasmatic nucleus (which relates to the control of circadian rhythms). There are no known monosynaptic projections from the retina to the nuclei of cranial nerves III and IV.

345. The answer is c. (*Kandel, pp 185-187. Siegel and Sapru, pp 263-264.*) Evidence indicates that within the dorsal horn of the spinal cord, descending pain-inhibitory fibers from the lower brain stem (serotonergic and noradrenergic fibers) synapse upon interneurons that are enkephalinergic. These enkephalinergic neurons then synapse upon both presynaptic terminals of primary pain-afferent fibers and the dendrites of dorsal horn projection (postsynaptic) neurons; which also receive inputs from the primary nociceptive afferent fibers. In this arrangement, by acting upon these neuronal processes, the descending fibers from the lower brain stem ultimately inhibit pain impulses that enter the substantia gelatinosa of the dorsal horn of the spinal cord.

346. The answer is c. (*Kandel, pp 629-632. Nolte, pp 330-339. Siegel and Sapru, pp 312-315.*) The olfactory receptor and its primary afferent fiber terminate upon dendrites of mitral cells. This relationship is of importance because it is the axon of the mitral cell that projects out of the olfactory bulb (forming the major component of the lateral olfactory stria). The granule cell processes make synaptic contact with dendrites of mitral cells, forming dendrodendritic synapses, but are not known to make synaptic contact with primary afferent terminals. Cells arising in the olfactory tubercle are not known to project to the olfactory bulb. Instead, projections of cells situated in the olfactory tubercle contribute fibers to the medial forebrain bundle and stria medullaris.

347. The answer is a. (*Kandel, pp 510-521. Siegel and Sapru, pp 274-278.*) When a cone is hyperpolarized by light, there is a reduction in the release of transmitter substance (glutamate). This reduced amount of transmitter results in excitation of the on-center bipolar cell and inhibition of the off-center bipolar cell (presumably because the two types of bipolar cells contain different postsynaptic receptors). Since bipolar cells excite the ganglion cells, an off-center bipolar cell will be inhibited when light is present and, thus, will be unable to excite the ganglion cell to which it is connected. On-center bipolar cells are excited when light is present and so are the ganglion cells to which they are connected. In addition, on-center bipolar cells inhibit ganglion cells that receive their primary input from off-center bipolar cells. This serves to increase the likelihood that these ganglion cells will remain inhibited when the light stimulus is present. A cone cell may make synaptic contact with two types of bipolar cells (on-center or off-center). Because they possess different postsynaptic receptor mechanisms, the two types of bipolar cells will respond differently to input from cones.

348. The answer is d. (*Afifi, pp 305-307. Kandel, p 633.*) Experimental evidence indicates the prefrontal cortex is a key region for the conscious perception of smell. This conclusion is based upon two observations. First, the prefrontal cortex receives major inputs from the olfactory bulb by the following routes: olfactory bulb to pyriform cortex to prefrontal cortex, or olfactory bulb to pyriform cortex (and olfactory tubercle) to mediodorsal thalamic nucleus to prefrontal cortex. Second, lesions of the prefrontal cortex result in a failure to discriminate odors. Olfactory functions are not known to be associated with any of the other choices. Instead, the primary auditory receiving area is located in the auditory cortex, the posterior parietal lobule is concerned with such processes as the programming mechanisms associated with complex motor tasks, the cingulate gyrus has been associated with such functions as spatial learning and the modulation of autonomic and emotional processes, and the precentral gyrus contains the primary motor area.

349. The answer is e. (*Kandel, pp 510-521.*) Lateral inhibition within the retina is generated most effectively by the horizontal cells. A horizontal cell receives inputs from a given receptor cell and, when activated, inhibits adjacent receptor cells. This mechanism is a primary basis for the establishment of form vision, and without the horizontal cell, form vision would be poor if present at all. It is possible for a given cone cell to differentially affect two neighboring bipolar cells and for an on-center bipolar cell to hyperpolarize an adjacent off-center ganglion cell. However, the primary flow of information through these neuronal elements is in the plane of orientation that most directly connects the receptor cell to the ganglion cell through a bipolar cell. Therefore, the contribution of these elements to lateral inhibition is relatively minimal (if at all) in comparison to the effects generated by horizontal cells. The ganglion cell is not known to play any role in lateral inhibition.

350. The answer is c. (*Kandel, pp 523-543. Siegel and Sapru, pp 274-278.*) Cells in the lateral geniculate nucleus respond very much like ganglion cells in the retina because of the point-to-point projection pathway from the retina to the lateral geniculate. Accordingly, lateral geniculate cells have small concentric receptive fields that are either on-center or off-center in which the cells respond best to small spots of light that are in the center of the receptive field. On the other hand, cells in the visual cortex display a much greater complexity in their responses to images in the visual field. Instead of responding to small spots of light, they respond to lines and borders in the different areas of the visual field. In particular, the simple cell responds as a function of the retinal position in which the line-stimulus is located, as well as its orientation (eg, whether it is in a vertical or horizontal position). As a result, when a bar of light is positioned in the appropriate part of the visual field with the appropriate orientation, the cells in area 17 will respond maximally. When either of these parameters is altered, the firing pattern of the cell will be reduced or totally inhibited. Complex cells lack clear excitatory and inhibitory zones (ie, these neurons respond to bars of light in a given orientation but they are not position specific).

Hypercomplex cells are stimulated by bars of light of specific lengths or by specific shapes.

351. The answer is e. (*Kandel, pp 625-634. Siegel and Sapru, pp 312-314.*) The olfactory cilia are extensions of the receptor cell, and it is this part of the cell that initially responds to an olfactory stimulus. The cilia contain protein membranes that bind with different odorants, which constitutes a necessary condition for excitation of the olfactory cell. Mitral and granule cells are situated in the olfactory bulb and, consequently, are not part of the receptor mechanism. Sustentacular cells are supporting cells and are not part of the receptor mechanism. Basal cells are the precursors for receptor cells and, thus, are also not directly part of the receptor mechanism.

352. The answer is b. (*Kandel, pp 626-636. Siegel and Sapru, pp 312-315.*) A number of recent studies have indicated that different olfactory glomeruli respond to different kinds of olfactory stimuli. In a sense, this represents a type of organization of the olfactory bulb that bears a functional similarity to the spatial organization that exists for other sensory systems and which is now disrupted by the continuous exposure to the strong odorant. There is no evidence that such a spatial arrangement exists for other components of the olfactory system, nor is there any evidence that temporal summation plays any role in the process of olfactory discrimination.

353. The answer is d. (*Nolte, pp 330-339. Siegel and Sapru, pp 312-315.*) The principal output pathways of the olfactory bulb arise from mitral cells and a related cell, called a tufted cell. The mitral cells project their axons out of the olfactory bulb to other regions of the forebrain associated with the transmission of olfactory information to the cerebral cortex. The major pathway subserving this is the lateral olfactory stria. Other cells that are mentioned in this question are either not present in the olfactory bulb (Golgi cells) or they have no known projections outside of the olfactory bulb. Receptor cells project only as far as the glomerulus. The granule cell has no axon. The periglomerular cell makes only local connections among neighboring glomeruli.

354. The answer is b. (*Kandel, p 633. Nolte, pp 330-339. Siegel and Sapru, pp 312-315.*) Mitral cell axons enter the lateral olfactory stria and project caudally through this bundle to supply the medial amygdala and pyriform cortex. Olfactory projections to other nuclei, such as the hippocampal formation, prefrontal cortex, medial thalamus, and septal area, require at least one additional synaptic connection such as in the pyriform cortex, amygdala, or olfactory tubercle.

355. The answer is a. (*Afifi, pp 259, 297, 323. Nolte, p 339. Siegel and Sapru, p 315.*) Uncinate fits (hallucinations) are characterized by seizure activity involving portions of the anterior aspect of the temporal lobe. The structures most often implicated include the uncus, parahippocampal gyrus, the region of the amygdala and adjoining tissue, and the pyriform cortex. During the occurrence of uncinate fits, a person experiences olfactory hallucinations of a highly unpleasant nature.

356. The answer is c. (*Nolte, pp 73-75, 243-248, 330-339. Siegel and Sapru, pp 281-283, 312-320.*) The pathway for conscious proprioception from the body utilizes the ventral posterolateral nucleus as its thalamic relay. Conscious proprioception from the head utilizes the ventral posteromedial nucleus as its relay. The taste pathway utilizes the ventral posteromedial nucleus as well. The visual system utilizes the lateral geniculate nucleus, and the auditory system utilizes the medial geniculate nucleus. In contrast, the olfactory system can transmit olfactory information to the prefrontal cortex without engaging thalamic nuclei. Thus, olfactory information reaches the pyriform cortex and amygdala from the olfactory bulb and then is transmitted directly to the prefrontal cortex. However, it should be noted that olfactory information also can reach the prefrontal cortex by virtue of projections from the olfactory tubercle and pyriform cortex via the mediodorsal thalamic nucleus. Thus, the olfactory system may utilize a parallel processing mechanism in transmitting inputs to the prefrontal cortex. Nevertheless, a tumor localized to the thalamus would leave intact the possibility for olfactory sensation to be spared in this patient.

Anatomy of the Forebrain

Questions

Questions 357 to 361

For each vignette, select the labeled structure in the figure that is most likely affected. Each lettered option may be used once, multiple times, or not at all.

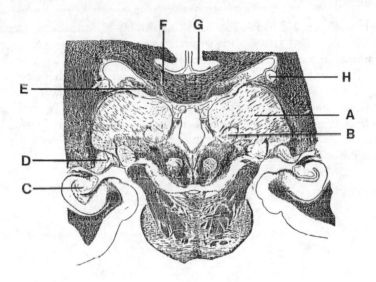

357. A 78 year old female was found unconscious in her home and then rushed to the emergency room of a local hospital. Upon waking, the patient was administered a neurological examination and MRI. The patient was shown to have had some cortical brain damage from the stroke. Consequently, she had difficulty in understanding language and was diagnosed with a form of receptive aphasia. Which neurons in this figure project their axons to the region of cortex affected by the stroke?

358. A patient presented with a movement disorder later diagnosed as Huntington disease. She subsequently passed away and an autopsy revealed brain damage in the forebrain. Which structure displays the location of brain damage?

359. A young man received a head injury in a football game, which later resulted in the development of seizure activity and the loss of his short-term memory. Which of the following is the most likely structure affected by this injury?

360. As a result of a vascular occlusion, a 64-year-old woman developed a homonymous hemianopsia. Which structure is most likely affected by this occlusion?

361. A 43-year-old female had been complaining of difficulty in sleeping along with mood changes for several weeks. Following a neurological examination, it was determined that the patient had a small tumor present in her brainstem reticular formation that could account for her sleep and mood disturbances. One of the routes by which the reticular formation could influence functions of the cerebral cortex, such as sleep-wakefulness cycles and mood, includes parts of the forebrain. From which region do neurons play an important role in transmitting information from the reticular formation to widespread areas of the cerebral cortex?

Questions 362 to 368

For each vignette, select the labeled structure in the figure that is most likely affected. Each lettered option may be used once, multiple times, or not at all.

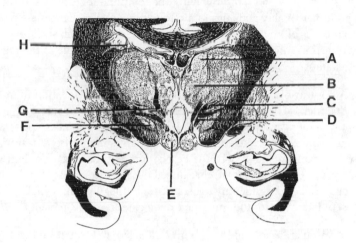

362. An elderly man suffered a stroke that was limited mainly to the globus pallidus, resulting in a hyperkinetic disorder. This was due mainly to the degeneration of fiber bundles that arise from the globus pallidus, which supply the ventrolateral (VL) and ventral anterior (VA) nuclei of the thalamus. Which structure was most likely affected by the stroke?

363. A 72-year-old male sustains a vascular occlusion involving a region of his forebrain. Afterward, he displays symptoms of dyskinesia, which is later diagnosed as hemiballism. Which structure is most likely damaged by the vascular occlusion?

364. A person has a stroke involving the ventral aspect of the diencephalon, resulting in significant damage to the mammillary bodies. As a result, there is considerable loss of input that normally supplies a major target region of the mammillary bodies. Which structure is now deprived of such input?

365. Concerning the patient described in Question 364, there is considerable degeneration in the major efferent pathway of the mammillary bodies. She also presented with disturbances in memory but otherwise appeared relatively normal. Which structure is most likely damaged?

366. As a result of an injury involving the temporal lobe, a person suffers changes in personality and autonomic functions. These changes are due in part to the loss of input to the medial hypothalamus. Which structure normally transmits information from parts of the temporal lobe to the medial hypothalamus?

367. A 53-year-old male presents with an unusual constellation of movement disorders. These include choreiform movements at rest as well as intention tremors and poor coordinated movements. The neurologist who examined the patient concluded that the patient suffered from movement disorders characteristic of both the cerebellum and basal ganglia and was probably due to a small stroke that affected a structure related to both of these neuronal groups. Identify the structure in the diagram, which if damaged, could account for the combined deficits seen in this patient.

368. A vascular lesion affecting a middle-aged woman resulted in the development of changes in affective responses and related aspects of emotionality, characterized by a flattened affect. The neurologist attributed the flattened affect to the loss of communication between the affected structure and the prefrontal cortex. Which of the structures was affected by the lesion?

Questions 369 to 375

For each vignette, select the labeled structure in the figure that is most likely affected. Each lettered option may be used once, multiple times, or not at all.

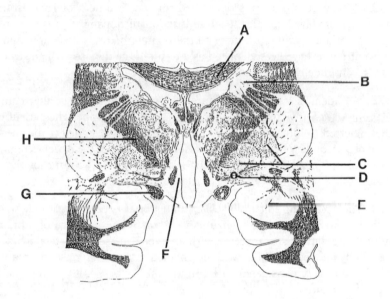

369. A 68-year-old male is taken to the emergency room after having a stroke while working in his office. Several days later, he presents to the emergency room with an upper motor neuron (UMN) paralysis of the right hand and right leg as well as a motor aphasia. An magnetic resonance imaging (MRI) indicates that the stroke involved structures situated within the forebrain. Which structure was most likely affected by the stroke?

370. A patient suffered from epilepsy for approximately 10 years and had been successfully treated with drugs. In recent months, the intensity of the seizures became significantly worse, spreading to both hemispheres of the brain, as drug treatment proved ineffective. In order to block the spread of the seizures, surgery was indicated. Which structure was now the subject of the surgical procedure?

371. A patient presented with a hypokinetic movement disorder. Both the neurosurgeon and the neurologist recommended a surgical lesion of the major output pathway of the basal ganglia in order to alleviate his condition. In which structure was the surgical lesion placed?

372. A new procedure was developed for the treatment of Parkinson's disease. It involved the direct administration of dopamine, a dopamine agonist, or a dopamine precursor to the brain structure whose dopamine concentrations have been depleted as a result of the disease. Which structure received delivery of these compounds?

373. A patient is sent to be examined by an endocrinologist after complaining of excessive thirst and increased excretion of urine. The patient is then referred to a neurologist and neuroradiologist, who detect the presence of a secondary brain lesion after viewing an MRI of the patient's brain. Where is the most likely locus of the lesion that could account for these deficits?

374. After receiving a neurological examination, a patient is told that he is suffering from psychomotor seizures induced by the presence of a brain tumor. The patient also presents with an altered personality state characterized by marked irritability with heightened anger in response to circumstances normally considered to be innocuous. Where is the most likely locus of the tumor?

375. A patient is referred to a neurologist after complaining that he cannot see out of the right half of each eye. The examination, coupled with an MRI, reveals the likely presence of a brain lesion causing the right homonymous hemianopsia. Which structure is most likely affected by the lesion?

Questions 376 to 379

For each vignette, select the labeled structure in the figure that is most likely affected. Each lettered option may be used once, multiple times, or not at all.

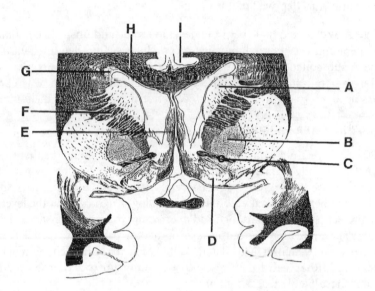

376. A patient who was suffering from Huntington disease died and an autopsy is performed. The neuropathologist notes marked degeneration in the forebrain. Which structure would be expected to show marked neuronal loss?

377. After displaying progressive memory loss over a period of several months, an elderly patient was referred to a neurologist, who concluded that the patient was suffering from Alzheimer disease. Several years later, the patient died and an autopsy was performed, indicating a significant loss of cholinergic neurons in specific regions of the forebrain. Which structure most likely exhibited the greatest loss of cholinergic neurons?

378. A 47-year-old male began to display marked involuntary movements at rest and a subsequent neurological examination revealed that he is suffering from a form of chorea. Chorea is believed to be due in part to a loss of GABAergic neurons in the neostriatum. Which structure normally receives major GABAergic input from neurons originating in the neostriatum but is now deprived of this input?

379. A 32-year-old male began to develop erratic and unstable emotional behavior and was referred initially to a psychiatrist and then to a neurologist. A subsequent MRI revealed the presence of a tumor in a region that receives significant input from the hippocampal formation and which projects its axons to the hypothalamus. Which structure contains the tumor?

Questions 380 and 381

380. A 32-year-old woman visits a gynecologist after noting that her menstrual cycle had stopped. She further complained of headaches, which had become more severe over the past several months and also reported difficulty with her peripheral vision. Her gynecologist told her that the level of the prolactin hormone was high and referred her to a neurologist. The neurological examination was normal except that the patient was unable to see fingers in the temporal fields (lateral half of each visual field) of both of her eyes. An MRI revealed the presence of a tumor. In which area would a tumor most likely cause a high prolactin level?

a. Adenohypophysis
b. Neurohypophysis
c. Amygdala
d. Hippocampus
e. Adrenal gland

381. In the patient from Question 380, which of the following types of visual loss will most likely occur?

a. Central scotoma
b. Superior quadrantanopsia
c. Bitemporal hemianopsia
d. Homonymous hemianopsia
e. Papilledema

382. A 76-year-old woman is admitted to a local hospital after complaining of a spiking fever. An MRI reveals a tumor in a region of the forebrain that is the cause of the spiking fever. Which of the following regions is the most likely site of the tumor?

a. Amygdala
b. Anterior hypothalamus
c. Ventromedial thalamus
d. Mammillary bodies
e. Hippocampus

383. A 37-year-old female was admitted to the hospital after she gained approximately 150 lb over an 8-month period. In addition, her behavior became quite erratic, in that she would scream and threaten someone who asked her an innocuous question. An MRI revealed the presence of what appeared to be a rapidly growing tumor that the neurologists believed could account for the increase in weight and aberrant emotional behavior. Which is the most likely site of this tumor?

a. Lateral hypothalamus
b. Dorsomedial thalamus
c. Mammillary bodies
d. Supraoptic nucleus
e. Ventromedial hypothalamus

384. A female patient experiences a significant disruption in the circadian rhythms for various sex hormones and corticosterone. A tumor is discovered in the forebrain of the patient. Which of the following structures most likely contains the tumor?

a. Posterior hypothalamic nucleus
b. Lateral hypothalamus
c. Ventromedial nucleus of hypothalamus
d. Suprachiasmatic nucleus of hypothalamus
e. Dorsomedial hypothalamic region

Questions 385 and 386

385. An 83-year-old female was admitted to the emergency room following a stroke. Sometime after she regained consciousness, a neurological examination revealed that the application of mild tactile stimulation on the right arm was extremely painful, while the remainder of the neurological examination was relatively normal for an individual of her age. Where was the most likely locus of the stroke?

a. Right precentral gyrus
b. Left precentral gyrus
c. Right ventroposterolateral thalamus
d. Left ventroposterolateral thalamus
e. Left ventroposteromedial thalamus

386. In the patient in Question 385, which of the following regions of the central nervous system constitutes the primary origin of the neurons that provide sensory input into the region affected by the stroke?

a. Lateral medulla
b. Medial medulla
c. Midbrain periaqueductal gray
d. Spinal cord
e. Dorsomedial pons

Questions 387 and 388

387. A 27-year-old female was suffering from excruciating pain that could not be reduced or eliminated through drug treatment. A decision was made by the neurosurgeon to attempt alleviate the pain by surgically cutting pathway mediating pain impulses to the thalamus. Which pathway did the neurosurgeon select to be cut in order to alleviate the pain?

a. Fasciculus gracilis
b. Fasciculus cuneatus
c. Spinocerebellar tract
d. Spinothalamic tract
e. Tectospinal tract

388. In a case similar to that described in Question 387, a patient was also suffering from excruciating pain. However, the neurosurgeon decided to try another approach to alleviate the pain. This approach involved the application of deep electrical stimulation to selected regions of the brain. Which of the following regions was selected for the application of stimulation in order to produce analgesia?

a. Anterior nucleus of thalamus
b. Caudate nucleus
c. Ventral horn of spinal cord
d. Dorsomedial hypothalamus
e. Periaqueductal gray

389. A patient suffering from significant pain is seen by a neurologist. He recommends a drug (or combination of drugs) that targets the primary neurotransmitters involved in the modulation of pain. Which of the following constitutes the most likely targets of such a pain-alleviating drug?

a. Aspartate and cholecystokinin
b. Glutamate and angiotensin
c. Epinephrine and γ-aminobutyric acid (GABA)
d. Dopamine and norepinephrine
e. Opioids and serotonin

Anatomy of the Forebrain

Answers

357 to 361. The answers are 357-A, 358-H, 359-C, 360-D, 361-B.
(Nolte, pp 280-287, 390-413, 558-563, 594-605. Siegel and Sapru, pp 204-220, 353-354, 415-418, 422-426, 447-453.) This section is taken at the level of the posterior thalamus and, because of the oblique cut, also includes parts of the midbrain and pons. The pulvinar (A), a very large nucleus situated at this level of the thalamus, projects extensively to wide regions of the inferior parietal lobule. Portions of the inferior parietal lobule and superior temporal cortex include the region referred to as Wernicke area, which is associated with receptive aphasia. The caudate nucleus (H) and putamen (not labeled), collectively referred to as the neostriatum, have been implicated in Huntington disease and show reduced levels of the neurotransmitter, GABA. The hippocampal formation (C) is associated with a number of different processes, including short-term memory and as a seizure focus during temporal lobe epilepsy. Thus, a lesion of this structure will likely produce deficits in short-term memory, and trauma to this region will result in temporal lobe epilepsy. The lateral geniculate nucleus (D), situated in the far ventrolateral aspect of the posterior thalamus, is a relay nucleus for the transmission of visual information to the cortex. Damage to this structure would result in a homonymous hemianopsia. The centromedian (CM) nucleus (B), identified by its encapsulated appearance, can be found in posterior levels of the thalamus, where it receives inputs from the brainstem reticular formation and projects to the neostriatum as well as to wide regions of the cerebral cortex. In this manner, it plays a role in the functions of the reticular formation, and presumably those associated with regulation of sleep-wakefulness and mood states.

362 to 368. The answers are 362-D, 363-F, 364-A, 365-G, 366-H, 367-C, 368-B. *(Nolte, pp 390-413, 479-492, 580-587, 596-602. Siegel and Sapru, pp 204-220, 346-354.)* This section is taken at the level of the mammillary bodies (at ventral levels) and includes parts of the anterior thalamus (at dorsal levels). The lenticular fasciculus (D), situated just below the thalamic fasciculus and immediately above the subthalamic nucleus at the level of this brain section, arises from the dorsomedial aspect of the medial pallidal segment and projects to the VL, VA, and CM nuclei of the thalamus. Damage to the neurons of the medial pallidal segment would cause degeneration of the efferent projections from this region, one pathway of which is the lenticular fasciculus. The subthalamic nucleus (F), which lies on the dorsal surface of the internal capsule, maintains reciprocal connections with the globus pallidus through a pathway called the *subthalamic fasciculus*. Damage to the subthalamic nucleus has been associated with the onset of hemiballism. The anterior nucleus of the thalamus (A), which lies at the rostral end of the thalamus in a dorsomedial position, receives a major input from the mammillary bodies via the *mammillothalamic tract*. The mammillary bodies (E), situated at the base of the posterior aspect of the hypothalamus, are the origin of the mammillothalamic (G) tract, which innervates the anterior thalamic nucleus. The region immediately below the tail and body of the caudate nucleus is occupied by a major output pathway of the medial amygdala (within the temporal lobe), the *stria terminalis* (H). It supplies the medial preoptic region, bed nucleus of the stria terminalis, and medial hypothalamus. The thalamic fasciculus can be seen in sections taken through the caudal half of the thalamus and is clearly visualized in a position dorsal to the subthalamic nucleus and lenticular fasciculus. The *thalamic fasciculus* (C) also projects to the ventral lateral and VA thalamic nuclei. While many of the fibers contained in this bundle arise from the medial pallidal segment, others arise directly from the dentate nucleus of cerebellum. Thus, damage to this pathway would most likely result in deficits characteristic of both the basal ganglia and cerebellum. A large nuclear mass situated in the medial aspect of the posterior two-thirds of the thalamus is the mediodorsal thalamic nucleus (B). This nucleus projects extensively to wide regions of the frontal lobe, including the prefrontal cortex. In turn, the prefrontal region of the cortex and adjoining regions of the frontal lobe project their axons back to the mediodorsal nucleus. Thus, there are reciprocal connections linking the mediodorsal nucleus and rostral portions of the frontal lobe. Because of the major input to the prefrontal cortex from the mediodorsal nucleus and since the prefrontal cortex plays an important role in the regulation of affective processes, damage to the mediodorsal nucleus would clearly alter emotional responses associated with the prefrontal cortex.

369 to 375. The answers are 369-H, 370-A, 371-D, 372-B, 373-F, 374-E, 375-G. *(Nolte, pp 390-412, 457-472, 474-492. Siegel and Sapru, pp 204-220, 288-289, 347-349, 434-436, 450-458.)* This section is taken from rostral levels of the diencephalon. Corticobulbar and corticospinal fibers contained within the internal capsule (H) arise from the deeper layers of the cerebral cortex (ie, layers V-VI). A lesion of the internal capsule would produce a UMN paralysis of the contralateral side of the body because of disruption of corticospinal fibers as well as damage to some corticobulbar fibers contained within the internal capsule. In this instance, there was damage associated with corticobulbar fibers descending from the motor speech area, resulting in a motor aphasia. Fibers associated with the corpus callosum (A) arise from more superficial layers of the cortex (ie, layers II-III) and project to the homotypic region of the contralateral cortex. Because this commissure represents the principal means by which one side of the cortex communicates with the other, surgical disruption of these fibers is carried out when all means of drug therapy have been shown to be ineffective and when seizures are shown to have spread to the cortices on both sides of the brain. Fibers of the ansa lenticularis (D) arise from the ventral aspect of the medial pallidal segment and can be visualized at more anterior levels of the pallidum. It represents a major output pathway of the basal ganglia and its axons supply the VL, VA, and CM nuclei of the thalamus. The neostriatum (ie, caudate nucleus [B] and putamen) receives dopaminergic inputs from the substantia nigra. Loss of dopamine levels in the caudate is associated with Parkinson disease, and experimental strategies have been applied to treat this disorder through replenishment of dopamine in the caudate nucleus. Different cells of the paraventricular nucleus of the hypothalamus (F), situated in the dorsomedial region at anterior levels, synthesize oxytocin and vasopressin. These hormones are transported down their axons to the posterior pituitary. Loss of vasopressin would result in excessive thirst and increased urine secretion (ie, diabetes insipidus), since vasopressin acts as an antidiuretic hormone. Although the marked changes in emotionality could be accounted for by damage to either the medial hypothalamus or the amygdala (E), psychomotor seizures are typically associated with temporal lobe structures and not with the hypothalamus. Thus, the correct answer in this case is E. Different fiber groups of the amygdala provide major inputs into the medial and lateral regions of the hypothalamus and thus constitute a significant modulator of hypothalamic functions, including rage and aggression. The optic tract (G) arises from the retina. Each optic tract represents fibers associated with the visual fields of the opposite side. Therefore, a lesion of the optic tract will result in a homonymous hemianopsia.

376 to 379. The answers are 376-A, 377-D, 378-B, 379-E. *(Nolte, pp 289, 474-492, 595-602. Siegel and Sapru, pp 204-220, 288-289, 347-349, 434-436, 450 458.)* This section is taken at the level of the septum pellucidum, the anterior commissure, and the substantia innominata. While a variety of structures may show degeneration in Huntington disease and other forms of chorea, it is generally agreed that Huntington disease and chorea are associated with loss of GABAergic neurons situated principally in the neostriatum (ie, caudate nucleus [A] and putamen). Fibers from the region of the basal nucleus of Meynert located in the substantia innominata (D) (at the base of the brain in the far rostral forebrain) send a cholinergic projection to wide areas of the neocortex. Loss of these cholinergic neurons has generally been associated with the presence of Alzheimer disease. The globus pallidus (B) receives GABAergic inputs from the neostriatum (ie, caudate nucleus and putamen), and these inputs represent the principal axonal projection of the neostriatum to the pallidum. Fibers from the region of the basal nucleus of Meynert located in the substantia innominata (D) (at the base of the brain in the far rostral forebrain) send a cholinergic projection to wide areas of the neocortex. Loss of these cholinergic neurons has generally been associated with the presence of Alzheimer disease. The septal area (E), seen at this level of the forebrain as a thin structure separated by the lateral ventricles on both sides, receives major inputs from the hippocampal formation, projects many of its axons to the hypothalamus, and is a principal component of the limbic system.

380 and 381. The answers are 380-a and 381-c. *(Ropper, pp 618-651. Afifi, pp 444-447, 582-592. Kandel, pp 544, 978-980.)* The MRI of the woman's head revealed a pituitary microadenoma, a benign tumor arising from the anterior pituitary or adenohypophysis. This particular tumor consisted of cells that secrete the hormone prolactin, which is not only the stimulating factor for production of milk (for lactation), but inhibits menstruation when levels are high. The symptoms related to this tumor are commonly manifest during the childbearing years. The visual problem is called *bitemporal hemianopsia*. Since the pituitary gland is in very close proximity to the optic chiasm, pituitary tumors often compress this structure. Since only the medial fibers (which perceive the temporal field of each eye) in each optic nerve cross, these are the fibers damaged by these tumors, and the patient will be unable to see either temporal visual field. Neither central scotoma (an island of visual loss surrounded by normal vision in one eye), which is usually seen with lesions of the retina or optic nerve, nor papilledema (blurring of the optic disc margin when viewed by fundoscopic examination due to increased intracranial pressure) would be caused by damage to the optic chiasm. The optic chiasm can be compressed by pituitary tumors, causing bitemporal hemianopsia (see the answer for the previous question). The prolactin-releasing factor is found in the arcuate nucleus of the hypothalamus and activates the lactotropic cells of the anterior pituitary gland. Several different peptides, including dopamine, have the capacity to raise the level of prolactin in the blood. Specifically, the tuberoinfundibular dopaminergic system regulates prolactin secretion through direct projection to the pituitary. For this reason, a newer treatment for prolactin-secreting microadenomas is the drug bromocriptine, a dopamine agonist commonly used in the treatment of Parkinson disease. By giving a dopamine agonist, serum prolactin increases, inhibiting production by the tumor cells, and eventually the tumor size shrinks. This has become either an alternative or a first-line treatment prior to trying radiation or surgery.

382. The answer is b. (*Siegel and Sapru, pp 437-438, 441.*) The anterior hypothalamus contains temperature-sensitive neurons referred to as "thermoreceptors" that respond to changes in blood temperature. These neurons also have the capacity to affect both endocrine (ie, secretion of thyroid-stimulating hormone to increase metabolic rates) and autonomic mechanisms that can cause dilation of peripheral blood vessels, thus affecting an overall heat loss process to compensate for the increase in body temperature. The presence of a tumor in the anterior hypothalamus would significantly distort this mechanism, leading to an increase in body temperature. (Opposing effects are typically seen with lesions of the posterior hypothalamus.)

383. The answer is e. (*Siegel and Sapru, pp 437-441, 442.*) Tumors of the region of the ventromedial nucleus have been associated with significant weight gain in both animals and in humans. It may be due to a disruption or activation of the mechanism regulating feeding behavior in neighboring regions of hypothalamus such as the paraventricular nucleus. The rage-like responses were probably also associated with the stimulation-like properties of the tumor upon neurons in the ventromedial hypothalamus, which constitutes a primary structure for the regulation of this form of emotional behavior. Other regions of hypothalamus do not relate to either of these defects.

384. The answer is d. *(Siegel and Sapru, p 441.)* The suprachiasmatic nucleus of the hypothalamus is of critical importance in the setting and regulation of biological rhythms. This is due to a considerable extent to the fact that it receives retinal inputs essential for the triggering of circadian rhythms for a number of sex hormones, corticosterone, and melatonin produced from the pineal gland. The other choices have no known relationship to the regulation of circadian rhythms for these hormones.

385 and 386. The answers are 385-d and 386-d. *(Kandel, pp 446-450, 454-460, 473-475, 480-487, 874-875. Siegel and Sapru, pp 264-265.)* A stroke involving the ventral posterolateral nucleus of the thalamus can produce an entity called the *Dèjèrine-Roussy syndrome, or thalamic pain syndrome.* There is contralateral pain or discomfort out of proportion to the stimulus on the affected side of the body. Emotional disturbance aggravates the response. Some patients describe the sensation as knifelike or hot. As the deficit (numbness) resolves, the pain may lessen. This syndrome may also occur in lesions of the parietal white matter and is thought to occur as a result of an imbalance of afferent sensory impulses. Sensation of the limbs and trunk are projected through the lateral spinothalamic tract (originating in the dorsal horn of spinal cord) through the ventral posterolateral nucleus of the thalamus to the somatosensory cortex. It is an area with a high density of opiate receptors and opioidergic neurons and is thought to represent a key area in gating pain.

387. The answer is d. *(Kandel, pp 446-450, 454-460, 473-475, 480-487, 874-875.)* The spinothalamic tract is the only sensory pathway listed that mediates pain. The fasciculus gracilis and cuneatus mediate conscious proprioception, not pain; the spinocerebellar tract mediates unconscious proprioception (muscle spindle and Golgi tendon organ inputs to cerebellum); and the tectospinal tract is a descending tract, mediating no sensory information to the brain.

388. The answer is e. *(Kandel, pp 446-450, 454-460, 473-475, 480-487, 874-875.)* The periaqueductal gray is an area that produces analgesia when stimulated in both animals and humans. It constitutes the origin of the descending pain inhibitory pathway that modulates pain inputs at the level of the dorsal horn of the spinal cord. Other choices listed in this question have little or no relationship to the control of pain.

389. The answer is e. (*Kandel, pp 446-450, 454-460, 473-475, 480-487, 874-875. Siegel and Sapru, pp 263-264.*) Many neurotransmitters have been implicated as pain modulators, including the opioids and enkephalins, norepinephrine, serotonin, substance P, GABA, and acetylcholine. Most analgesic medications are designed to target a particular aspect of the pain pathway. In more recent years, the advent of a class of drugs called *tricyclic antidepressants* has added another dimension to medical pain treatment. The methylated forms of these medications are useful blockers of serotonin reuptake. Since serotonin is known to be a pain modulator, it is thought that blocking the reuptake of serotonin enhances its action and facilitates the action of intrinsic opiates to relieve pain. This is a common class of drugs used to treat chronic pain, since these medications are not addictive.

Motor Systems

Questions

390. A patient delays initiation of movement, displays an uneven trajectory in moving her hand from above her head to touch her nose, and is uneven in her attempts to demonstrate rapid alternation of pronating and supernating movements of the hand and forearm. Which of the following regions most likely contains the lesion?

a. Hemispheres of the posterior cerebellar lobe
b. Flocculonodular lobe of the cerebellum
c. Vermal region of the anterior cerebellar lobe
d. Fastigial nucleus
e. Ventral spinocerebellar tract

391. A 59-year-old male suffered a stroke and later presented with a spastic paralysis. Which of the following structures affected by the stroke most likely accounts for the spasticity?

a. Ventral horn cells
b. Corpus callosum
c. Postcentral gyrus
d. Internal capsule
e. Substantia nigra

392. A 74-year-old woman with a history of hypertension suddenly displays loss of consciousness. Sometime later, the patient presents with weakness of her left body, including upper and lower limbs, weakness of her face, and slurred speech. The diffusion weighted MRI of this patient is shown here, in which the high signal reflects vascular occlusion of a region of the brain. Which of the following best characterizes what happened to this patient?

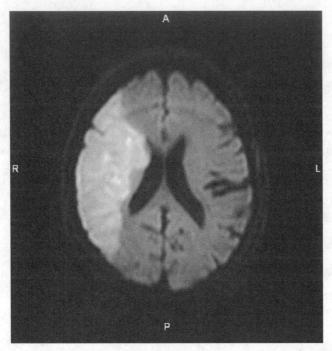

(Reproduced, with permission, from Anschel DJ, Romanelli P, Mazumdar A. McGraw-Hill Specialty Board Review: Clinical Neuroimaging. New York: McGraw-Hill; 2008:45.)

a. A stroke involving the right anterior cerebral artery
b. A stroke involving the right middle cerebral artery
c. Occlusion of the right anterior communicating artery
d. Occlusion of the right posterior communicating artery
e. A stroke of the posterior cerebral artery

393. A 50-year-old male presents with dizziness, headaches, and ataxia of the limbs. He was given an MRI, shown on the figure here and a hemangioblastoma was noted (indicated by the white arrow). Where is the tumor most likely located?

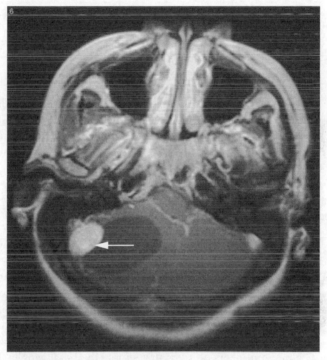

(Reproduced, with permission, from Anschel DJ, Romanelli P, Mazumdar A. McGraw-Hill Specialty Board Review: Clinical Neuroimaging. New York: McGraw-Hill; 2008:79.)

a. Midbrain
b. Cerebellum
c. Rostral pons
d. Caudal pons
e. Medulla

394. A patient who suffered a stroke presents with a paralysis of the right side of the lower face, right spastic paralysis of the limbs, deviation of the tongue to the right with no atrophy, and no loss of taste from any region of the tongue. Which of the following structures was most likely affected by the stroke?

a. Internal capsule of the right side
b. Internal capsule of the left side
c. Right pontine tegmentum
d. Base of the medulla on the right side
e. Base of the medulla on the left side

395. A 74-year-old female was brought to the hospital after she suffered a stroke. Several days later, a neurological examination revealed that she was unable to perform certain types of learned, complex movements (referred to as apraxia). Which of the following regions of the cerebral cortex was most likely affected by the stroke?

a. Precentral gyrus
b. Postcentral gyrus
c. Premotor cortex
d. Prefrontal cortex
e. Cingulate gyrus

396. A 58-year-old male complained of a severe headache and was taken to the emergency room of a local hospital, where the patient had impaired consciousness. A few days later, the patient presented with signs of choreiform movements at times of rest. An MRI suggested the presence of a vascular occlusion of wide areas of the frontal and parietal lobes that damaged the overwhelming numbers of fibers that supply the basal ganglia. Which of the following regions constitute the receiving area of the overwhelming majority of fibers that supply the basal ganglia?

a. Paleostriatum
b. Neostriatum
c. Subthalamic nucleus
d. Substantia nigra
e. Claustrum

397. A 47-year-old male is admitted to a hospital after he presented with writhing, wild, flinging-like movements of his left arm that became progressively worse over time. An MRI revealed the presence of a tumor present over the caudate and putamen on the right side of the brain. The neurologist concluded that the tumor caused significant damage to neurons in this region, thus disrupting their normal functions. Which of the following best characterizes neurons in the neostriatum that were disrupted by the tumor?

a. Inhibited by γ-aminobutyric acid (GABA) released at corticostriate terminals
b. Inhibited by GABA released at nigrostriatal terminals
c. Inhibited by substance P released at corticostriate terminals
d. Excited by acetylcholine (ACh) released from hypothalamic-caudate terminals
e. Excited by glutamate released at corticostriate terminals

398. A child is suffering from a developmental abnormality that affects the primary transmitter released from terminals of both neostriatal and paleostriatal neurons. Which neurotransmitter is most likely affected by this abnormality?

a. Glycine
b. Enkephalin
c. Dopamine
d. GABA
e. Glutamate

399. A 46-year-old female received a diagnosis of having a movement disorder associated with disturbances of the basal ganglia. In particular, she presents with writhing, uncoordinated movements at rest of her left arm and leg. An MRI revealed the presence of a tumor affecting mainly the right caudate nucleus and putamen. Which of the following best explains why the dysfunction is expressed on the side of the body contralateral to the region of the basal ganglia directly affected by the stroke?

a. Fibers from the basal ganglia to the spinal cord are crossed.
b. Fibers from the basal ganglia project to motor nuclei of the brainstem whose axons then project to the contralateral spinal cord.
c. Fibers from the basal ganglia project to the ipsilateral motor cortex.
d. Axons from the basal ganglia project to the cerebellum, whose outputs are known to modulate the contralateral side of the body.
e. Fibers from the basal ganglia project directly to the contralateral motor cortex.

400. A 30-year-old male suffers a serious injury of the central nervous system that results from an industrial accident. A neurological evaluation suggests that the major input to the flocculonodular lobe is damaged. Which of the following structures that provides the major input to the flocculonodular lobe was damaged?

a. Nucleus dorsalis of Clarke
b. Red nucleus
c. Vestibular nuclei
d. Cerebral cortex
e. Midbrain reticular formation

401. A 43-year-old male who began to display marked involuntary movements at times of rest was seen by a neurologist, who concluded that he was suffering from Huntington disease. Which of the following neurotransmitters was lost or reduced in this individual?

a. Dopamine in the neostriatum
b. Substance P in the substantia nigra
c. ACh and GABA in intrastriatal and cortical neurons
d. Serotonin in the neostriatum
e. Histamine in subthalamic nucleus

402. A patient is admitted to the local hospital for treatment of a vascular occlusion within the forebrain. A magnetic resonance imaging (MRI) indicates that the damage is limited to the subthalamic nucleus. As a result of this lesion, which of the following disorders is likely to be present in the patient?

a. Torsion dystonia
b. Tremor at rest
c. Hemiballism
d. Spastic paralysis
e. Tardive dyskinesia

403. A patient presents with a movement disorder which includes most prominently chorea-like symptoms. In treating this patient, the neurologist adopts a strategy based upon our current level of knowledge of neuro science of this region of the brain. Which of the following strategies is the neurologist most likely to apply?

a. ACh blockers because there is an excess of this transmitter in the caudate nucleus
b. Dopamine blockers because there is too low a ratio of ACh to dopamine in the neostriatum
c. Serotonin blockers because there is too low a ratio of serotonin to ACh and dopamine in the neostriatum
d. Substance P antagonists because the ratio of substance P to ACh is too high in the neostriatum
e. Norepinephrine antagonists because the ratio of norepinephrine to ACh is too high in the subthalamic nucleus

404. A 65-year-old male has been under long-term treatment for an anxiety disorder. Recently, the psychiatrist observed that he began to develop symptoms of tardive dyskinesia. This disorder is most likely the result of which of the following alterations?

a. A reduction in serotonin receptors in the neostriatum
b. A change in ACh receptors that causes a hypersensitivity to ACh
c. A change in enkephalin receptors that causes a hypersensitivity to enkephalin
d. A change in GABA levels in the basal ganglia
e. A change in dopamine levels in the limbic system

405. Two 18-year-old boys were experimenting with designer drugs and after they took the drugs, each of them presented with a movement disorder associated with basal ganglia dysfunction. The drug was later identified as the neurotoxin 1-methyl-4-phenyl-1,2,3,6-tetrahydropyridine (MPTP) and has recently been applied experimentally with considerable success as a model for the study of which of the following diseases?

a. Huntington disease
b. Hemiballism
c. Parkinson disease
d. Tardive dyskinesia
e. Dystonia

406. A 25-year-old man, who began to have difficulty in walking, is examined by a neurologist and neurosurgeon. They conclude that a tumor is compressing upon the lateral aspect of his spinal cord, affecting primarily the spinocerebellar tracts. Which of the following structures is the principal region within the cerebellum that receives these fibers?

a. Anterior lobe
b. Posterior lobe
c. Flocculonodular lobe
d. Fastigial nucleus
e. Dentate nucleus

407. A middle-aged male is diagnosed with a rare form of encephalopathy, which mainly causes demyelination of cerebral cortical neurons that project to the cerebellum. Which of the following best describes the distribution of these fibers?

a. Somatotopically distributed only to the anterior lobe
b. Somatotopically distributed only to the vermal region of the anterior and posterior lobes
c. Somatotopically distributed to the cerebellar hemispheres
d. Not somatotopically organized but do project to the hemispheres of the anterior and posterior lobes
e. Distributed mainly to the interposed and dentate nuclei

408. As a result of a dysfunction in development, a 4-year-old boy has difficulty walking and maintaining balance. It is later determined that there is significant loss of neurons in the cerebellum that disrupts the neuronal organization of the cerebellar glomerulus. Which of the following best characterizes this glomerulus?

a. Mossy fiber terminals, Golgi axons, and axon terminals of granule cells
b. Climbing fiber terminals, Golgi axons, and granule cell dendrites
c. Mossy fiber terminals, Purkinje cell axons, and granule cell dendrites
d. Mossy fiber terminals, Golgi and granule cell dendrites, and Golgi cell axon terminals
e. Climbing fiber terminals, Golgi cell dendrites, Purkinje cell dendrites, and axon terminals of parallel fibers

Questions 409 to 410

409. A 55-year-old male had been complaining about having difficulty in coordinating the use of his arms in meaningful ways. For example, when examined by a neurologist, the patient was unable to move his finger accurately to his nose from his side when requested to do so but instead would undershoot or overshoot the target. He also had difficulty in making rapid alternating rotational movements of the hand. The neurologist believed that the patient was suffering from a disorder that resulted in a lesion of a region of the cerebellum or structures related to it. Which of the following regions most likely contained this lesion?

a. Fastigial nucleus
b. Vermal region
c. Cerebellar hemispheres
d. Inferior cerebellar peduncle
e. Vestibular nuclei

410. In the patient in Question 409, the neurologist believed that the neurological deficit was due to the lack of feedback from the affected structure to its target region elsewhere in the central nervous system. Which region is most likely devoid of this critical input?

a. Reticular formation
b. Vestibular nuclei
c. Basal ganglia
d. Cerebral cortex
e. Inferior olivary nucleus

411. A 23-year-old female was exposed to a neurotoxin that selectively destroyed the Purkinje cell layer of the cerebellum, resulting in loss of balance and coordination. Of the structures or regions indicated below, which one was most directly affected by the loss of Purkinje cells?

a. Red nucleus
b. Deep cerebellar nuclei
c. Reticular formation
d. Ventrolateral (VL) nucleus (thalamus)
e. Spinal cord

412. A 64-year-old male who had been an alcoholic patient for many years died from a myocardial infarction. A CT scan of his brain taken through the level of the cerebellum as well as one showing the hemispheres and sulci are shown here. Which of the following clinical signs would this patient be most likely to display?

a. Intention tremor
b. Spasticity
c. Rigidity
d. Ataxia of legs
e. Movement disorder at rest

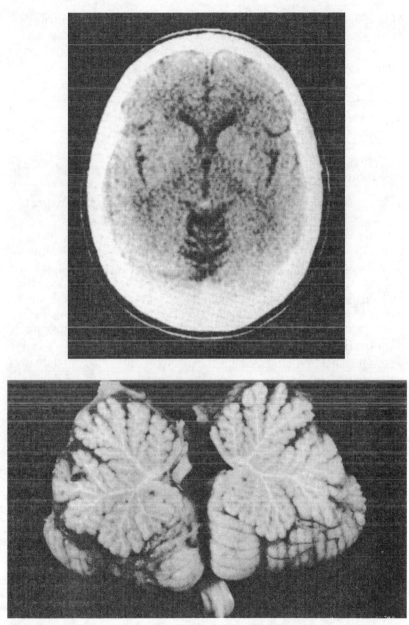

(Reproduced, with permission, from Ropper AH, Samuels MA. Adams & Victor Principles of Neurology, 9th ed. New York: McGraw-Hill, 2009.)

413. A man presents with a wide-based, ataxic gait during his attempts at walking. He is also unsteady, sways when standing, and displays a tendency to fall backward or to either side in a drunken manner. In which of the following structures is a lesion most likely located?

a. Hemispheres of the posterior cerebellar lobe
b. Anterior limb of the internal capsule
c. Dentate nucleus
d. Anterior lobe of the cerebellum
e. Flocculonodular lobe of the cerebellum

Questions 414 and 415

414. A previously healthy 62-year-old man is brought to a neurologist by his daughter because of increasing difficulty in walking. His daughter noticed that for the past year, he had difficulty getting out of a chair and took a lot of time to begin to walk. When he did walk, he walked with a slow, shuffling gait. In addition, she had noticed some changes in his face, and that he had been drooling excessively. His signature on checks became progressively smaller from the beginning of his name to the end, and he had developed a new tremor. She brought him in to make sure this was not just "aging." The neurologist examines the patient and notices immediately that his facial expression was masklike, with few eyeblinks. When asked to write a sentence, the letters become progressively smaller toward the end of the sentence. His speech is soft and monotonous, and he has a slow, resting pill-rolling tremor in both of his hands. He has very little spontaneous movement, and his arms, legs, and trunk were stiff. When the neurologist tries to flex his arm, he feels many catches, similar to a cog-wheel. There is no weakness, sensory problems, or abnormalities in his reflexes. When asked to walk, the patient takes many tries to rise from his chair. When he finally stands up, his posture is stooped and flexed. His gait is slow, his feet shuffle when he walks, and his arms do not swing with his steps. The neurologist tells the patient's daughter that she is correct that this is not just aging and explains to her all of the details about a new medication that her father needs to take. Damage to which of the following structures most likely causes this patient's problem with movement?

a. Substantia gelatinosa
b. Substantia nigra, pars reticularis
c. Substantia nigra, pars compacta
d. Caudate nucleus
e. Thalamus

415. In the patient in Question 414, the blood supply of which of the main structure is damaged?

a. Lenticulostriate branches of the middle cerebral and anterior cerebral arteries
b. Perforating branches of the basilar and vertebral arteries
c. Anterior choroidal artery and anterior cerebral artery
d. Branches of posterior cerebral and posterior communicating arteries
e. Anterior cerebral and anterior communicating arteries

416. A 65-year-old male is informed by his neurologist that he has Parkinson disease. Which of the following neurotransmitters is deficient in this patient?

a. Norepinephrine
b. Glutamate
c. Dopamine
d. ACh
e. GABA

417. A patient suffers from Parkinson disease. His neurologist prescribes a drug, which constitutes a precursor to the neurotransmitter deficient in this individual, as a medication for his disorder. Which of the following precursors to the deficient neurotransmitter was administered as a medication to improve the condition of this patient?

a. Tyrosine
b. Choline
c. Acetyl-CoA
d. Tryptamine
e. L-dihydroxy phenylalamine (L-DOPA)

418. A 67-year-old male has been suffering from Parkinson disease for a number of years and every current drug administered to the patient ultimately was unsuccessful in alleviating the symptoms. Since drug treatment with this patient is typical of the unsuccessful treatment given to many other patients, a pharmaceutical company attempts to develop a new drug for the treatment of Parkinson disease. The approach utilized by this company involves the application of a drug that will block the action of a certain enzyme that normally functions to destroy a specific neurotransmitter. Such a drug would effectively increase the amount of the deficient neurotransmitter in the brain. Which of the following enzymes would be targeted by this drug?

a. Choline acetyltranferase
b. Monoamine oxidase
c. GABA transaminase
d. Acetylcholinesterase
e. Tyrosine hydroxylase

Questions 419 and 420

419. A 57-year-old man who has always been a very heavy drinker, often consuming two pints of whiskey per day, for many years, notices that he now needs to stand with his feet far apart in order to maintain his balance and that he waddles when he walks. The doctor who evaluates him tests his memory and speech carefully, as well as his cranial nerves, and is unable to find any deficits. There is no weakness, sensory loss, or abnormalities in his reflexes. When asked to touch the doctor's finger and then his nose, the patient misses his nose slightly, but rapidly corrects the movement on both sides. When asked to slide his right heel down his left shin, his heel slides sideways and clumsily across the bone until it reaches his ankle. The response with the left heel is similar. When asked to walk, the patient walks with his feet very far apart. If he tries to walk in a tandem fashion, with one heel in front of the other toe, he begins to fall, and the doctor has to catch him. The doctor orders an MRI of the patient's head. Which of the following terms best describes the patient's gait?

a. Stiff
b. Festinating
c. Ataxic
d. Spastic
e. Shuffling

420. In the patient in Question 419, a gait problem of this type could be caused by lesions in which of the following systems?

a. Cerebellar tracts only
b. Posterior columns only
c. Corticospinal tracts
d. Both the cerebellar and the posterior column systems
e. Spinothalamic system

421. A 18-year-old male with a history of alcohol and drug abuse was admitted to a local hospital after he was observed to have consistently lost his balance upon attempting to walk. In his attempt to retain his balance, he would walk with a wide, ataxic gait. In which of the following structures did an MRI scan identify the locus of the lesion?

a. Red nucleus
b. Cerebellar vermis
c. Substantia nigra
d. Internal capsule
e. Basilar pons

422. A patient presents with nystagmus and a gait ataxia. An MRI detects the presence of a lesion in the region of the cerebellum. With which functional division of the cerebellum is most likely the affected region associated?

a. Cerebrocerebellum
b. Spinocerebellum
c. Dentate nucleus
d. Middle cerebellar peduncle
e. Interposed nuclei

423. A patient presents with cerebellar ataxia and nystagmus. An MRI later identifies the site of the lesion. To which of the following deep cerebellar nucleus or related structure do the neurons in the damaged region project?

a. Globose nucleus
b. Emboliform nucleus
c. Fastigial nucleus
d. Dentate nucleus
e. Superior cerebellar peduncle

424. A patient with a long history of alcoholism with a dramatic gait ataxia and nystagmus dies 2 months after he is admitted to a local hospital. Following an autopsy, the neuropathological examination reveals significant loss of which of the following cells?

a. Schwann cells
b. Pyramidal cells
c. Spindle cells
d. Anterior horn cells
e. Purkinje cells

Questions 425 and 426

425. An 86-year-old woman has had difficulty with high blood pressure, high cholesterol, diabetes, strokes, and blood clots in her legs for many years. One day, her grandson arrived at her apartment in a senior citizen center for his weekly visit and found her lying unconscious on the floor. He immediately called an ambulance. The paramedics in the ambulance gave her some medications, including glucose, but she did not awaken. She was taken to the nearest emergency room, where a physician was called to evaluate her. She was breathing on her own and had a pulse, but could not be aroused to any stimulus. Her arms and legs were stiff and would not move in response to a painful stimulus. Her eyes moved in response to moving her head. Finally, in response to a very loud shout and pinch on the arm, she briefly opened her eyes; however, she immediately shut them again. Further attempts to arouse the patient were unsuccessful. She was taken for a CT scan of her head, and then taken to an intensive care unit. An acute stroke in which portion of the CNS would most likely cause this scenario?

a. Right frontal lobe
b. Left frontal lobe
c. Right temporal lobe
d. Pons and midbrain
e. Right occipital lobe

426. In the patient in Question 425, which of the following is the most likely cause of the stiffness in her arms and legs?

a. Infarction of the corticospinal tracts bilaterally in the pons
b. Damage to the basal ganglia
c. Infarction of the precentral gyrus
d. Infarction of the internal capsules bilaterally
e. Thalamic infarction

Questions 427 and 428

427. An elderly male who had been living in a nursing home was found unconscious by a nurse. He was rushed to a hospital and remained unconscious for approximately 24 hours. When he recovered consciousness, he was examined by a neurologist. The patient was unable to move his left leg or arm. He also experienced double vision and was unable to move his right eye medially when requested to follow the movement of the neurologist's finger, when it was moved into a medial position. It was concluded that the stroke involved an occlusion of an artery in the brain. Which of the following arteries or branches of an artery were most likely occluded in this case?

a. Anterior cerebral artery
b. Middle cerebral artery
c. Posterior cerebral artery
d. Superior cerebellar artery
e. Posterior inferior cerebellar artery

428. In the patient in Question 427, which of the following structures were most likely affected by the stroke?

a. Nucleus of facial nerve and basilar pons
b. Nucleus of trochlear nerve and dorsal midbrain tegmentum
c. Nucleus of oculomotor nucleus and cerebral peduncle
d. Nucleus of trigeminal nucleus and basilar pons
e. Internal capsule and optic tract

429. A 62-year-old male is hospitalized for a stroke, which caused an inability to move his right eye to the right, and a partial paralysis of the limbs on the left side. Which of the following combinations of structures were most likely affected by this cerebral occlusion?

a. Cranial nerve VI and basilar pons
b. Cranial nerve VI and pontine tegmentum
c. Cranial nerve III and cerebral peduncle
d. Cranial nerve III, red nucleus, and cerebral peduncle
e. Motor regions of the cerebral cortex and frontal eye field

Motor Systems

Answers

390. The answer is a. (*Nolte, pp 520-521. Siegel and Sapru, pp 360-376.*) The classic appearance of a patient with a lesion of the cerebellar hemispheres is one in which voluntary and skilled movements are affected. They are uncoordinated, and there are errors in the range, force, and direction of movement. The relationships between the cerebellum and the motor regions of the cerebral cortex have been disrupted. Lesions of other regions, such as the flocculonodular lobe, vermal region of the anterior cerebellar cortex, or fastigial nucleus, produce different symptoms (disturbances of balance and nystagmus associated with the flocculonodular lobe and vermal regions, disturbances of muscle tone associated with the anterior cerebellar cortex). Although pure lesions limited to the ventral spinocerebellar tract have not been reported, it is likely that such a lesion could not account for the symptoms indicated in this question. Information carried by this tract concerns activity of Golgi tendon organs of muscles of the lower limbs.

391. The answer is d. (*Nolte, pp 467-470. Siegel and Sapru, pp 329-339, 351-353.*) An upper motor neuron (UMN) paralysis occurs following a lesion of the internal capsule. Such a lesion disrupts not only fibers destined for the spinal cord, but others that project to parts of the reticular formation and activate inhibitory reticulospinal mechanisms. Loss of such inhibitory input to spinal cord motor neurons then leads to increased levels of excitation of these neurons. The behavioral manifestation of this process is spasticity. Lesions of ventral horn cells produce a flaccid paralysis. Lesions of the postcentral gyrus primarily produce sensory loss, not spasticity. Since the corpus callosum is concerned with interhemispheric transfer of information, a lesion of this bundle will not produce spasticity. A lesion of the substantia nigra will result in Parkinson disease, which is associated with tremors at rest and rigidity, but not spasticity.

392. The answer is b. (*Anschel, p 45. Ropper, pp 667-673.*) This patient suffered a stroke of the middle cerebral artery and from the appearance of the MRI, the damage was quite extensive. It resulted in both an upper motor neuron disorder of the body and weakness of the muscles of the face, which in addition, affected speech patterns (ie, slurred speech). A stroke of the anterior communicating artery would not likely produce damage limited to one side of the brain and would also affect the blood supply to the most anterior regions of brain that were spared in this patient. A stroke of the anterior cerebral artery would likewise affect more anterior regions of the brain. The posterior communicating and posterior cerebral arteries would have affected other regions of the brain, including internal structures such as hypothalamus (with respect to the posterior communicating artery).

393. The answer is b. (*Anschel, p 79. Ropper, pp 986-987.*) The location of the tumor is the cerebellar hemisphere. This type of tumor occurs most often in association with von Hippel-Lindau disease and has signs of increased intracranial pressure, headache, and because of its location, cerebellar dysfunction such as ataxia. The other choices given in this question include regions distant from the location shown in the figure. Moreover, it is quite unlikely that any of the other choices could be associated with the symptoms and signs indicated in this patient.

394. The answer is b. (*Kandel, pp 1306-1309. Siegel and Sapru, pp 334-336.*) This constellation of deficits, including paralysis of the lower right face, paralysis of the lower right limbs, and right deviation of the tongue, requires a lesion located in the left internal capsule. Since the motor fibers from the cortex that supply all three of these regions (ie, limbs, lower face, and tongue) are all crossed, a lesion of the internal capsule will produce each of these deficits. Also, recall that the tongue will deviate to the side of the lesion when the lesion affects the lower motor neuron (LMN) (ie, cranial nerve XII) directly. When it affects the UMN (ie, fibers in the internal capsule), inputs into the contralateral nucleus of cranial nerve XII are affected. Thus, the tongue in this instance will deviate to the side opposite to the lesion. A lesion of the pontine tegmentum will not affect descending corticospinal or corticomedullary fibers, since these fibers are contained in the basilar part of the pons. A lesion of the medulla would be too caudal to affect cortical fibers that terminate on cells of the facial nucleus whose axons innervate muscles of the lower face.

395. The answer is c. (*Kandel, pp 654-672, 770-777. Siegel and Sapru, pp 330-333.*) The premotor areas play an important role in the programming or sequencing of responses that compose complex, learned movements.

They receive significant inputs for this process from the posterior parietal lobule and, in turn, signal appropriate neurons in the brain stem and spinal cord (both flexors and extensors). Lesions of the postcentral gyrus produce a somatosensory loss. Lesions of the precentral gyrus produce paralysis. Neither lesions of the prefrontal cortex nor those of the cingulate gyrus have been reported to produce apraxia.

396. The answer is b. *(Kandel, pp 853-864. Siegel and Sapru, pp 343-351.)* The neostriatum (ie, caudate nucleus and putamen) constitutes the principal, if not exclusive, receiving area for afferent fibers to the basal ganglia. Loss of such input could interfere with the functions of the neocortex and thus produce signs of dysfunction associated with this region such as choreiform movements at rest. The subthalamic nucleus and the substantia nigra share reciprocal connections with the paleostriatum (ie, globus pallidus) and the neostriatum, respectively. However, these areas receive few, if any, fibers from the cerebral cortex or the CM nucleus of the thalamus, which are the major afferent sources to the basal ganglia. Functions of the claustrum are not well understood, but it is believed to be more closely associated with the neocortex than with the basal ganglia.

397. The answer is e. *(Kandel, pp 853-864. Siegel and Sapru, pp 343-351.)* The cerebral cortex is a principal source of afferent fibers to the neostriatum and utilizes glutamate as its transmitter, which is excitatory to caudate neurons. Thus, a tumor of the neostriatum would disrupt both the inputs to it from the cerebral cortex as well as its outputs to the globus pallidus and substantia nigra and therefore account for the disorder described in this patient. Neither GABA nor substance P is a transmitter from the cortex to the neostriatum; nor is GABA a transmitter released from the nigrostriatal terminals. Projections from the hypothalamus to the caudate nucleus have never been demonstrated and, presumably, do not exist.

398. The answer is d. *(Kandel, pp 853-861. Siegel and Sapru, pp 313-351.)* The major transmitter released at terminals of neostriatal and paleostriatal fibers is GABA. Thus, the output of the basal ganglia is mainly inhibitory. This suggests that thalamic influences upon the cortex are generated through the process of disinhibition, whereby neurons of the basal ganglia are inhibited. The presence of glycine in striatal neurons has yet to be demonstrated. Enkephalins are released from terminals of neostriatal-pallidal fibers but not from other efferent neurons of the striatum. Dopamine is released from the brain stem and some adjoining hypothalamic neurons but certainly not from striatal neurons. The neostriatum receives cortical inputs that utilize glutamate, but glutamate is not typically released from efferent fibers of the neostriatum.

399. The answer is c. (*Kandel, pp 853-864. Siegel and Sapru, pp 343-351.*) The basic principle governing how the basal ganglia control motor activity is that they do so by modulating neurons of the motor cortex and premotor areas (of the ipsilateral side) via synaptic connections in the VL and ventral anterior (VA) nuclei of the thalamus. One can see from the circuits

globus pallidus (medial segment) → VL nucleus → area 4 of cortex
globus pallidus (medial segment) → VA nucleus → area 6 of cortex

that damage to the basal ganglia on one side of the brain will affect cortical neurons on the same side. This will result in dyskinesia expressed on the contralateral side of the body because the corticospinal tract is crossed. The other possibilities listed in the question are not viable. Projections of the basal ganglia to the brain stem nuclei are minimal. The basal ganglia do not project fibers down to the spinal cord, nor do they project to the cerebellum.

400. The answer is c. (*Kandel, pp 833-846. Siegel and Sapru, pp 360-366.*) The principal source of afferent fibers to the flocculonodular lobe is the vestibular complex, in particular, the inferior and medial vestibular nuclei. For this reason, this lobe of the cerebellum is sometimes referred to as the vestibulocerebellum. The red nucleus and cerebral cortex project topographically (via relays in the inferior olivary nucleus and deep pontine nuclei, respectively) to the anterior and posterior lobes. Pathways arising from the spinal cord, such as the spinocerebellar tract, project to the anterior lobe. Other fibers arising from the spinal cord enter the cerebellum through a relay in the inferior olivary nucleus. Such fibers terminate in both anterior and posterior lobes.

401. The answer is c. (*Kandel, pp 864-866. Siegel and Sapru, pp 353-354.*) In Huntington disease, the essential neurochemical change is in the basal ganglia, where there is a significant reduction in the two transmitters ACh and GABA. In particular, there are reduced levels of enzymes associated with the synthesis of ACh and GABA (ie, choline acetyltransferase, glutamic acid decarboxylase, respectively), and GABA, directly.

402. The answer is c. *(Kandel, pp 864-866. Siegel and Sapru, p 354.)* A lesion of the subthalamic nucleus results in hemiballism, a form of dyskinesia in which the patient displays severe involuntary movements. It is believed to occur as a result of an imbalance in the output signals of the basal ganglia. There is a change in the relationship between efferent pathways associated with the two pallidal segments (ie, a direct pathway from the neostriatum [inhibiting the medial pallidal segment] to the VL and VA nuclei of the thalamus versus indirect pathways, involving connections between the lateral pallidal segment through the subthalamic nucleus [which is excitatory to the medial pallidal segment], as well as projections via the substantia nigra to the thalamus and neostriatum). Thus, in hemiballism the indirect pathway is disrupted, resulting in a change in the output signals of the pallidum to the thalamus.

403. The answer is b. *(Kandel, pp 861-866. Siegel and Sapru, p 354.)* Choreiform movements have generally been associated with damage to the neostriatum (the cortex and the globus pallidus have occasionally been implicated). Normally, there is a balance in what seems to be opposing effects of ACh, dopamine, and GABA in the neostriatum. In this disorder, the levels of ACh and GABA are significantly reduced. This creates an imbalance in which dopamine levels now become (relatively) too high. Accordingly, effective pharmacological treatment involves the use of dopamine receptor blockers.

404. The answer is d. *(Kandel, p 1201. Aminoff, pp 251, 257-258. Siegel and Sapru, p 354.)* Tardive dyskinesia, a disorder involving involuntary movements of the mouth, face, and tongue, is caused by long-term treatment with antipsychotic drugs. This treatment is likely to involve GABA neurons in the basal ganglia because both GABA and the enzyme that synthesizes it, glutamic acid decarboxylase, are depleted after long-term treatment with antipsychotic drugs. It was previously thought that dopamine receptor hypersensitivity could account for the appearance of this disorder because it could be brought on with haloperidol treatment. However, a dopamine receptor hypothesis is not probable because this form of dyskinesia does not always appear when supersensitivity is present following long-term drug treatment. Moreover, supersensitivity can be reversible following discontinuation of the drug, while tardive dyskinesia would still be present. Other transmitter systems have not been implicated in this disorder.

405. The answer is c. *(Kandel, pp 862-864. Siegel and Sapru, pp 351-353.)* MPTP was discovered by accident when drug abusers who were using a synthetic heroin derivative developed signs of Parkinson disease. It was discovered that their drug included the contaminant MPTP. As a consequence, MPTP has been applied systemically in a number of experimental animals, resulting in significant decreases in dopamine content of the brain due to the loss of dopaminergic neurons in the substantia nigra. These animals also developed symptoms similar to those seen in Parkinson patients. For these reasons, this drug is currently being used for research purposes in order to develop a better understanding of this disease and to establish possible drug therapies for its treatment and eventual cure.

406. The answer is a. *(Nolte, pp 494-521. Siegel and Sapru, pp 360-364.)* One of the most important features of the anterior lobe of the cerebellum is that it receives major inputs from structures that mediate information concerning muscle spindle and Golgi tendon organ activity (sometimes referred to as unconscious proprioception). The pathways that mediate unconscious proprioception include the dorsal and ventral spinocerebellar tracts and the cuneocerebellar tract. Accordingly, the cerebellar anterior lobe is sometimes referred to as the spinocerebellum. The fastigial and dentate nuclei receive their principal inputs from the cerebellar cortex, and their axons project out of the cerebellum. The posterior lobe receives few, if any, inputs from pathways that mediate unconscious proprioception information.

407. The answer is c. *(Kandel, pp 833-846. Nolte, pp 502-510. Siegel and Sapru, pp 364-365.)* A unique feature of the connections between the cerebral cortex and the cerebellum is the somatotopically organized projection from the cerebral cortex largely to the cerebellar hemispheres (some fibers terminate in the vermis). The somatotopic maps are arranged in both anterior and posterior lobes in a manner that has the distal musculature functionally represented in the lateral aspect of the hemispheres, while the proximal musculature is represented toward or in the vermal region. Because of this somatotopic arrangement, the lateral hemispheres are concerned with functions associated with detailed movements of the limbs, while more medial regions are concerned with regulation of the proximal musculature (eg, postural mechanisms).

408. The answer is d. (*Kandel, pp 835-837. Siegel and Sapru, pp 367-371.*) The cerebellar glomerulus consists of mossy fiber terminals, Golgi dendrites, axon terminals of Golgi cells, and granule cell dendrites. The flow of information in the glomerulus is as follows: (1) Information reaches the cerebellar cortex through mossy fibers. (2) Axon terminals of mossy fibers terminate upon dendrites of either granule or Golgi cells. (3) Collaterals of parallel fibers (axons of granule cells) may contact dendrites of Golgi cells, whose axons then feed back onto the granule cells. (4) Mossy fiber terminals synapse with Golgi cell dendrites, whose axons then make synaptic contact with the granule cell (feed forward mechanism). The axons of the granule cells run parallel to the cortex and perpendicular to the orientation of the Purkinje cell dendrites with which they synapse. The circuitry for feedback and feed-forward mechanisms is as follows:

Feedback mechanism
Mossy fiber axon terminal → granule cell dendrites → granule cell axon
  → Golgi cell dendrites → Golgi cell axon → (inhibits) granule cell

Feed-forward mechanism
Mossy fiber axon terminal → Golgi cell dendrites → Golgi cell axon
  → (inhibits) granule cell

409. The answer is c. (*Siegel and Sapru, pp 357-376.*) This patient presented with a disorder associated with a lesion of the cerebellar hemisphere. This region of the cerebellar cortex is linked anatomically and functionally with the cerebral cortex. Its linkage is through the dentate nucleus, whose axons project to the VL thalamic nucleus, which in turn, project to the motor and premotor regions of the cerebral cortex. This feedback is essential for producing smooth, accurate movements of the limbs that are well coordinated. Loss of such feedback thus results in the deficits seen in this patient. Other regions listed in this question bear no relation to this disorder but relate to other functions such as balance, modulation of muscle tone, and posture.

410. The answer is d. (*Siegel and Sapru, pp 357-376.*) As noted in the explanation to the previous question (Question 409), the cerebellar cortex projects to the motor and premotor regions of the cerebral cortex as part of an important feedback pathway linking the cerebral and cerebellar cortices.

411. The answer is b. *(Siegel and Sapru, pp 367-370.)* Purkinje cells are inhibitory neurons whose axons supply the deep cerebellar nuclei. The Purkinje cells of the lateral aspects of the hemispheres supply the dentate nucleus; those in the intermediate region supply the interposed nuclei; and those situated in the vermal region supply the fastigial nucleus. The outputs of the cerebellum to the other regions (with the exception of spinal cord) listed in this question receive their direct inputs from deep cerebellar nuclei. The spinal cord receives its inputs from cerebellum only indirectly, via cerebellar projections to such regions as the red nucleus, cerebral cortex, vestibular nuclei, and reticular formation.

412. The answer is d. *(Ropper, pp 1124-1126. Siegel and Sapru, pp 375-376.)* The CT scan revealed the presence of significant alcoholic cerebellar degeneration showing folial atrophy of the anterior aspect of the cerebellar vermis, which is characteristic of this disorder. Damage to this region of cerebellum typically induces a broad-based gait ataxia of the legs. The other choices are not correct. Spasticity is characteristic of an upper motor neuron disorder involving the corticospinal tract; rigidity is associated mainly with decerebration (at pontine or midbrain levels of brainstem); an intention tremor is associated with the cerebellar hemispheres, and not the vermal region; a movement disorder at rest is associated with damage to the basal ganglia.

413. The answer is e. *(Nolte, pp 505-517. Siegel and Sapru, pp 375-376.)* Since the flocculonodular lobe receives and integrates inputs from the vestibular system, it is understandable why lesions that disrupt this integrating mechanism for vestibular inputs would result in difficulties in maintaining balance. Indeed, this is a classic feature of lesions of the flocculonodular lobe but is not associated with lesions in the hemispheres of the posterior lobe, the anterior limb of the internal capsule, or the dentate nucleus, which are functionally linked to the frontal lobe. Lesions of the anterior lobe also do not affect mechanisms of balance.

414 and 415. The answers are 414-c and 415-d. *(Ropper, pp 1033-1045. Kandel, pp 861-866, 1306-1309. Siegel and Sapru, pp 350-353.)* The patient has Parkinson disease, a degenerative condition caused by progressive loss of dopaminergic cells in the substantia nigra, pars compacta. This is an area that controls the speed and spontaneity of movement, so damage to this area can produce deficits that include a slow, shuffling gait with a tendency to move progressively faster (festinating gait); problems with maintaining size in handwriting, with a tendency to write with small letters (micrographia); masklike facial expression with a paucity of eyeblinks; and difficulty getting out of a chair. Other problems include a soft, monotonous voice; muscle rigidity (lead-pipe rigidity); a tremor at rest that is "pill-rolling"; and a combination of a tremor and rigidity, especially in the arms, which, when flexion is attempted, elicits a "cogwheeling" property. Failure to swallow with a normal frequency makes drooling a problem. Dementia (senility) is also a problem with Parkinson patients, especially later in the course of the disease. The blood supply to the substantia nigra arises from the posterior circulation, specifically the posteromedial branches of the posterior cerebral artery and branches of the posterior communicating artery. The lenticulostriate branches of the middle cerebral artery supply other portions of the basal ganglia, such as the striatum and the globus pallidus. The anterior choroidal artery also supplies some of the telencephalic nuclei of the basal ganglia.

416. The answer is c. *(Ropper, pp 1033-1045. Kandel, pp 861-866, 1306-1309. Siegel and Sapru, pp 350-353.)* The majority of cells that are lost in this disease are dopaminergic cells in the substantia nigra, pars compacta. Only the pars compacta region of the substantia nigra contains dopaminergic neurons. Glutamate, norepinephrine, and GABA have not been implicated in Parkinson disease. While some treatment strategies for Parkinson disease involve regulation of acetylcholine in the neostriatum, deficiencies in this neurotransmitter have not been linked to this disorder.

417. The answer is e. *(Ropper, pp 1033-1045. Kandel, pp 861-866, 1306-1309. Siegel and Sapru, pp 350-353.)* Medications are currently available to lessen the symptoms of Parkinson disease. Some of these medications contain various concentrations of L-DOPA, an immediate precursor to dopamine which can cross the blood-brain barrier. Dopamine itself does not cross the blood-brain barrier, so it cannot be directly replaced.

418. The answer is b. *(Ropper, pp 1156-1157. Kandel, pp 861-866, 1306-1309. Siegel and Sapru, pp 350-353.)* Medications that antagonize the breakdown of catecholamines by monoamine oxidase can increase the amount of dopamine available for the remaining cells in the substantia nigra.

419 and 420. The answers are 419-c and 420-d. *(Kandel, pp 833-849, 879-885. Ropper, pp 84-86, 112-115. Siegel and Sapru, pp 360-376.)* An ataxic gait is an unsteady gait. Gaits due to motor weakness or spasticity tend to involve circling of the weak leg (circumduction); festinating or shuffling, which are often due to parkinsonism or disease of the basal ganglia, involve a stooped posture with shuffling of the feet and very small steps. An ataxic gait may result from motor incoordination due to cerebellar disease or from lack of proprioception in the lower extremities due to disease in the posterior column system (gait becomes unsteady when a patient is unable to detect the location of his or her feet). Degeneration of both systems may occur due to alcoholism, although in this case we are told that the patient does not have any sensory deficits when this modality is tested in isolation. This is an example of alcoholic cerebellar degeneration.

421. The answer is b. *(Ropper, pp 1124-1126. Kandel, pp 861-866, 1306-1309. Siegel and Sapru, pp 360-376.)* As noted in Answers 419 and 420, chronic alcoholism can lead to degeneration (probably through nutritional deficiency) of neurons in the cerebellar cortex, particularly of the Purkinje cells, and is usually restricted to anterior and superior parts of the vermis, as well as anterior portions of the anterior lobes. For this reason, most of the deficits in this syndrome involve midline structures such as the trunk, which are represented mainly in the vermis (whose major projection is to the fastigial nucleus). Trunk instability usually causes problems with gait. In addition, because the cerebellar homunculus represents the legs in the anterior portion of the anterior lobe, the legs are affected more than the arms. Loss of volume within the vermis of the cerebellum is readily visualized, especially on an MRI of the brain, because this technique allows good visualization of the posterior fossa. If these changes are visualized, then the condition is most likely chronic (as also indicated by the history) and most likely irreversible. However, it is important to make sure that the patient is well nourished, takes vitamins, (especially vitamin B_1 [thiamine]), and stops drinking in order to prevent other neurological problems from occurring. Damage to other brain regions listed does not cause such effects.

422. The answer is b. (*Ropper, pp 78-83. Kandel, pp 861-866, 1306-1309. Siegel and Sapru, pp 360-376.*) The spinocerebellum receives sensory inputs from the spinal cord and is instrumental in controlling posture and movement. It includes the vermis and the intermediate hemisphere. The cerebrocerebellum consists of the lateral hemispheres and is instrumental in the planning of movement. The dentate nucleus comprises the cell bodies that form the superior cerebellar peduncle. The middle cerebellar peduncle transmits signals from the cerebral cortex to the cerebellar hemispheres and is not linked to this disorder.

423. The answer is c. (*Ropper, pp 78-83. Kandel, pp 861-866, 1306-1309. Siegel and Sapru, pp 360-376.*) The spinocerebellar cortical (Purkinje) cells project mainly to the fastigial nucleus. The interposed nuclei receive inputs from the intermediate zone of the hemispheres; the dentate nucleus receives inputs from the lateral aspect of the hemispheres; the superior cerebellar peduncle contains the axons of the interposed and dentate nuclei.

424. The answer is e. (*Ropper, pp 78-83. Kandel, pp 861-866, 1306-1309. Siegel and Sapru, pp 360-376.*) Purkinje cells are found in the cerebellar cortex. None of the other choices are cells that are found in the cerebellum.

425 and 426. The answers are 425-d and 426-a. (*Ropper, pp 339-344, 346-355. Kandel, pp 887-888, 898-902, 1307-1311. Siegel and Sapru, p 424.*) The CT scan of the woman's brain revealed a large, acute stroke of her upper pons and midbrain. Strokes of these areas often result from occlusion of the basilar artery and can produce coma or a variant of hypersomnia called *akinetic mutism* or *coma vigil*. An electroencephalogram (EEG) of a patient like this shows a pattern associated with slow-wave sleep, but eye movements are preserved. It is likely that the corticospinal tracts within the pons were damaged during this very large stroke, causing the increased tone from lack of inhibition, as well as the lack of movement in the patient's arms and legs.

427. The answer is c. (*Siegel and Sapru, pp 500-501.*) The stroke involved branches of the posterior cerebral artery that supply the midbrain, and in particular, the structures affected in this case (see explanation for Question 428). The anterior and middle cerebral arteries supply the forebrain and not the midbrain. The superior cerebellar artery supplies the dorsolateral aspects of the rostral pons and caudal midbrain and does not affect the structures damaged in this stroke. Likewise, the posterior inferior cerebellar artery supplies the dorsolateral medulla and the structures affected by this artery cannot account for the deficits seen in this patient.

428. The answer is c. (*Siegel and Sapru, pp 500-501.*) This constellation of deficits point to Weber syndrome (or superior alternating hemiplegia) in which there is inability to move the eye medially coupled with contralateral limb paralysis. The structures affected include the oculomotor nerve and cerebral peduncle. The other choices were incorrect because none included damage to the oculomotor nerve, which was affected by the stroke in this case.

429. The answer is a. (*Siegel and Sapru, pp 500-502.*) This case is an example of a caudal basal pontine syndrome. The constellation of deficits were due to damage from a stroke involving the medial branches of the basilar artery affecting axons of cranial nerve VI, which pass ventrally through the basilar pons before exiting the brain stem. In addition, parts of the basilar pons containing the descending corticospinal fibers, which control movements of the contralateral limbs, were also affected. The other choices are incorrect because they do not include all of these structures which were damaged by the stroke.

Higher Functions

Questions

Questions 430 and 431

430. A 67-year-old man suffers an infarct of the geniculothalamic branch of the posterior cerebral artery. In particular, there is involvement of nuclei of the posterior thalamus. Which of the following is the most likely effect of such an infarct?

a. Emotional volatility in response to an innocuous statement
b. Short-term memory loss that occurs about 1 week following the infarct
c. Long-term memory loss that occurs about 1 month following the infarct
d. Severe pain triggered by cutaneous stimuli applied to the patient
e. Spastic paralysis of the contralateral limbs

431. In the patient in Question 430, which of the following regions would the neurons affected by this infarction normally project?

a. Hypothalamus and midbrain
b. Parietal and occipital cortices
c. Precentral and postcentral gyri
d. Basal ganglia and premotor cortex
e. Prefrontal cortex and medial aspect of the frontal lobe

432. A 52-year-old woman has an infarct involving a branch of the posterior communicating artery, causing damage to the ventral anterior (VA), ventrolateral (VL), dorsomedial, and anterior thalamic nuclei. Which of the following is the most likely clinical manifestation of this infarct?

a. Hemiparesis and neuropsychological impairment
b. Loss of sleep and apnea
c. Loss of appetite and thermoregulation
d. Total blindness of the contralateral eye
e. Marked endocrine dysfunction

433. A 55-year-old female experienced a sudden onset of a new, unusually severe headache of a generalized nature, the type of which she previously never experienced. The patient was admitted to a local hospital and it was noted that she appeared to have an acute elevation of blood pressure. Which of the following is the most likely source or basis for the headache experienced by this patient?

a. Trigeminal neuralgia
b. An intracranial mass
c. Migraine
d. Subarachnoid hemorrhage
e. Tension

434. A 21-year-old male is examined by a neurologist after complaining of headaches. He complains of throbbing pain in his head that comes on over a period of minutes, affecting mainly one side of his head, and then dissipating, only to return later in the week. This type of headache had been bothering this patient for approximately 5 years. The neurologist concluded that the patient suffered from migraine. Which of the following drugs might he have recommended that the patient be given?

a. Haloperidol
b. Sumatriptan
c. Topiramate
d. Carbamazepine
e. Vigabatrin

Questions 435 and 436

435. A patient has an infarct involving the medial branches of the basilar root of the posterior cerebral artery. The primary region affected includes nuclei of the medial thalamus. Which of the following effects would most likely result from the infarct?

a. Grand mal epilepsy
b. Severe acute depression and hyperphagia
c. Drowsiness and abnormalities in memory and attention
d. Marked somatosensory loss, including pain and temperature
e. Upper motor neuron (UMN) paralysis

436. Concerning the patient described in Question 435, the most likely basis for the behavioral and neurological effects of the infarct is the loss of processing of information from which of the following structures?

a. Hypothalamus
b. Parietal cortex
c. Reticular formation
d. Amygdala
e. Hippocampal formation

437. A patient is admitted to a local mental health clinic after experiencing significant loss of emotional affect. An MRI reveals an infarct that affects a region of the thalamus. Which of the following structures is consequently deprived of significant input as constitutes the major output of the mediodorsal thalamic nucleus?

a. Precentral gyrus
b. Postcentral gyrus
c. Prefrontal cortex
d. Posterior parietal lobe
e. Temporal lobe

438. A 67-year-old female suffers a stroke limited to a region of the superior temporal gyrus. Which of the following structures provides the primary input to the superior temporal gyrus?

a. Centromedian (CM) thalamic nucleus
b. Medial geniculate thalamic nucleus
c. Lateral geniculate thalamic nucleus
d. Dorsomedial thalamic nucleus
e. Anterior thalamic nucleus

439. A 69-year-old female suffered an infarction on the left side of her brain and presented with the following signs: sensory loss on the right side of her body, paresthesia, and thalamic pain. Which of the following regions were affected by the infarction?

a. Posterior thalamic nuclei
b. Anterior thalamic nuclei
c. Medial hypothalamic nuclei
d. Lateral hypothalamus
e. Neostriatum

440. A patient was diagnosed with having a brain infarct and presented primarily with contralateral hemiparesis and dysarthria. Which of the following regions were affected by the infarct?

a. Medial thalamic nuclei
b. Lateral thalamic nuclei
c. Dorsomedial thalamus
d. Ventromedial thalamus
e. Medial hypothalamus

441. A middle-aged male was having difficulty sleeping and was referred to a sleep clinic. The diagnostician specifically sought to determine whether the patient showed rapid eye movement (REM) sleep on the recorded electroencephalogram (EEG) activity. What kind of activity should the diagnostician look for in order to determine the presence of REM sleep?

a. Slow-wave EEGs
b. Sleep spindles
c. Rapid low-voltage EEGs
d. High-voltage biphasic waves
e. An increase in most skeletal muscle tone

442. A 47-year-old male had difficulty in sleeping and was sent to a sleep clinic where he was seen by a neurologist. An analysis of his sleep patterns revealed a relative absence of an REM sleep throughout the course of the study of her sleep states. A subsequent MRI revealed the presence of a small vascular lesion in the brain that the neurologist believed accounted for the absence of his REM sleep patterns and poor overall sleep. Which of the structures listed below is likely to be damaged and thus account for his loss of REM sleep?

a. Spinal cord—medulla border
b. Rostral aspect of the medulla
c. Rostral aspect of the pons
d. Tectal aspect of the rostral midbrain
e. Hypothalamic-thalamic border

443. A study was conducted using a first-year medical student as a subject in order to identify the EEG pattern present during relaxed periods of wakefulness. Assuming that the student was "normal," which of the following EEG rhythms would most likely be present during this period?

a. α-Rhythms (8-13 Hz)
b. β-Rhythms (13-30 Hz)
c. θ-Rhythms (4-7 Hz)
d. δ-Rhythms (0.5-4 Hz)
e. Spike and wave activity

444. A patient is confused and displays localized jerks in his right hand, which progress to jerks of the entire arm with a brief loss of consciousness. Which of the following best characterizes this disorder?

a. Generalized seizure
b. Absence seizure
c. Simple partial seizure
d. Complex partial seizure
e. Petit mal epilepsy

445. A 45-year-old male had been receiving drug therapy for the treatment of complex partial seizures when he suffered a deterioration of his condition. One day he fell to the ground with a further loss of consciousness in which all of his extremities were extended and rigid, and jerks of these limbs were displayed as well. Which of the following best characterizes his new condition?

a. Generalized seizure
b. Absence seizure
c. Simple partial seizure
d. Complex partial seizure
e. Petit mal epilepsy

446. A middle-aged male patient was referred to an endocrinologist by his family physician after displaying excessive urination and thirst. He was diagnosed as having diabetes insipidus probably induced by a cranio-pharyngioma of the posterior aspect of the pituitary, thus impairing the release of vasopressin from the posterior pituitary. However, it is synthe-sized elsewhere. In which of the following structures is it synthesized?

a. Mammillary bodies
b. Lateral hypothalamus
c. Supraoptic hypothalamic nucleus
d. Ventromedial hypothalamic nucleus
e. Posterior hypothalamus

447. An 18-year-old female was seen by several specialists in endocrinol-ogy and neurology after reporting chronic hypothermia. An MRI revealed the presence of a small tumor in the brain. Which of the following is the most likely location of this tumor?

a. Septal area
b. Hippocampal formation
c. Amygdala
d. Anterior hypothalamus
e. Posterior hypothalamus

448. A 34-year-old female developed a tumor that impinged upon the supraoptic nucleus. Which of the following functions was affected by this tumor?

a. Feeding behavior
b. Temperature regulation
c. Sexual behavior
d. Short-term memory functions
e. Water balance

449. Following a routine examination, a tumor was detected mainly in the lateral hypothalamus in a 26-year-old male. Sometime afterward, he began to display a significant change in behavior. Which of the following disorders best characterizes this behavior?

a. Hyperphagia
b. Alcoholism
c. Hypersexuality
d. Aphagia
e. Hypertension

450. A child of 10 years was suffering from growth retardation. An endocrinological and neurological examination suggested a dysfunction in hypothalamic neurons that regulate growth hormone. The most likely locus of these neurons that are incapable of releasing growth hormone is which of the following?

a. Supraoptic nucleus
b. Paraventricular nucleus
c. Lateral hypothalamus
d. Arcuate nucleus
e. Mammillary bodies

451. A 49-year-old male showed changes in emotional behavior over the past few months. Several characteristics of his behavior included heightened sexuality, a very placid appearance, and making physical contact with almost anything that he could touch. The neurologist's diagnosis was that the patient was exhibiting Klüver-Bucy syndrome. A magnetic resonance imaging (MRI) was performed on the patient and a small vascular lesion was detected. Which of the following structures most likely contains the lesion?

a. Septal area
b. Amygdala
c. Cingulate gyrus
d. Medial hypothalamus
e. Lateral hypothalamus

452. A middle-aged female, who was suffering from a rare autosomal recessive condition that results in calcification and degeneration of specific regions of the forebrain, was seen by a psychiatrist. The patient was given a battery of tests and was found to be unable to recognize fear in pictures presented to her. Nor was she able to draw a picture depicting fear while she was capable of drawing pictures depicting other emotions. An MRI indicated significant atrophy of tissue in a specific region of the brain. Which of the regions indicated below is the most likely target of this rare autosomal recessive condition?

a. Mammillary bodies
b. Septal area
c. Amygdala
d. Cingulate gyrus
e. Lateral hypothalamus

453. A 19-year-old male began to have delusional thoughts which increased progressively over time. He was seen by a psychiatrist who concluded that he was suffering from a form of schizophrenia. In terms of our present understanding of schizophrenia, which of the following is believed to be linked most closely to the development of this disorder?

a. Environmental factors rather than genetic ones
b. Increases in brain dopamine levels
c. Increases in brain serotonin levels
d. Decreases in brain endorphin levels
e. Decreases in brain neuropeptide levels

454. A 62-year-old male had been a chronic alcoholic for approximately 25 years. He was tested by a psychologist and was found to be unable to form new declarative memories. In effect, the deficit involved severe anterograde and retrograde amnesia and confabulation. Which of the structures listed below is most closely associated with the locus of the lesion?

a. Superior parietal cortex
b. Habenular nucleus
c. Lateral thalamic nuclei
d. Mammillary bodies
e. Caudate nucleus

455. A boy was severely bitten by a dog and later developed a rabies infection which was not treated. The infection affected and destroyed a group of anatomical structures subserving short-term memory functions, thus resulting in severe memory deficits. Which of the following groups of structures were most likely destroyed?

a. Hippocampal formation, mammillary bodies, anterior thalamic nucleus, prefrontal cortex
b. Hippocampal formation, septal area, hypothalamus, midbrain periaqueductal gray
c. Hippocampal formation, mammillary bodies, anterior thalamic nucleus, cingulate gyrus
d. Amygdala, hippocampal formation, mammillary bodies, septal area, prefrontal cortex
e. Prefrontal cortex, hippocampal formation, septal area, medial hypothalamus, prefrontal cortex

Question 456 and 457

456. The T2-weighted MRI scan on the left side of the figure below is of a normal patient. In the CT scan on the right side, the patient sustained a right cerebral hemorrhage, indicated by the large white area. Which of the following deficits most likely resulted from the cerebrovascular accident?

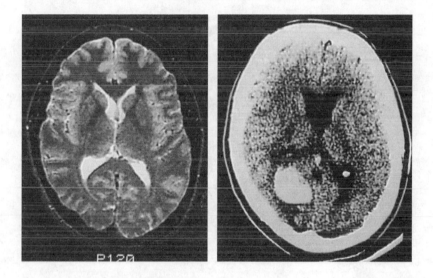

a. Right homonymous hemianopsia
b. Left homonymous hemianopsia
c. Loss of intellectual and emotional processes
d. Aphasia
e. Hemiparesis of the right side of the body

457. Based on the figure in Question 456, which of the following blood vessels was affected by the cerebrovascular accident?

a. Anterior cerebral artery
b. Middle cerebral artery
c. Posterior cerebral artery
d. Superior cerebellar artery
e. Striate arteries

Questions 458 and 459

458. The CT scan shown in the accompanying figure below reveals that the patient has a glioma (T) on the right side of the brain. Which of the following has the patient most likely sustained?

R   L

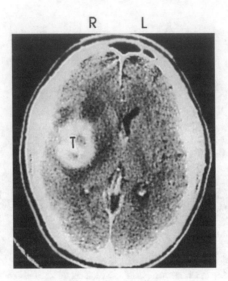

a. A UMN paralysis of the left side
b. Dyskinesia
c. Intention tremor
d. Upper left quadrantanopia
e. Upper right quadrantanopia

459. In the figure in Question 458, which of the following structures was most likely damaged by the tumor?

a. Lentiform nucleus only
b. Internal capsule only
c. Thalamus only
d. Lentiform nucleus and internal capsule
e. Lentiform nucleus, internal capsule, and thalamus

Questions 460 and 461

460. The patient, whose CT scan is shown in the figure, sustained an occlusion of a major artery on the left side of the brain. Which of the following deficits is most likely present in this patient?

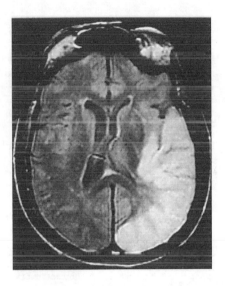

a. A right homonymous hemianopsia only
b. Aphasia only
c. A right homonymous hemianopsia coupled with aphasia
d. Marked intellectual deficits
e. Marked intellectual deficits coupled with hemiballism

461. In the figure in Question 460, which of the following blood vessels is occluded?

a. Anterior cerebral artery
b. Middle cerebral artery
c. Posterior cerebral artery
d. Posterior choroidal artery
e. Superior cerebellar artery

Questions 462 and 463

462. The vertebral angiogram in the given figure reveals the effects of a severe motorcycle accident upon a 21-year-old woman. As a result of the accident, from which of the following does she most likely suffer?

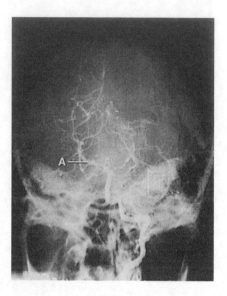

a. A UMN paralysis of the right side of the body
b. A right homonymous hemianopsia
c. A left upper quadrantanopia
d. Aphasia
e. Dyskinesia

463. In the figure in Question 462, which of the following arteries was occluded on the left side and labeled in the figure on the normal side as A?

a. Vertebral
b. Basilar
c. Middle cerebral
d. Anterior cerebral
e. Posterior cerebral

464. The MRI scan in the following figure reveals a large chromophobe adenoma (T) of the pituitary that impinges on the adjoining brain tissue. The patient suffered pituitary insufficiency as well as visual deficits. Which of the following dysfunctions is the result of this tumor?

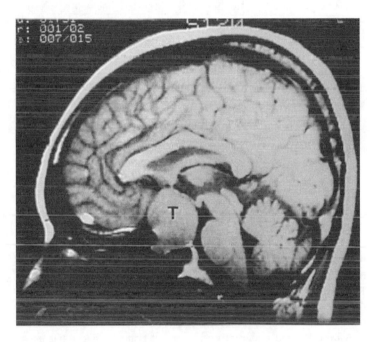

a. Binasal hemianopsia
b. Bitemporal hemianopsia
c. Loss of the accommodation reflex
d. Loss of the pupillary light reflex
e. Loss of conjugate gaze

Questions 465 and 466

465. A previously healthy 68-year-old woman experienced twitching of her left finger that soon extended to her hand, arm, shoulder, and then to her leg. At this point, she became unconscious. Her legs and arms began to jerk for several minutes and her neck extended backward. She did not respond to comments or requests by people who were near her. She was admitted to a hospital, at which time, she regained consciousness but was able to answer some questions such as identifying the present month. She had better movement of right side of her body than her left but was some-what ineffective in following commands given by her physician. From which area of the brain did the seizure most likely begin?

a. Left precentral gyrus
b. Right precentral gyrus
c. Right temporal lobe
d. Left temporal lobe
e. Thalamus

466. In the patient in Question 465, which of the following most likely accounts for her loss of consciousness following the seizure?

a. Involvement of the reticular activating system
b. Head trauma
c. Bilateral postictal suppression
d. Thalamic involvement
e. Brain hemorrhage from the seizure

467. A middle-aged male with a history of epilepsy had what began as a focal seizure, but which led to clonic motor activity that spread in a systematic fashion from thumb, finger, wrist, arm, and then to the leg. Which of the following best explains the spread of this clonic activity?

a. Proximity of the body part to the spinal cord
b. Proximity of the body part to the cerebral cortex
c. Somatotopic representation within the brain stem
d. Somatotopic representation within the basal ganglia
e. Somatotopic representation within the precentral gyrus

468. A patient with temporal lobe epilepsy is treated with a drug designed to inhibit the principal cell type responsible for the seizures. Which of the following cell types is targeted by this drug?

a. Basket cell
b. Purkinje cell
c. Stellate cell
d. Schwann cell
e. Pyramidal cell

469. An animal preparation was used for the study of the electrophysiological properties associated with epileptic seizures in which the type of potentials essential for the initiation of seizures was identified. Which of the following bursts of potentials noted in this study is linked to the initiation of seizures?

a. Inhibitory postsynaptic potentials (IPSPs)
b. Membrane potentials
c. Resting potentials
d. Excitatory postsynaptic potentials (EPSPs)
e. Nernst potential

470. A 32-year-old male was suffering from epilepsy and was administered a drug that could antagonize the basic neurochemical process associated with the generation of seizures. Which of the following is the most likely mechanism for the generation of seizures for which drug therapy could apply?

a. Na^+ channel blockade
b. γ-Aminobutyric acid (GABA) inhibition
c. Glutamate inhibition
d. Aspartate inhibition
e. Substance P inhibition

Questions 471 and 472

471. A 76-year-old woman who has a 10-year history of high blood pressure and diabetes was reaching for a jar of flour to make an apple pie, when her right side suddenly gave out, and she collapsed. While trying to get up from the floor, she noticed that she was unable to move her right arm or leg. She attempted to cry for help because she was unable to reach the telephone; however, her speech was slurred and rather unintelligible. She lay on the floor and waited for help to arrive. Her son began to worry about his usually prompt mother when she did not arrive with her apple pie. After several attempts to telephone her apartment without getting an answer, he drove there and found her lying on the floor. She attempted to tell him what had happened, but her speech was too slurred to comprehend. Assuming that his mother had had a stroke, the son called an ambulance. A neurology resident was called to see the patient in the emergency room because the physicians there likewise thought that she had a stroke. The resident noted that she followed commands very well, and, although her speech was very slurred, it was logical in organization. The lower two-thirds of her face drooped on the right. Her tongue pointed to the right side when she was asked to protrude it. Her right arm and leg were severely, but equally, weak; her left side had normal strength. She felt a pin and a vibrating tuning fork equally on both sides. Where in the central nervous system (CNS) did her stroke most likely occur?

a. Left precentral gyrus
b. Right precentral gyrus
c. Left basilar pons or left internal capsule
d. Right putamen or globus pallidus
e. Left thalamus

472. In the patient in Question 471, a CT scan revealed a new infarct in the left internal capsule. Which of the following arteries was occluded, causing the stroke?

a. Lenticulostriate branches of the middle cerebral artery
b. Posterior cerebral artery
c. Anterior cerebral artery
d. Vertebral artery
e. Posterior choroidal artery

473. An elderly male patient in a hospital suffered an extensive stroke following a procedure to repair a defect in a heart valve. When the patient regained consciousness, a neurological examination revealed a paralysis of his left arm and leg, as well as inability to recognize a pin prick or tuning fork on his left leg or arm. Other sensory and motor functions of the face appeared normal. Which of the following constitutes the most likely regions damaged by the stroke?

a. Prefrontal and primary motor cortices
b. Primary motor and somatosensory cortices
c. Premotor and posterior parietal cortices
d. Genu of internal capsule
e. Inferior and middle frontal gyri

474. An 86-year-old female suffered a stroke that left her paralyzed over her right side of the body, including both arm and leg. In addition, the lower jaw deviated to the right and her tongue also extended to the right when asked to protrude it. When she was asked to raise her eyebrows, her forehead appeared symmetric. Which of the following best explains why her forehead was spared from weakness?

a The forehead is innervated by different fibers originating in the postcentral gyrus.
b. There are two cranial nerves innervating the forehead.
c. The forehead is represented bilaterally at the cortical level.
d. The forehead is stronger than the rest of the face.
e. Thalamic regions receiving inputs from the forehead contain few inhibitory neurons.

475. An elderly male suffered a stroke that appeared to involve the left internal capsule rather than the cerebral cortex. It resulted in paralysis of the right arm and leg, the tongue deviated to the right side when he was asked to protrude it; lower (jaw) facial expression on the right side was lost, and his speech was slurred, but fluent and grammatically correct. Which of the following best describes the speech deficit in this patient?

a. Wernicke aphasia
b. Broca aphasia
c. Anomia
d. Dysarthria
e. Conduction aphasia

Questions 476 and 477

476. A 12-year-old girl has no history of medical problems. One day, while in the kitchen with her mother, she told her mother that she felt very frightened all of a sudden and had a funny feeling in her stomach. Immediately after this, she turned her head to the right, stared persistently, and began to chew. Her mother called her name several times, but the girl who was usually very obedient, did not answer. After approximately 1 minute of staring, she slowly turned her head back to her mother. Apparently confused, she asked her mother where she was. Over the next 10 to 15 minutes, she became less and less confused, and by the time she was in the car being driven to the pediatrician by her mother, she felt like she was back to normal. The pediatrician listened to patient's mother's story when they arrived. He examined the patient and could find no abnormalities on general physical examination or on neurological examination. The pediatrician told her mother that he would refer her daughter to a pediatric neurologist for further evaluation, as well as further evaluation of the need for medication. Which of the following is the most likely diagnosis?

a. Attention deficit disorder (ADD)
b. Temporary psychosis
c. Conversion disorder
d. Epilepsy
e. Schizophrenia

477. In the diagnosis in Question 476, from which area of the brain is this problem most likely emanating?

a. Medulla
b. Occipital lobe
c. Temporal lobe
d. Thalamus
e. Midbrain

478. A 67-year-old male has been treated by drugs for complex partial seizures for the past 5 years. Recently, his behavior appeared more irrational. He displayed an erratic temperament, in which he would scream at people for little or no reason, and also showed "road rage" that he had not displayed before. He was treated by both a neurologist and psychiatrist and given an MRI, which revealed a tumor situated in the medial aspect of the left midtemporal lobe. Both the neurologist and psychiatrist believe that the tumor is responsible for the irrational behavior because it has an excitatory effect upon neurons that innervate and influence the hypothalamic functions. If this hypothesis is correct, which of the following pathways is activated as a result of the presence of the tumor?

a. Stria medullaris
b. Medial forebrain bundle
c. Stria terminalis
d. Mammillothalamic tract
e. Ansa lenticularis

Questions 479 and 480

479. A patient had been suffering from a rare degenerative disorder that selectively destroyed neurons of the hippocampal formation. As a result, there was a significant loss of inputs into regions of the forebrain that normally receive information from the hippocampal formation. Which of the following groups of structures are directly affected by the loss of neurons in the hippocampal formation?

a. Septal area, anterior thalamic nucleus, mammillary bodies
b. Cingulate gyrus, amygdala, mediodorsal thalamic nucleus
c. Habenular complex, globus pallidus, caudate nucleus
d. Septal area, olfactory tubercle, cingulate gyrus
e. Mammillary bodies, mediodorsal thalamic nucleus, paraventricular nucleus

480. In the patient in Question 479, which of the following deficits is most likely to develop?

a. Hemiparesis
b. Diminished memory function
c. Diminished sensation
d. Improved attention
e. Dyslexia

Questions 481 and 482

481. One morning, an 82-year-old male found that it was difficult for him to walk as his left foot collapsed. He called 911 for assistance and noticed that his speech was slurred. The emergency room physician noted, in addition to his speech, the following deficits: his left arm and leg were markedly weak and muscle tone was flaccid. Reflexes were depressed on the left side but normal on the right side. All sensory modalities were depressed on the left side. The left side of his face drooped and he consistently looked to the right side. When asked to look to the left, his eyes would not move beyond the midline. Likewise, when asked to raise his left hand, he raised his right hand. When asked if his left hand belonged to him, he replied that it did not. The physician drew a circle depicting a clock and the patient was asked to fill in the numbers in the clock. The numbers 1 through 12 were all placed on the right side of the clock. The physician also asked the patient to draw a vertical line that bisected a horizontal line drawn by the physician. The patient drew a vertical line on the right side of the line. When the physician waved his hand in front of the temporal visual field of the left eye or the nasal visual field of the right side, the patient did not blink. Aside from the drooping of the left side of the face (in which the forehead was spared), other cranial nerve functions appeared normal. The physician ordered a CT scan of the patient's head and then admitted him to the hospital for further testing. Which of the following neurological deficits did the patient display?

a. Left hemiparesis, hemineglect, left homonymous hemianopsia, left hemisensory loss
b. Left hemiparesis, right superior quadrantanopsia
c. Left hemiparesis, left hemisensory loss, hemineglect, left superior quadrantanopsia
d. Left hemisensory loss, hemineglect, bitemporal hemianopsia
e. Left hemisensory loss, hemineglect, left superior quadrantanopsia

482. In the patient in Question 481, where in the nervous system has the damage most likely occurred?

a. Left temporal and parietal lobes
b. Right frontal and temporal lobes
c. Right frontal and parietal lobes
d. Left frontal and parietal lobes
e. Left occipital lobe

483. An elderly female patient suffered a stroke resulting in weakness of her left limbs, reduced reflexes in those limbs, inability to gaze to the left and loss of facial expression on the left side, and failure to verbally acknowledge that anything was wrong with the left arm or leg. In this patient, which of the following was most likely occluded?

a. Right anterior cerebral artery
b. Left anterior cerebral artery
c. Right posterior cerebral artery
d. Right middle cerebral artery
e. Left middle cerebral artery

484. A patient is unaware that he cannot move his limbs on the left side of his body and he does not blink his eye in response to the waving of the neurologist's hand in his left upper temporal visual field. Damage to which of the following nerve fibers most likely accounts for this component of the overall deficit?

a. Left facial nerve
b. Right oculomotor nerve
c. Left optic nerve
d. Optic chiasm
e. Right optic radiations

485. A patient is diagnosed with sensory neglect because he is unable to notice the left side of his body. Which of the following regions of the cerebral cortex is most likely damaged in this patient?

a. Left anterior frontal cortex
b. Right anterior frontal cortex
c. Right posterior frontal cortex
d. Right posterior parietal cortex
e. Right anterior parietal cortex

Questions 486 and 487

486. A 79-year-old man was brought to the emergency room because his family was worried that he suddenly was not using his right arm and leg and seemed to have a simultaneous behavior change. He was unable to write a reminder note to himself, even with his left hand, and he put his shoes on the wrong feet. A neurologist was called to the emergency room to examine the patient. A loud bruit was heard with a stethoscope over the left carotid artery in his neck. When asked to show the neurologist his left hand, he pointed to his right hand, since it could not move. The neurologist asked him to add numbers, and he was unable to do this, despite having spent his life as a bookkeeper. The patient was unable to name the fingers on either hand, and he could not form any semblance of a letter using his left hand. The patient's eyes did not blink when the neurologist waved his hands close to them in the left temporal and right nasal visual fields. The right lower two-thirds of his face drooped. There was some asymmetry of his reflexes between the right and left sides, and there was a positive Babinski response of his right toe. Where in the CNS is the damage located?

a. Right frontal and parietal lobes
b. Left frontal and parietal lobes
c. Right frontal lobe
d. Left frontal lobe
e. Right temporal lobe

487. Assuming that the patient in Question 486 had a stroke, which of the following arteries has become occluded?

a. Left anterior cerebral
b. Right anterior cerebral
c. Right middle cerebral
d. Left middle cerebral
e. Left posterior cerebral

488. A 42-year-old male, previously in good health, suddenly became interested in child pornography, showed diminished impulse control, sought sexual favors from office employees, and was later charged with molesting a child. At the urging of his family, he sought the help of a psychiatrist who subsequently referred him to a neurologist. The patient showed evidence of constructional apraxia and agraphia, but other neurological tests appeared normal. An MRI was given and a brain tumor was discovered. Which of the following regions is likely to contain the tumor?

a. Precentral gyrus
b. Orbitofrontal cortex
c. Angular gyrus
d. Superior temporal gyrus
e. Supramarginal gyrus

489. A 73-year-old male is admitted to a local hospital after he first began complaining of headaches, which were then followed by a significant weakness in his right arm and leg, slurred speech, and lack of expression on the right side of the jaw. An MRI reveals the presence of a well-defined brain tumor (shown here). Which of the following structures or regions damaged by the tumor best accounts for the observed deficits?

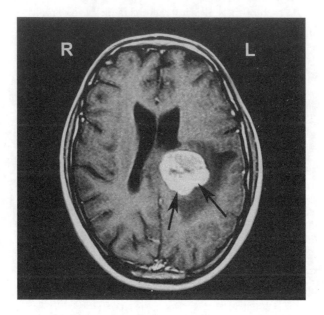

a. Caudate nucleus
b. Globus pallidus
c. Internal capsule
d. Temporal neocortex
e. Dorsal thalamus

490. The family of a 67-year-old female noticed that she was experiencing headaches, having difficulty completing mechanical tasks such as tying her right shoelace, and inability to voluntarily move her eyes to the right. After being hospitalized, an MRI (shown here) revealed the presence of a glioblastoma. Which of the following regions was primarily affected by the tumor that best accounts for the observed deficits?

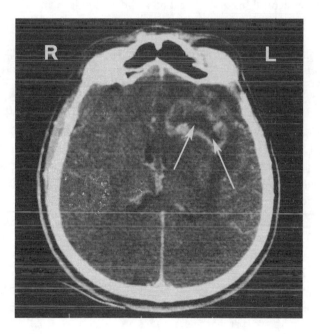

a. Prefrontal cortex
b. Premotor region
c. Precentral gyrus
d. Basal ganglia
e. Posterior limb of internal capsule

Questions 491 and 492

491. A 75-year-old male college graduate, is brought to a neurologist by his family because he is having problems with his gait, suffers from urinary incontinence (for the past 6 months), and recently began to have problems with his short-term memory and paying his bills. The gait problem manifests itself mainly as difficulty climbing stairs and frequent falls. The patient has no past medical history other than a subarachnoid hemorrhage resulting from a ruptured cerebral aneurysm many years earlier. When the neurologist examines him, she finds he cannot remember three objects 5 minutes after they are shown to him, even when prompted. He is unable to figure out how many quarters are in $1.75, and he spells the word "world" incorrectly. A grasp reflex (squeezing the examiner's hand as a reflex reaction to stroking of the palm) is present. Although his motor strength is full in all of his extremities, when asked to walk, he takes many steps in the same place without moving forward, and then starts to fall. His cranial nerve, sensory, and cerebellar examinations are normal. The patient has a grasp reflex and dementia. A lesion in which of the following regions would most likely cause this deficit?

a. Occipital lobe
b. Frontal lobe
c. Medulla
d. Thalamus
e. Pons

492. You are asked to evaluate the patient with the neurologist. The nurse in the office asks if you would like to order a CT scan, and you request one. The CT scan shows that all the ventricles are dilated, especially the frontal horns of the lateral ventricles, without any evidence of obstruction by a tumor. Which of the following is the most likely mechanism underlying the enlargement of the ventricles?

a. Decreased cerebrospinal fluid (CSF) absorption
b. Low blood pressure
c. Decreased CNS blood flow
d. Decreased intracranial pressure
e. High blood pressure

Questions 493 and 494

493. A 38-year-old male is admitted to a hospital after losing consciousness on a number of occasions. During the periods in which consciousness is lost, it is reported that he displays stereotyped motor responses such as lip smacking and scratching. The patient reports to the neurologist that he seems to be in a "dreamy" state. He seems to experiences an altered level of consciousness and feels as if he were detached from his presence state of consciousness. At the same time, the patient has difficulty speaking, displays intense feelings of anxiety, and shows further signs of hallucinations such as flashing lights, voices of unknown people, or unpleasant smells. An MRI is taken (shown here) and a diagnosis is made. An EEG shows the presence of focal spikes, and high-voltage, slow-wave discharges. Which of the following is the most likely diagnosis?

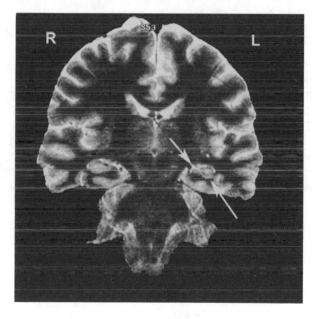

a. Absence seizures
b. Tonic-clonic seizures
c. Pseudoseizures
d. Complex partial seizures
e. Frontal lobe seizures

494. Which of the following regions of the brain, indicated by the arrows, is associated with these seizures?

a. Amygdala
b. Hippocampus
c. Globus pallidus
d. Temporal neocortex
e. Entorhinal cortex

Questions 495 and 496

495. A 75-year-old man, who is right-handed, was told in the past by his internist that he has an irregular heartbeat. The patient decided that he did not wish to learn anything further about this condition, so he did not return to this physician, and it remained untreated. One morning, he awoke to find that his face drooped on the right side and that he could not move his right arm or right leg. When he tried to call an ambulance for help, he had a great deal of difficulty communicating with the operator because his speech was slurred, nonfluent, and missing some pronouns. The call was traced by the police; an ambulance arrived at his house and took him to an emergency room. A neurologist was called to see the patient in the emergency room. When he listened to the patient's heart, he detected an irregular heartbeat. It was very difficult to understand his speech because it was halting, with a tendency to repeat the same phrases over and over. He had difficulty repeating specific sentences given to him by the neurologist, but he was able to follow simple commands such as "Touch your right ear with your left hand." His mouth drooped on the right when he attempted to smile, but his forehead remained symmetric when he wrinkled it. He could not move his right arm at all, but he was able to wiggle his right leg a little bit. Which of the following language problems does this patient have?

a. Dysarthria
b. Wernicke aphasia
c. Broca aphasia
d. Alexia
e. Pure word deafness

496. In the patient in Question 495, which area of the brain was most likely damaged?

a. Internal capsule and thalamus
b. Right occipital lobe
c. Pontine reticular formation
d. Corpus callosum
e. Left precentral gyrus and Broca area

497. A 69-year-old male was admitted to the emergency after losing consciousness. When he regained consciousness, he was examined by a neurologist who concluded that there was an occlusion of one of the arteries supplying the brain. In addition, the neurologist recorded that the patient presented with a marked motor aphasia. Which of the following arteries was most likely occluded in this patient?

a. Anterior cerebral artery
b. Posterior cerebral artery
c. Anterior inferior cerebellar artery
d. Middle cerebral artery
e. Basilar artery

Questions 498 and 499

498. A 49-year-old male began to act in ways that could be described as "anti-social," coupled with what appeared to be intellectual deficits. He was sent for a neurological examination, given an MRI (shown in the figure), and then sent to a neuropsychologist for further examination. The patient was given a card-sorting task in which he was asked to sort the cards on the basis of color, shape, or number. The patient was unable to shift the categorization from shape to number when requested to do so. The patient also continued to perseverate in the use of original strategies in other problem-solving tasks even though those strategies were incorrect. The MRI (shown here) revealed the presence of a brain tumor. Which of the following regions most likely contained the tumor?

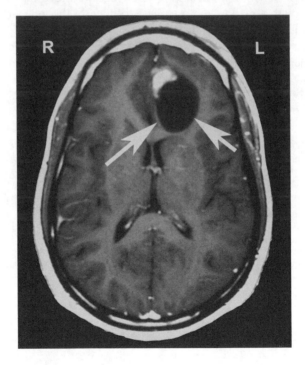

a. Precentral gyrus
b. Prefrontal cortex
c. Premotor cortex
d. Parietal cortex
e. Head of caudate nucleus

499. In the patient in Question 498, what is the primary source of thalamic afferent fibers which project to the region containing the tumor?

a. Anterior thalamic nucleus
b. VA thalamic nucleus
c. Dorsomedial thalamic nucleus
d. Pulvinar nucleus
e. Reticular nucleus

500. A 60-year-old man went to a sleep clinic after he had repeated episodes of loud snoring during sleep, coupled with sudden periods of restlessness, and cessation of breathing. After extensive analysis, the physicians concluded that the patient's problem was not a result of obstructive sleep. Instead, it was judged that this condition reflected central sleep apnea due to loss of chemoreceptor sensitivity of the neuronal control mechanisms governing respiration. Which of the following sites within the CNS is most closely associated with these effects?

a. Dorsal horn of the thoracic spinal cord
b. Reticular formation of the medulla
c. Midbrain periaqueductal gray
d. Hippocampal formation
e. Border of occipital and parietal lobes

Higher Functions

Answers

430 and 431. **The answers are 430-d, 431-b.** *(Afifi, pp 163-168. Ropper, pp 138, 159-160. Siegel and Sapru, pp 264-265, 471-472.)* The infarct caused damage to posterior thalamic nuclei, which may also include VPL and VPM (Dejerine Roussy disease). When these structures are damaged, a disorder referred to as thalamic pain can ensue. In this condition, light cutaneous stimulation is sufficient to produce severe pain. The projections from nuclei situated in this region project principally to the parietal and occipital lobes and play a role in the regulation of pain (although the precise mechanisms remain unknown). The projections to the occipital cortex relate to visual functions of the neurons of the posterior thalamus that are unrelated to pain. The other processes offered as alternate choices have not been shown to be related to functions of the posterior thalamus.

432. **The answer is a.** *(Afifi, pp 157-165, 180-190. Siegel and Sapru, pp 470-475.)* Damage to the VA, VL, dorsomedial, and anterior thalamic nuclei would most likely result in motor impairment such as a hemiparesis (because of the connections of these nuclei with the motor and premotor cortices). Damage to the dorsomedial nucleus could also be linked with neuropsychological impairment because of its connections with the prefrontal cortex and adjoining regions of the frontal lobe. The other processes mentioned in Question 432 have not been shown to be related to these groups of nuclei.

433. **The answer is d.** *(Aminoff, pp 74-92. Ropper, pp 808-816.)* The patient experienced a subarachnoid hemmorrhage in which the headache is typically sudden in onset, very intense, and generalized. The other choices involved sources of headaches which are different; they are either subacute or chronic and typically involve specific anatomical regions.

434. **The answer is b.** *(Aminoff, pp 88-89. Ropper, pp 166-168.)* Sumatriptan, a 5-HT agonist, administered through a nasal spray, is typically given for the treatment of migraine. The other choices involve drugs generally given for the treatment of psychiatric disorders or epilepsy. Haloperidol is a neuroleptic that has sedative properties and is a central dopamine antagonist. Topiramate, carbamazepine, and vigabatrin are anticonvulsant drugs used for the treatment of seizures.

435 and 436. The answers are 435-c and 436-c. *(Afifi, pp 155-168, 350-352.)* An infarct that affects the medial thalamus, which includes the dorsomedial nucleus and midline thalamic and intralaminar nuclei, can result in abnormalities in memory, attention, and drowsiness. The other choices offered for Question 435 have not been shown to be related to functions associated with medial thalamic structures. A key input into the medial thalamus is the reticular formation. In this manner, the medial and intralaminar thalamus represent a relay from reticular formation to the cerebral cortex. Since a major function of the reticular function is to regulate states of sleep and wakefulness, these thalamic nuclei thus contribute to these states. When these nuclei are damaged, this mechanism is affected, resulting in drowsiness.

437. The answer is c. *(Afifi, pp 158-159. Siegel and Sapru, pp 470-475.)* The medial thalamus supplies much of the frontal lobe, and in particular, the prefrontal cortex. In this manner, the medial thalamus would affect the functions of these cortical regions, which involve memory and other cognitive processes as well as affective processes.

438. The answer is b. *(Afifi, p 250. Siegel and Sapru, p 484.)* The superior temporal gyrus is the primary auditory receiving area in the cerebral cortex. Accordingly, the primary afferent source to this region arises from the medial geniculate nucleus, which constitutes a specific thalamic relay for processing of auditory information.

439. The answer is a. *(Afifi, pp 157-170, 172-173. Siegel and Sapru, pp 264-265.)* The primary feature of an infarct of the posterolateral territory (associated with branches of the posterior cerebral artery) is pansensory loss contralateral to the lesion, paresthesia, and thalamic pain. The anterior thalamus and hypothalamus are not involved in this constellation of symptoms. Neither is the neostratum.

440. The answer is b. *(Afifi, pp 157-170, 172-173. Siegel and Sapru, pp 470-475.)* The lateral region of thalamus as well as the posterior limb of internal capsule are supplied by choroidal branches of the internal carotid artery. Infarct of this artery most frequently results in contralateral hemiparesis and dysarthria. Although lesions associated with this artery may affect only motor functions, they may also cause loss of pain, touch, and sometimes visual functions. The other choices given in this question are not associated with this constellation of deficits.

441. The answer is c. (*Kandel, pp 937-940. Siegel and Sapru, pp 422-424.*) REM sleep is characterized by a low-voltage EEG pattern typical of an alert person. For this reason, REM sleep is sometimes referred to as *paradoxical sleep*. Other EEG patterns, such as slow waves, high-voltage EEGs, and sleep spindles, occur at other stages of sleep. In addition, REM sleep is characterized by a general loss of skeletal muscle tone, with the exception of the eye muscles, which govern the REMs.

442. The answer is c. (*Kandel, pp 940-943. Siegel and Sapru, pp 422-423.*) Animal research studies have indicated that the region of the rostral pons bordering on the caudal midbrain contains special sets of cholinergic neurons that are maximally active during REM sleep (and during wakefulness, as well). These neurons are located in the reticular formation. One group of neurons has been identified as the nucleus reticularis pontis oralis. Other neurons include the region of the pedunculopontine nucleus. It appears that these cholinergic neurons depolarize GABAergic neurons, which prevent rhythmic firing of reticular formation neurons. This latter effect allows for the asynchronous firing of thalamocortical neurons that take place during periods of wakefulness and REM sleep.

Therefore, damage to this region would most likely disrupt the REM sleep patterns seen in this patient.

443. The answer is a. (*Kandel, pp 916-917. Siegel and Sapru, pp 422-423.*) During states of quiet wakefulness or drowsiness, the EEG pattern becomes slower (8-13 Hz; average amplitude of 50 V) than what is seen during an alert state. This pattern is called an α-wave.

444. The answer is d. (*Kandel, pp 910-918. Siegel and Sapru, pp 460-463. Aminoff, p 43.*) This person displays a complex partial seizure, which is characterized by a confusional state with brief losses of consciousness. It is called a partial seizure because the seizure involves a localized region, reflected by jerks of the muscles of a specific part of the body. The focus of this seizure is typically in the temporal lobe, such as the amygdala, hippocampal formation, or adjoining cortical regions. A simple partial seizure does not involve loss of consciousness. Absence seizures are nonconvulsive seizures are also called *petit mal epilepsy*. Generalized seizures typically involve many areas of the brain simultaneously and typically involve all of the limbs. The patient falls to the ground and loses consciousness.

445. The answer is a. *(Kandel, pp 910-918. Aminoff, p 43. Siegel and Sapru, pp 460-463.)* The seizure described in this patient has progressed from a complex partial seizure to a generalized seizure. As indicated previously, this type of seizure involves all of the limbs. The patient falls to the ground and typically loses consciousness. As stated in the answer to Question 444, the other choices involve seizures that are characterized differently than what was described in the progression of this case.

446. The answer is c. *(Kandel, p 979. Siegel and Sapru, pp 432-434.)* Certain magnocellular neurons of the hypothalamus synthesize the hormones vasopressin and oxytocin. These include the paraventricular and supraoptic nuclei. The cell bodies of the magnocellular neurons that produce vasopressin are found mostly within the supraoptic nucleus. Vasopressin (antidiuretic hormone) is important because it makes the membranes of the convoluted tubules and collecting ducts of the kidneys more permeable to water. This results in water conservation. Damage to this nucleus or to the posterior pituitary, the target region of the vasopressin neurons, often as the result of a tumor, will induce a disorder called diabetes insipidus, characterized by polyuria and polydipsia.

447. The answer is e. *(Afifi, p 277. Kandel, pp 1000-1002. Siegel and Sapru, p 437.)* The process of temperature regulation requires the integration of autonomic, skeletomuscular, and endocrine responses. For example, dilation of blood vessels of the skin (an autonomic response) facilitates heat loss, while constriction of these vessels helps to conserve heat. Panting and shivering (skeletomuscular responses) aid in the processes of heat loss and conservation (heat generation), respectively. Finally, when an organism is exposed to cold for long periods of time, there is an increase in thyroxine release from the anterior pituitary gland, which helps to increase body temperature by increasing metabolism. The classic interpretation of the role of the hypothalamus in temperature regulation has been that the anterior hypothalamus constitutes a heat loss center, while the posterior hypothalamus is a heat conservation center. Although such a generalization is somewhat oversimplified, the general phenomenon has been demonstrated. Thus, a lesion or tumor of the posterior pituitary will most likely induce a form of disorder of thermoregulation, in this case, hypothermia. Lesions located at other sites, indicated by other choices in this question, would not produce hypothermia. Lesions of the limbic system (ie, septal area, hippocampus, amygdala) have not been reported to produce hypothermia. Lesions of the anterior hypothalamus have been reported to induce hyperthermia.

448. The answer is e. (*Kandel, p 979. Siegel and Sapru, pp 432-434.*) The supraoptic nucleus, like the paraventricular nucleus, contains magnocellular neurons that synthesize vasopressin and oxytocin and transport these hormones down their axons to the posterior pituitary. For this reason, the supraoptic nucleus plays a significant role in the regulation of water balance. There is no evidence to support the notion that the supraoptic nucleus has a role in feeding behavior, temperature regulation, sexual behavior, or short-term memory functions.

449. The answer is d. (*Kandel, pp 1002-1003. Siegel and Sapru, pp 437-438.*) Lesions of the lateral hypothalamus are likely to produce aphagia. Feeding behavior is elicited by stimulation of the lateral hypothalamus. Neurons in this region respond to the sight or taste of food. Since drinking is also associated with lateral hypothalamic functions, a lesion of this structure would also disrupt this behavior. Lesions of the lateral hypothalamus do not produce either hypertension or sexual behaviors. The neurons regulating these functions are situated elsewhere within the hypothalamus.

450. The answer is d. (*Ropper, pp 540-546. Siegel and Sapru, pp 435, 442.*) Growth hormone—releasing hormone is located mainly in the arcuate and tuberal region of the ventromedial hypothalamus. Damage to neurons in this region would affect the release of this hormone and its influence in producing growth hormone in the anterior pituitary. Other regions of hypothalamus listed in this question are not known to contain growth hormone—releasing factor.

451. The answer is b. *(Kandel, p 988. Siegel and Sapru, p 457.)* In this syndrome, produced experimentally in monkeys and also seen in cats, there is an extreme change in the personality of the animal. Its responses to emotion-laden stimuli are much reduced. It appears very tame. Aggressive tendencies are not evident. It also manifests oral tendencies and displays hypersexuality This syndrome is the result of lesions of the temporal lobe in which parts of the amygdala are involved. Lesions of other regions such as the hypothalamus, cingulate cortex, or septal area do not produce the Klüver-Bucy syndrome.

452. The answer is c. *(Purves, pp 742-747.)* Studies conducted on fear conditioning in rats have demonstrated that the amygdala plays a very important role in this process. Rare evidence obtained from patients have shown that individuals suffering from a rare autosomal recessive condition called "Urbach-Wiethe" disease, in which there is bilateral atrophy of the portion of the temporal lobe which includes the amygdala, have no sense of the emotion of "fear." They are unable to recognize it; nor are they capable of depicting it in a drawing. Other regions listed in this question have not been linked to the emotion of fear.

453. The answer is b. *(Kandel, pp 1200-1204. Siegel and Sapru, pp 509-512.)* There have been a variety of neurochemical and related theories of schizophrenia that have evolved over the past three decades. Unfortunately, each of these theories has had its limitations. Nevertheless, one of the more popular theories has been that schizophrenia is linked to increased levels of brain dopamine. The hypothesis suggests that schizophrenia results from overstimulation of the brain by the dopaminergic system. Support for this view comes from the observation that antipsychotic agents are known to block dopamine receptors. Co-twin behavioral and developmental studies have shown that, while environmental factors are certainly important in the ontogeny of schizophrenia, genetic factors are also quite significant in the development of this disease. Other researchers have suggested that schizophrenia may bear some relationship to decreased levels of serotonin in the brain, as evidenced by the hallucinogenic effects of lysergic acid diethylamide (LSD), which binds to serotonin receptors. Other investigations have shown that opioid peptide blockade by naloxone is effective in reducing hallucinations, which suggests that increased levels of endorphins may be linked to this disorder. Investigations involving neuropeptides have indicated that neuropeptides such as cholecystokinin (CCK) is colocalized with dopamine in brain neurons. In this fashion, CCK may function as a neuromodulator for dopamine, in which case increased levels of CCK may be linked with schizophrenia in the same fashion as are increased levels of dopamine.

454. The answer is d. *(Afifi, pp 298-299. Nolte, pp 625-626. Purves, pp 799-800. Siegel and Sapru, pp 450-452.)* Chronic alcoholism can result in a disorder called Korsakoff syndrome. This disorder is characterized as a memory disorder involving loss of both retrograde and anterograde memories, including consolidation of declarative memories. Such patients also produce a confabulatory response to cover up their memory failure. The disorder is caused by a vitamin B (thiamine) deficiency associated with alcoholism, and the general consensus is that the mammillary bodies are one of the structures affected by the destructive effects of alcohol. The other structures listed as choices in this question have not been reported to be linked to Korsakoff syndrome.

455. The answer is c. *(Kandel, pp 987-988. Nolte, pp 624-626. Siegel and Sapru, pp 450-452.)* For many years, it was believed that a neural circuit composed of the hippocampal formation → mammillary bodies → anterior thalamic nucleus → cingulate gyrus hippocampal formation played a major role in the regulation of emotional behavior. More recent studies by a number of investigators have revealed that neither the mammillary bodies nor the anterior thalamic nucleus appears to contribute to the regulation of emotional behavior. Instead, it is believed that this circuit may subserve functions more closely related to short-term memory.

456. The answer is b. *(Kandel, pp 544, 1306-1309. Nolte, pp 418-424. Siegel and Sapru, p 288.)* The cerebrovascular accident produced damage of the right primary visual cortex. Therefore, this would result in a homonymous hemianopsia of the left visual fields. Since the damage was confined to the occipital lobe, there would be little effect upon other processes such as speech, motor functions, or intellectual activities.

457. The answer is c. *(Kandel, pp 544, 1306-1309. Nolte, pp 125-140, 445-450. Siegel and Sapru, pp 500-501.)* The occipital lobe is supplied by the posterior cerebral artery. The calcarine cortex (primary visual cortex) is supplied by a branch of this artery, the calcarine artery. The anterior cerebral artery supplies the medial aspect of the frontal lobe and the anterior-medial aspect of the parietal lobe. The middle cerebral artery supplies the lateral aspect of the frontal and parietal lobes. The superior cerebellar artery supplies the dorsolateral aspect of a portion of the pons and the cerebellum. The striate arteries arise from the anterior and middle cerebral arteries and supply portions of the internal capsule and neostriatum.

458. The answer is a. *(Kandel, pp 854-857. Nolte, pp 474-491. Siegel and Sapru, pp 338-339.)* The tumor is situated in the lentiform nucleus and internal capsule. Therefore, corticospinal fibers will be affected, causing a UMN paralysis of the left side. Dyskinesia would not be seen because any effects normally seen in association with damage to the basal ganglia would be masked by the effects of the damage to the internal capsule. Since the cerebellum was not involved, there would be no intention tremor. Neither would there be any visual deficits from this glioma since optic nerve fibers are not involved.

459. The answer is d. *(Kandel, pp 854-857. Nolte pp 474-491. Siegel and Sapru, p 205.)* As noted in Answer 458, the tumor involves the lentiform nucleus of the basal ganglia and the internal capsule as well. At the stage when the CT scan was taken, the tumor had not involved the thalamus.

460. The answer is c. *(Nolte, pp 125-140, 445-450, 560-570.)* The arterial occlusion involves both the temporal and the occipital regions of the cortex. Therefore, it would affect Wernicke area as well as primary visual areas of the occipital lobe. The patient would most likely present with receptive aphasia as well as a right homonymous hemianopsia. The lesion would not likely produce marked intellectual deficits, since the prefrontal cortex was spared; nor would it produce hemiballism, since there was no damage to the subthalamic nucleus.

461. The answer is b. *(Kandel, pp 125-140, 1305-1309. Siegel and Sapru, pp 500-501.)* Although the tissue affected involves parietal, temporal, and occipital lobes, the primary artery affected is the middle cerebral artery. The unusual feature of this occlusion is that it appears that the middle cerebral artery extends more caudally than usual. Nevertheless, the middle cerebral artery is the only one of the choices presented that could account for the damage to the temporal and parietal cortices. The anterior cerebral artery supplies the medial aspects of the frontal and parietal lobes; the posterior cerebral artery supplies the occipital cortex (visual areas); the posterior choroidal artery mainly supplies part of the tectum, the medial and superior aspects of the thalamus, and the choroid plexus of the third ventricle. The superior cerebellar artery supplies the dorsolateral aspect of a portion of the pons and the cerebellum.

462. The answer is b. *(Kandel, pp 1305-1309. Nolte, pp 125-140, 445-450. Siegel and Sapru, pp 500-501.)* An arterial occlusion compromised the blood supply to the occipital lobe on the left side of the brain. Therefore, it would result in a right homonymous hemianopsia with no motor deficits (since no motor regions of the brain are affected).

463. The answer is e. *(Kandel, pp 1303-1311. Nolte, pp 125-140. Siegel and Sapru, pp 500-501.)* This vertebral angiogram is an anterior view of the back of the brain. It reveals an occlusion of the left posterior cerebral artery (A). It should be noted that the posterior cerebral arteries are formed from the bifurcation of the basilar artery. As the basilar artery runs in a caudal direction, it passes laterally to form the vertebral artery on each side.

464. The answer is b. *(Kandel, p 544. Nolte, pp 445-450, 555-556. Siegel and Sapru, pp 287-289.)* This large pituitary tumor is seen to compress the optic chiasm. Damage to the chiasm affects the crossing fibers of the nasal retina, which convey information from the temporal visual fields. This results in a bitemporal hemianopsia. Since some parts of the optic nerves are spared, pupillary reflexes are preserved. The neuroanatomic substrates for conjugate gaze (ie, frontal eye fields, pontine gaze center, medial longitudinal fasciculus, and nuclei of cranial nerves III, IV, and VI) are unaffected by the tumor; the mechanism of conjugate gaze remains intact.

465. The answer is b. *(Kandel, pp 388, 759, 920. Siegel and Sapru, pp 460-462.)* The patient had a seizure, which began focally on the left motor strip (the left precentral gyrus), moved up the motor strip, then secondarily generalized, or spread throughout the cortex. The phenomenon whereby there is twitching of an extremity that spreads to other areas on that extremity or other areas of the body is called a *Jacksonian march*. This phenomenon is named for Hughlings Jackson, a neurosurgeon who was instrumental in mapping out the cerebral cortex and describing the somatotopic organization of the cortex of the prefrontal gyrus called a *homunculus* (meaning "little man"). Observing patients with a Jacksonian march helped him to identify areas represented at each location of the motor strip. Seizures originating in the temporal lobe are typically different; they are generally absence seizures or complex-partial seizures, but do not display a *Jacksonian march*. A seizure from the left precentral cortex would have movements on the opposite side of the body than what was described in this patient. Seizures of the thalamus are not common.

466. The answer is c. *(Kandel, pp 919-927. Siegel and Sapru, pp 460-462.)* Very often, there is inhibition following a seizure, which accounts for drowsiness or a postictal state after the seizure has finished. Sometimes, epileptic discharges spread to other areas of the cortex, recruiting contiguous areas of the cortex through callosal, commissural, and sometimes thalamic circuits to eventually involve a large area of the cortex, causing the movements of the entire body. This occurs with a generalized seizure. If the cortices of both hemispheres become involved, there may be impairment or loss of consciousness. The cells (often pyramidal cells) in the cortex can generate a seizure through high-frequency, synchronous discharges in large groups. If the seizure begins focally, as this one did, there may be a *Todd paralysis*, as June had, where there is transient paralysis of the involved motor area during the postictal period.

467. The answer is e. *(Kandel, pp 759, 919-927. Siegel and Sapru, pp 460-462.)* There is somatotopic organization of the motor strip, and cortical neurons are included among the most likely to generate seizures, making this area the most likely to cause such a pattern.

468. The answer is e. *(Kandel, pp 919-927. Siegel and Sapru, pp 468-470.)* The pyramidal cell is a cell in the cortex that uses glutamate, an excitatory neurotransmitter, whereas most other types of cortical neurons use GABA, an inhibitory neurotransmitter. The spike, one identifying feature of an epileptic seizure seen on an EEG recorded on the scalp, is initiated by a depolarization shift, which is thought to be generated by EPSPs.

469. The answer is d. *(Kandel, pp 925-927. Siegel and Sapru, pp 460-462.)* EPSPs are considered to be an initiating cellular event for a seizure. To become a seizure, however, the cellular discharges require enhancement and synchronization.

470. The answer is b. *(Kandel, pp 922-925.)* Since seizure generation requires excitation, or a loss of inhibition, the only correct choice is the inhibition of GABA, an inhibitory neurotransmitter. All the other choices cause inhibition only. Many new anticonvulsant medications are currently being designed to either enhance GABA activity or inhibit the excitatory neurotransmitter, glutamate.

471. The answer is c. *(Kandel, pp 758-765. Siegel and Sapru, pp 329-330.)* A CT scan of the patient's head was done in the emergency room, which showed a new infarct or stroke in the genu and anterior portion of the posterior limb of the left internal capsule. This is the region of the internal capsule through which most of the fibers of the corticospinal and corticobulbar tracts pass in a somatotopically organized fashion before entering the brain stem. Because most of these fibers pass through a very small region, a small infarct can cause deficits in a wide distribution of areas. In this case, the patient had weakness in her face and tongue, causing her slurred speech, in addition to weakness of her arm and leg. Since somatosensory fibers destined for the postcentral gyrus occupy a position in the internal capsule caudal to the corticospinal tract fibers, these fibers were spared and she had no sensory deficits. The only other area in the CNS that can cause a pure motor hemiparesis is the basilar pons, an area through which corticospinal and corticobulbar fibers also run. The vascular supply of this region consists of perforators from the basilar artery, which are small and subject to atherosclerotic disease.

472. The answer is a. *(Kandel, pp 1303-1307. Siegel and Sapru, pp 48-49.)* The internal capsule is supplied primarily by the lenticulostriate branches of the middle cerebral artery. In addition, portions of the posterior limb of the internal capsule are supplied by the anterior choroidal artery, a branch of the internal carotid artery. Both the lateral striate branches and the anterior choroidal artery are small branches of larger arteries and are more susceptible to damage (atherosclerosis) from high blood pressure and diabetes than the larger vessels. The posterior cerebral artery supplies mainly the occipital lobe and parts of the midbrain; the anterior cerebral artery supplies mainly the medial aspect of the frontal and parietal lobes; the vertebral artery supplies the lower brainstem; and the posterior choroidal artery supplies the medial and superior surfaces of the thalamus, choroid plexus of the third ventricle, and parts of the tectum.

473. The answer is b. (*Kandel, pp 757-763. Siegel and Sapru, pp 328-333, 470-477.*) The corticospinal tracts contain motor fibers originating in the precentral gyrus, mediating voluntary motor function of the arms, legs, and trunk. They pass through the internal capsule to the crus cerebri in the midbrain. The postcentral gyrus is the receiving area for somatosensory information from the body and head regions. In order to account for the deficits described in this case, the stroke had to involve the precentral and postcentral gyri, which would affect both motor and sensory functions. Other choices in the question did not relate to these two regions of cortex.

474. The answer is c. (*Afifi, pp 236-237. Siegel and Sapru, pp 334-336.*) The patient's forehead was unaffected by the lesion because the forehead is bilaterally represented on the cortex, so the right side retains innervations and functions despite a lesion in the left internal capsule. Motor fibers from each side pass into the internal capsule ipsilaterally, so a lesion in the internal capsule will not affect the forehead.

475. The answer is d. (*Ropper, pp 466, 475-477.*) Dysarthria is slurred speech, occurring from lesions affecting innervation of the tongue, lips, and palate. We are given evidence that his tongue was weak in that it pointed to the right. The interruption of fibers traveling to the hypoglossal nerve from the left side eventually innervates the right genioglossus muscle, which pulls the tongue to the left. Dysarthria is a motor phenomenon, unlike aphasia, which is a disruption of language. Language is primarily generated in the cerebral cortex; therefore, because the lesion spares the cortex, there were no signs of aphasia. Broca aphasia is called nonfluent because it is difficult for words to be expressed, although language may be understood. Wernicke aphasia is called fluent because words can be expressed but with impaired comprehension. Conduction aphasia is rare; the patient will display frequent errors during spontaneous speech and will substitute or transpose sounds. Anomia is a severe condition in which the patient has great difficulty in recalling names or words.

476. The answer is d. (*Ropper, pp 310-313.*) This is an example of a complex partial seizure, most likely originating in the temporal lobe. A seizure is a paroxysmal derangement of the CNS due to rhythmic, synchronous discharges from cerebral neurons, causing changes in consciousness, sensation, and/or behavior. Complex partial seizures often start with a warning, or "aura." Since limbic structures are often involved, the seizure can include emotions, feelings of deja vu or jamais vu, or gastrointestinal sensations. Because olfactory pathways end in the temporal lobe, patients may experience smells as well. The seizure itself involves impairment of consciousness of some form, often manifested as staring, in addition to various stereotyped, automatic behaviors called *automatisms*. The latter may be manifested as chewing, repetitive swallowing, hand gestures, or vocalizations. These usually occur during the seizure, but may occur after it. After the seizure ends (the seizures usually last 1-2 minutes), the patient is often in a confused or postictal state for several minutes, or even up to several hours. Occasionally, a patient may manifest aggressive behavior while in the postictal state. Unless a structural lesion, such as a tumor, is present, the physical examination is usually normal. Verification of the diagnosis of epilepsy is done with the help of an EEG, which records potential differences of summed cortical action potentials over the scalp of a patient. Often, an epileptic spike, or sharp wave, is seen over the area from which the seizures arise. Epilepsy patients usually also have a CT scan or MRI to make certain that there is no structural lesion causing the seizures.

477. The answer is c. (*Ropper, pp 310-313, 317.*) Seizures similar to this one often begin with abnormal neuronal discharges in temporal lobe structures, which include the amygdala or hippocampus. These structures tend to have a lower threshold for this type of activity than other structures in the brain.

478. The answer is c. (*Afifi, pp 291-292. Siegel and Sapru, pp 449, 456-458.*) The major efferent pathway from the amygdala that projects to the medial hypothalamus is the stria terminalis and it is through this pathway that the amygdala can significantly modulate functions of the hypothalamus. The medial forebrain bundle is a major pathway of the lateral hypothalamus. The mammillothalamic tract and stria medullaris do not involve the amygdala.

479. The answer is a. (*Afifi, pp 286-288. Siegel and Sapru, pp 447-452.*) The hippocampal formation includes the hippocampus, the dentate gyrus, and the subiculum. Much of the output of the hippocampal formation arises from pyramidal cells of the subiculum and cornu ammonis fields. The major projections include the anterior thalamic nucleus, mammillary bodies, and septal area. Each of the other choices in this question include one or more structures that do not receive direct inputs from the hippocampal formation.

480. The answer is b. (*Kandel, pp 988-992, 1228-1237. Siegel and Sapru, pp 450-452.*) Since one form of memory, namely, "short-term" memory, is a function that is mediated by the hippocampal formation, loss of hippocampal neurons will result in significant deficits in "short-term" memory.

481. The answer is a. (*Kandel, pp 1306-1309. Ropper, pp 229-232, 241-246. Siegel and Sapru, pp 330-336.*) The patient was not only unable to move his left side (hemiparesis), but ignored its existence (anosagnosia or the syndrome of hemineglect, see answer to Question 485). Even though he neglected his left side, the blink reflex should still be intact if he only neglected the side. Therefore, a visual field deficit, called a *homonymous hemianopsia*, was present on the left side, in which the left temporal and right nasal fields were damaged. There may also have been some degree of primary sensory loss, which can be difficult to evaluate when a patient neglects the same side.

482. The answer is c. (*Ropper, pp 46-56, 437-453. Siegel and Sapru, pp 287-289, 330-336.*) The patient's deficits resulted from lesions of the posterior aspect of the frontal cortex, as well as from some contribution of corticospinal tract fibers from the parietal lobe and deeper motor cortical structures. In addition, the neglect and hemisensory loss resulted from damage to the posterior parietal cortex. The homonymous hemianopsia resulted from damage to the deep portion of the parietal lobe where the optic radiations pass to the superior and inferior banks of the visual cortex, causing the visual field defect. Choices other than (c) are incorrect for the following reasons: The temporal lobe is associated with auditory functions, movements of objects across the visual field, and facial recognition, and damage to this region is not associated with hemineglect or hemianopsia (although it is associated with quadrantanopia). Likewise, the occipital lobe is associated with visual functions and thus a lesion limited to the visual cortex could only account for the hemianopsia and not for hemineglect.

483. The answer is d. *(Kandel, pp 1303-1307. Siegel and Sapru, pp 48-49, 500.)* The posterior frontal lobe, as well as the parietal lobe, is supplied by the middle cerebral artery. Areas supplied by this artery, such as primary and supplementary motor areas, and the primary and secondary somatosensory cortices may be affected. As a result, the patient may have left-sided weakness, UMN facial weakness that spares the forehead, and hemisensory loss.

484. The answer is e. *(Kandel, pp 544-545, 1303-1307. Siegel and Sapru, pp 287-289.)* If the lesion is deep enough, the patient may have a visual field cut, called a *homonymous hemianopsia*, where fibers traveling from the optic chiasm to the occipital cortex within the optic radiations are interrupted. In this instance, the patient does not see the left temporal and the right nasal visual field. It is common for patients with neglect not to notice the areas of blindness because they ignore the left side. Patients with this problem are usually advised not to drive a car.

485. The answer is d. *(Kandel, pp 1303-1307. Ropper, pp 446-451. Siegel and Sapru, pp 333-334.)* The patient's problem is an example of the syndrome of hemineglect, which arises from a lesion of the posterior parietal lobe. This area is essential for spatial organization. If this area, usually on the nondominant (right) side, is no longer functioning, the patient will live in a world that consists solely of right side. Patients with the syndrome of hemineglect will look only to the right side (if the lesion is on the right), and when asked to look to the left, often will not cross the midline with their eyes. Especially when the lesion is acute, these patients will not acknowledge any person or objects on their left side, and it is not unusual for a patient to, for example, complain of losing his glasses when they are on a table on the left side. Since these patients see only the right side of everything, they will put all of the numbers of a clock on the right side of the clock and will bisect a line on its right side. In addition, they will comb only the right side of their hair, dress the right side of their bodies, and shave the right side of their faces. When confronted with a left-sided entity, such as a left arm, they will often ignore the question or may even go as far as claiming it belongs to someone else. In resolving lesions where the patient now has sensation and acknowledgment on the left side, he may still display extinction to double simultaneous stimuli where, if both sides are touched simultaneously, the patient feels the touch only on the right side and "extinguishes" the stimulus on the left. However, it is important to remember that neglect can resemble weakness because the patient will not move the left side.

486. The answer is b. (*Ropper, pp 446-451. Siegel and Sapru, pp 475-478.*) This case is an example of a lesion of the left (usually dominant) parietal lobe, most often in the angular gyrus, with some involvement of the precentral gyrus in the posterior frontal lobe. There is contralateral UMN weakness (with a positive Babinski sign), as well as several cortical sensory defects—specifically, right-left confusion, agraphia (inability to write, independent of motor weakness), acalculia (the inability to calculate), and finger agnosia (the inability to designate the fingers). The latter four elements are sometimes referred to as the *Gerstmann syndrome* by neurologists, and all represent spatial discriminatory functions of the parietal lobe (often the dominant parietal lobe, which is usually the left). The parietal lobe also subserves other visual-spatial functions such as construction of complex drawings. There are other locations within the CNS where UMN weakness can occur; however, the combination with parietal lobe signs can occur only in this location. If the damage was slightly more extensive, it may have involved Broca area, causing aphasia.

487. The answer is d. (*Kandel, pp 1303-1309. Siegel and Sapru, pp 48-50, 500-501.*) The artery serving this region (both posterior frontal and parietal lobes) is the left middle cerebral artery, which originates at the circle of Willis. Because it continues in a nearly straight line from the internal carotid artery, it is a common route for small emboli formed from blood clots in the internal carotid artery. The bruit noted over the right common carotid artery in this patient is most likely a result of a thrombus (clot) that occludes part of the lumen of the artery. These emboli can occlude the middle cerebral artery because it is considerably smaller than the internal carotid artery. Since the middle cerebral artery has many branches through which an embolus may travel, but the territory of this stroke is large, it is likely that the embolus lodged in a more proximal location in this case.

488. The answer is b. (*Kandel, pp 993-994. Ropper, pp 437-445. Siegel and Sapru, p 487.*) The orbitofrontal cortex plays an important role in intellectual functions, acquisition of skilled motor and other tasks, social integration, impulse control. Damage to this region (eg, a tumor) has been shown to be associated with diminution of these functions, including normal sexual behavior. A tumor of this region has been associated with diminished social forms of behavior. For example, such individuals express inappropriate social behaviors, an example of which is pedophilia. Constructional apraxia has on a number of occasions been associated with lesions of the prefrontal cortex. This deficit may be due to the disruption of the connections between the prefrontal cortex and the parietal lobe, which is normally linked with this dysfunction. Lesions or tumors of the other regions listed in this question have not been associated with dysfunctions in emotional and related functions.

489. The answer is c. (*Siegel and Sapru, pp 331-336, 338-339.*) The deficits observed in this patient were due to damage to the left internal capsule. The tumor impinged upon both genu and posterior limbs of the internal capsule, thus affecting corticospinal and some corticobulbar fibers. Such damage would account for both the contralateral limb paresis (due to damage to the corticospinal tract) and the loss of expression of the contralateral lower jaw (due to damage to corticobulbar fibers that supply the ventral aspect of the facial nucleus, whose axons innervate the lower jaw).

490. The answer is b. (*Siegel and Sapru, pp 334-336, 485-487.*) The tumor involved the region of the premotor cortex and the adjoining frontal eye field. The damage to the premotor region (a region that synchronizes the sequences necessary for the occurrence of complex movements) could account for the right motor apraxia observed in this patient and the damage to the frontal eye field affected the patient's ability to voluntarily gaze to the right. None of the other choices relate to the processes that were affected in this patient.

491. The answer is b. (*Rowland, pp 349-356.*) This case is an example of a condition called *normal-pressure hydrocephalus*. This may be caused by various nonprogressive meningeal and ependymal diseases, such as chronic meningitis and subarachnoid hemorrhages, which can initially block CSF absorption. Initially, the CSF pressure is high, which results in the enlargement of the ventricles. The CSF pressure becomes normal because the CSF absorption begins again. However, the enlarged ventricles, despite normal CSF pressure, cause hydrostatic impairment to the central white matter surrounding the ventricles. Maximal ventricular expansion is usually located in the frontal lobes with preservation of the cortical gray matter and other subcortical structures. As a result, patients with this condition have diminished frontal lobe functions, namely, gait problems without any weakness, as well as urinary incontinence and dementia. Frontal lobe dysfunction can also cause the reappearance of primitive reflexes, which disappear shortly after birth, such as the grasp reflex. Late in the course of normal-pressure hydrocephalus, the patient may develop *frontal lobe incontinence*, where he or she becomes indifferent to the incontinence, much like a very small child. Headaches are rare in this particular type of hydrocephalus. Normal-pressure hydrocephalus is usually diagnosed with a thorough neurological examination, in addition to a head CT, which shows enlarged ventricles and, occasionally, interstitial fluid within the white matter adjacent to the lateral ventricles. (Measurement of CSF pressures with a lumbar puncture and radionuclide cisternography—a procedure where a radionuclide is injected intrathecally, and its distribution is observed over a period of 24 hours—is also helpful.) Occasionally, shunting procedures, which allow the CSF to drain into the peritoneal cavity or the blood, are helpful if performed early in the course of this condition.

492. The answer is a. (*Rowland, pp 349-356.*) The major mechanism underlying hydrocephalus is decreased absorption of CSF. In the case of normal-pressure hydrocephalus, the problem is described in the answer for Question 491. Another cause of decreased absorption is obstruction of CSF flow by a tumor. Low blood pressure does not cause enlarged ventricles. High blood pressure causes hydrocephalus only as a result of hypertensive crisis, but not chronically. Decreased blood flow in the brain can actually be used as a temporizing measure to acutely decrease intracranial pressure in emergencies in order to make room for expanding tissue through the mechanism of decreasing carbon dioxide partial pressure (PCO_2) in the brain with a ventilator.

493. The answer is d. (*Aminoff, pp 265-277.*) The patient was suffering from complex partial epilepsy. Complex partial epilepsy is characterized by impairment of consciousness, some cognitive disturbances such as perception of a dream, stereotyped behavior, speech, and affective disturbances.

494. The answer is b. *(Ropper, pp 310-313, 318-319.)* The affected region is the hippocampus. Complex partial seizures arise from temporal lobe structures, although they may spread to other regions. With respect to the MRI for this patient, the arrows clearly point to the hippocampus and not to any of the other choices listed in this question.

495. The answer is c. *(Rowland, pp 8-13. Siegel and Sapru, p 484.)* The language problem is an example of Broca aphasia, a deficit seen with lesions of Broca area and manifested by defects in the motor aspect of speech, leaving the patient's speech halting and nonfluent. People with Broca aphasia tend to repeat certain phrases, as well as leave out pronouns. Since the language centers are usually located on the dominant side of the brain (the left side for a right-handed person), this lesion must be on the left side of the patient's brain. Wernicke aphasia is a problem with the sensory aspect of speech, where the patient can speak fluently, but the speech sounds like gibberish. The area of disruption in this type of aphasia is usually in Wernicke area, a region of the posterior superior temporal lobe. Dysarthria is slurred speech, but makes grammatical sense. Alexia is the inability to read. Pure-word deafness is a type of sensory aphasia whereby language, reading, and writing are only mildly disturbed, but auditory comprehension of words is very abnormal. This arises from lesions of the posterior temporal lobe.

496. The answer is e. *(Rowland, pp 7-13.)* The patient's condition is an example of a left inferior frontal lobe cortical stroke, including the region of Broca area and the left precentral gyrus. The weakness on his right side confirms this, since the left side of the brain controls the right side of the body. The right leg is most likely less involved than the arm because the leg area of the precentral gyrus extends onto the medial aspect of the frontal lobe, an area served by a different artery than that serving the arm and face areas. The internal capsule contains motor fibers traveling to the cortex, but usually does not involve language. The thalamus contains many sensory, motor, and association areas, but only rarely causes language problems. Functions of the pontine reticular formation do not include language. The corpus callosum is a white matter structure that connects the hemispheres. Lesions of the posterior aspect may cause language problems, such as alexia without agraphia (the ability to write, but not to read), but would not cause both an aphasia and weakness.

497. The answer is d. *(Rowland, pp 7-13, 295-296. Siegel and Sapru, pp 487, 500.)* The middle cerebral artery subserves the precentral gyrus, the area that has been damaged (Broca "motor speech" area). The damage can be more widespread, depending upon which portion of the vessel becomes occluded. The anterior cerebral artery supplies the orbitofrontal cortex, deep limbic structures, as well as the cingulate gyrus. The posterior cerebral artery supplies the thalamus, portions of the temporal lobes, and portions of the midbrain. The anterior inferior cerebellar artery supplies the lateral inferior pons and portions of the cerebellum. Perforating branches of the basilar artery supply medial portions of the brain stem.

498. The answer is b. *(Siegel and Sapru, pp 458-459, 487.)* The disorder described in this case is a classical prefrontal cortical syndrome and, accordingly, the tumor shown in the accompanying MRI includes parts of the prefrontal cortex. Prefrontal cortical disorders typically involve alterations in both affective and intellectual states. Such individuals display personality and mood changes as well as intellectual deficits. The intellectual deficits can be demonstrated in card sorting and other tasks which require problem solving, allowing for perseverative responses to occur.

499. The answer is c. *(Siegel and Sapru, pp 458-459, 471-474, 487.)* A major afferent source of the prefrontal cortex is the mediodorsal thalamic nucleus as it projects massively to wide areas of this region of cortex.

500. The answer is b. *(Kandel, pp 951-953.)* Sleep apnea can occur for several reasons. One common basis is an obstruction of the airways (called *obstructive sleep apnea*). In this case, as indicated in the statement of the question, the physicians ruled out this possibility. Another possible cause involves central sleep apnea. This is due to disruption of the mechanism involving chemoreceptors in the carotid body that monitors carbon dioxide and oxygen levels in the blood. Axons in the carotid body project via the glossopharyngeal nerve (IX) to the reticular formation of the medulla. Therefore, disturbances involving the carotid body could result in central sleep apnea. Here, inappropriate signals are sent to the medullary reticular formation, which, in part, projects caudally to ventral horn sites in the spinal cord, governing such muscles as those that regulate the diaphragm and, therefore, disrupt the normal breathing process.

Bibliography

Afifi AK, Bergman RA. *Functional Neuroanatomy*. 2nd ed. New York, NY: McGraw-Hill; 2005.

Aminoff MJ, Greenberg DA, Simon RP. *Clinical Neurology*. 6th ed. New York, NY: McGraw-Hill; 2005.

Anschel DJ, Romanelli P, Mazumdar A. *Clinical Neuroimaging: Cases and Key Points*. New York, NY: McGraw-Hill; 2008.

Brunton LL, Lazo JS, Parker KL. *Goodman and Gilman's The Pharmacological Basis of Therapeutics*. 11th ed. New York, NY: McGraw-Hill; 2006.

Cooper JR, Bloom FE, Roth RH. *The Biochemical Basis of Neuropharmacology*. 8th ed. New York, NY: Oxford University Press; 2003.

DeArmond SJ, Fusco MM, Dewey MM. *Structure of the Human Brain: A Photographic Atlas*. 3rd ed. New York, NY: Oxford University Press; 1989.

Kandel ER, Schwartz JH, Jessel TM. *Principles of Neural Science*. 4th ed. New York, NY: McGraw-Hill; 2000.

Martin JH. *Neuroanatomy*. 3rd ed. New York, NY: McGraw-Hill; 2003.

Nolte J. *The Human Brain: An Introduction to Its Functional Anatomy*. 6th ed. Philadelphia, PA: Mosby (Elsevier); 2009.

Purves D, Augustine GJ, Fitzpatrick D, et al. *Neuroscience*. 4th ed. Sunderland, MA: Sinauer Associates, Inc.; 2008.

Ropper AH, Samuels MA. *Adams and Victor's Principles of Neurology*. 9th ed. New York, NY: McGraw-Hill; 2009.

Rowland, LP, ed. *Merritt's Neurology*. 11th ed. Philadelphia, PA: Lippincott, Williams & Wilkins; 2005.

Siegel A, Sapru HN. *Essential Neuroscience*. Revised 1st ed. Philadelphia, PA: Lippincott, Williams & Wilkins; 2006.

Siegel GJ, Albers RW, Brady ST, Price DL. *Basic Neurochemistry*. 7th ed. Burlington, MA: Elsevier Academic Press; 2006.

Villiger E, Ludwig E, Rasmussen AT. *Atlas of Cross Section Anatomy of the Brain*. New York, NY: McGraw-Hill; 1951.

Index

A

Abducens nerve, 71, 81, 230, 231-232, 242, 255
Absence seizures, 363
Acetylcholine (ACh), 19, 22-23, 33t, 34, 48, 252
  Alzheimer disease and, 135
  autonomic nervous system and, 43t
  basal ganglia and, 320-321
  EPP and, 131
  heart and, 177
  ligand-gated channels and, 98
  myasthenia gravis and, 132
Acetylcholinesterase, 133
ACh. See Acetylcholine
Action potential, 18-19, 98-99, 102
  ganglion cells and, 269
  potassium and, 176-177
Active transport, 16
Adenohypophysis, 295
Adenosine, 33t
Adenosine receptors, 36
Adenosine triphosphate (ATP), 30, 110
Adenylyl cyclase, 35, 140
ADH. See Antidiuretic hormone
Adrenal medulla, 46, 80
β-adrenergic antagonists, 93
Adrenergic receptors, 35, 48
β-adrenergic receptors, 35, 111, 176
AIDS, 160
Akinetic mutism, 327
Alar plate, 10t, 81
Alcohol, 324, 326
Alpha motor neurons, 164, 167

Alpha-ketoglutaric acid, 24
ALS. See Amyotrophic lateral sclerosis
Alternating hypoglossal hemiplegia, 248
Alzheimer disease, 12, 23, 134, 135, 295
Amacrine cells, 269
α-amino-3-hydrxyl-5-methyl-4-isoxazole propionic acid (AMPA), 33, 113, 140
γ-aminobutyric acid (GABA), 19, 24-25, 33t, 111, 319
  basal ganglia and, 320-321
  chloride and, 110
  glutamic acid decarboxylase and, 134
  Huntington chorea and, 68
  seizures and, 370
  substantia nigra and, 246
  type II synapses and, 109
AMPA. See α-amino-3-hydrxyl-5-methyl-4-isoxazole propionic acid
Amygdala, 6, 55, 294
  central nucleus of, 177
  mitral cells and, 278-279
  stria terminalis and, 372
Amyloid, 135
Amyotrophic lateral sclerosis (ALS), 24, 42, 160-161
Analgesia, 274
Anencephaly, 82
Aneurysm, 253
Angular gyrus, 375
Anhydrosis, 252

Anions, 15
Ansa lenticularis, 294
Anterior cerebral artery, 8, 9*f*, 368
Anterior cingulate gyrus, 2
Anterior commissure, 6
Anterior communicating arteries, 8, 9*f*, 318
Anterior corticospinal tract, 166
Anterior flocculonodular lobe, 7
Anterior funiculus, 166
Anterior lobe, 54, 81, 322
Anterior neuropore, 80
Anterior spinal artery, 8
Anterior spinocerebellar tract, 37, 162
Anterior spinothalamic tract, 37, 166
Anterograde tracing, 13
Antidiuretic hormone (ADH), 139, 363
Antiports, 15
Anxiety disorders, 136
Aortic arch, 228
Aphagia, 364
Aphasia, 371
Aphonia, 227
Apomorphine, 240
Apoptosis, 82, 269
Apraxia, 56, 319
Arachidonic acid, 111
Arcuate nucleus, 26
Area 8, 254
Area 17, 277
Area post, 240
Argyll Robertson pupil, 50, 243-244
Arnold-Chiari malformation, 82
Astereognosia, 56
Astigmatism, 269
Astrocytes, 13
Ataxia, 234, 236

Ataxic gait, 54, 83, 161, 163, 247, 277, 324, 326
Atherosclerosis, 9*f*, 246, 370
Athetosis, 54
ATP. *See* Adenosine triphosphate
Auditory system, 52, 241, 246
Auerbach plexus, 47
Automatisms, 372
Autonomic nervous system, 42-50, 176-178
Axon hillock, 101
Axonal transport, 12-13
Axons, 11, 12, 162

B
Babinski sign, 56, 171, 375
Bacterial meningitis, 72
Barbiturates, 25, 34
Baroreceptor reflex, 49, 228
Barr body, 12
Basal cells, 278
Basal ganglia, 6, 53-54, 67, 319, 320-321
Basal nucleus of Meynert, 23, 134, 295
Basal plate, 10*t*, 81
Basal pontine syndrome, 245
Basilar artery, 8, 244-245, 250-251
Basilar pons, 68-69, 250
Basilar region, 7
Bell palsy, 248-249
Benedikt syndrome, 251-252
Benzodiazepine, 136, 141
Biceps muscle, 159
Bicuculline, 33
Bipolar cells, 269, 276, 277
Bipolar disorders, 140-141
Bitemporal hemianopsia, 72, 270, 295-296

Bladder, 177
Blinking response, 225
Blood pressure, 228, 229
Blood supply, 8, 9f
Blood-brain barrier, 72, 73, 137
Botzinger complex, 49
Brachial plexus, 94, 159
Bradykinesia, 27
Brainstem, 8, 41f, 50-51, 68, 225-255
  dopamine and, 320
  Horner syndrome and, 251
  trochlear nerve and, 254
Branchial arch, 225
Broca aphasia, 56, 69, 375, 378
Bromocriptine, 296
Brown-Séquard syndrome, 39-41,
  163, 168, 170

C
Calcarine cortex, 366-367
Calcarine fissure, 272
Calcium, 16t, 99, 111, 112, 176
  internal carotid artery and, 270
  Lambert-Eaton syndrome and,
  132
  voltage gating of, 21
cAMP, 110
Carbamazepine, 135, 361
Carbidopa (Sinemet), 27
Carbon dioxide, 243
Carbon dioxide partial pressure
  (PCO_2), 377
Carotid body, 379
Carotid sinus reflex, 176, 228, 229
Carpal tunnel syndrome, 94
Carrier proteins, 15
Catecholamines, 26-28, 130,
  132, 133

Catechol-O-methyltransferase
  (COMT), 26, 140
Cations, 15, 98, 111
Caudal basal pontine syndrome, 328
Caudal tegmental pontine syndrome,
  250
Caudal ventral respiratory group
  (cVRG), 49
Caudal ventrolateral medullary
  depressor area (CVLM), 49
Caudate nucleus, 6, 53, 67, 292
Cavernous sinus, 230
CCK. See Cholecystokinin
Central canal, 166
Central nucleus, 177
Central scotoma, 296
Cerebellar ataxia, 93
Cerebellar glomerulus, 323
Cerebellar peduncles, 6-7
Cerebellar vermis, 82
Cerebellum, 6-7, 54-55, 322-323
Cerebral aqueduct, 7
Cerebral artery, 317-318
Cerebral cortex, 1-6, 56, 66, 67, 319,
  322-323
Cerebral peduncle, 71, 253
Cerebrospinal fluid (CSF), 72, 81, 83,
  161, 376-377
Cervical disk prolapse, 160
cGMP. See Cyclic guanosine 5'-
  monophosphate
Channel proteins, 15
Chemical synapses, 20, 109-110
Chlordiazepoxide, 136
Chloride, 11, 16t, 96, 110, 112
Cholecystokinin (CCK), 140, 366
Cholera, 13
Choline, 22

Choline acetyltransferase, 130, 140
Chorda tympani nerve, 249
Chorea, 53-54
Choreiform movements, 321
Choroid plexus, 72, 81
Chromaffin cells, 80
Chromatin, 12
Ciliary body, 44-45
Cingulate gyrus, 6, 277, 319
Circle of Willis, 8, 9*f*
Circumventricular organ, 240
Claustrum, 319
Clonidine, 135, 136-137
Clonus, 93
Cogwheeling, 325
Combined systems disease, 42
Complex cells, 277
Complex partial epilepsy, 138, 362,
    363, 377-378
COMT. *See* Catechol-*O*-
    methyltransferase
Cones, 269, 276, 277
Constructional apraxia, 376
Contralateral cortex, 162
Contralateral hemiplegia, 242
Corneal reflex, 225
Cornu ammons, 372
Corpus callosum, 69, 81, 294, 378
Corpus striatum, 26
Corticobulbar fibers, 294, 370
Corticospinal fibers, 42, 166-167,
    237, 294, 328
Corticospinal tract, 171, 228, 371
Corticosterone, 297
Cough, 226
Cranial nerves, 10*t*, 50-51, 225-255.
    See also specific nerves

Cranial nerve I, 8
Cranial nerve III, 8, 44, 51, 71, 239,
    242, 243, 245, 252-253,
    255
Cranial nerve IV, 8, 51, 230, 238, 243,
    253, 254, 255
Cranial nerve IX, 226, 229, 231, 233,
    236, 240-241, 243, 248
Cranial nerve V, 8, 225, 237, 239,
    241, 242, 244, 250
Cranial nerve VI, 51, 242, 243, 249,
    250
Cranial nerve VII, 8, 160, 231, 233,
    241, 243, 249, 250
Cranial nerve VIII, 8, 241
Cranial nerve X, 8, 231, 240-241,
    243, 248
Cranial nerve XI, 8, 176, 178,
    226-227, 232, 241, 379
  infection of, 232-233
  parotid glands and, 226
  pharynx and, 225
  taste and, 249
Cranial nerve XII, 8, 51
Crus cerebri, 238, 245
CSF. *See* Cerebrospinal fluid
Cuneocerebellar tract, 37
Curare, 132, 176
CVLM. *See* Caudal ventrolateral
    medullary depressor area
cVRG. *See* Caudal ventral respiratory
    group
Cyclic guanosine 5'-monophosphate
    (cGMP), 31, 138
Cytoplasm, 12
Cytoskeleton, 12, 95
Cytosol, 95

D

DAG. *See* Diacylglycerol

Dandy Walker syndrome, 00, 02, 03

DBH. *See* Dopamine-β-hydroxylase

Decarboxylase, 130, 134

Dèjèrine-Roussy syndrome, 297, 360

Delta (δ) receptors, 36

Deltoid muscles, 159

Demyelination, 103, 160, 161, 168-169

Dendrites, 11, 12

Dentate gyrus, 372

Dentate nucleus, 54, 235, 322, 324, 327

Deoxyribonucleic acid (DNA), 12

Depression, 28, 133-134, 135

Dermatomes, 169

Descending colon 47

Diabetes, 94, 248

Diacylglycerol (DAG), 34, 111

Diazepam (Valium), 33

Diencephalon, 6, 294

Diffusion, 141

Digitalis glycosides, 240

Dihydroxyphenylalanine (DOPA), 26

Diplopia, 166

DNA. *See* Deoxyribonucleic acid

DOPA. *See* Dihydroxyphenylalanine

L-DOPA, 130

    for Parkinson disease, 325

    tyrosine and, 134

DOPA-carboxylase, 26-27

Dopamine, 26-27, 33*t*, 130, 246, 320

    Parkinson disease and, 68, 294

    pars compacta and, 246

    substantia nigra and, 68, 325

    tyrosine and, 134

Dopamine agonists, 296

Dopamine receptor blockers, 321

Dopamine receptors, 33, 239

Dopamine-β-hydroxylase (DBH), 27, 130, 140

Doral gray columns, 10t

Dorsal columns, 37, 161, 167, 170, 272-273

    first-order neurons and, 167, 237, 272

    medial lemniscus and, 237

Dorsal funiculus, 166

Dorsal horn, 165, 275

Dorsal motor nucleus, 176

Dorsal pons, 230

Dorsal respiratory group (DRG), 50

Dorsal root ganglia, 80, 166, 170

Dorsal spinocerebellar pathway, 162

Dorsal spinocerebellar tract, 165

Dorsolateral medulla, 241

Dorsomedial nucleus, 360, 361

Dorsomedial pontine tegmentum, 93

DRG. *See* Dorsal respiratory group

Drinking, 55

Dynamic nuclear bag, 167

Dynorphins, 31

Dysarthria, 162, 245, 248, 371, 378

Dyskinesia, 367

Dysphagia, 229, 245

Dystonia, 93

E

Ecstasy. *See* 3,4, methylene-deoxy-methamphetamine

Edinger-Westphal nucleus, 45, 253-254

Electrical synapses, 20, 109
Emboliform, 235-236
Emotion, 55, 71, 293
End plate potential (EPP), 21, 130-131
Endocrine functions, 55
Endomorphin, 36
β-Endorphin, 30
Enkephalin, 19, 30, 238, 274, 275, 298, 319-320
Enteric nervous system, 44
Enzymatic degradation, 141
Ependymal cells, 14
Epiglottis, 240
Epilepsy, 12, 69, 138, 139-140
Epinephrine, 28, 33*t*, 130
EPP. *See* End plate potential
EPSP. *See* Excitatory postsynaptic potential
Erb palsy, 159
Essential tremor, 93
Excitatory amino acids, 19, 274
Excitatory focus-and-surround inhibition, 51
Excitatory postsynaptic potential (EPSP), 21, 35, 110, 369-370
Excitotoxicity, 24
Exocytosis, 110
Extracellular space, 16, 16*t*, 136

F

Facial nerves, 71, 225, 230, 231, 245, 249
Farsightedness, 269
Fasciculus cuneatus, 37, 161, 170, 171, 297
Fasciculus gracilis, 37, 164, 170, 171, 297

Fastigial nucleus, 54, 228, 322
  ataxia and, 236
  nystagmus and, 236
Fear, 365
Female reproductive system, 48
Femoral neuropathy, 94
First-order neurons, 164-165
  dorsal columns and, 167, 237, 272
  inferior vestibular nucleus and, 236
  nTS and, 236, 244
Flexor carpi radialis, 159
Flocculonodular lobe, 7, 55, 320, 324
Floor plate, 10*t*
Fluoro-Gold, 13
Fluoxetine (Prozac), 29, 133-134
Foramen of Luschka, 81
Foramen of Magendie, 81
Forebrain, 6, 292-298
  cranial nerves of, 8
Fornix, 6, 67, 68
Fourth ventricle, 7
Frey syndrome, 50
Frontal eye fields, 254

G

GABA. *See* γ- aminobutyric acid
GABA$_A$ receptors, 33, 136
GABA$_B$ receptors, 35
GABA-oxoglutarate transaminase (GABA-T), 25
Gabapentin, 135, 138
GABA-T. *See* GABA-oxoglutarate transaminase
GAD, *See* L-glutamic acid-1-decarboxylase
Gag reflex, 226
Gamma globulin, 169

Gamma motor neurons, 164
Ganglion cells, 269
  lateral inhibition and, 277
  in retina, 269, 275
Gap junction, 109, 110
Gaseous neurotransmitters, 31-32
Gastrointestinal tract (GIT), 46-47
Gated channels, 17
Gaze palsy, 253-254
General visceral efferent, 71
Generalized seizures, 363
Geniculate ganglion, 225, 233
Gerstmann syndrome, 70
GIT. *See* Gastrointestinal tract
Glaucoma, 269
Glial cells, 13-14
  glutamate and, 24
Globose, 235-236
Globus pallidus, 6, 53, 325
Glossopharyngeal nerve. *See* Cranial
  nerve IX
Glucose, 24, 72
Glutamate, 24, 33t, 111, 113, 133,
  136, 320
  cones and, 276
  epilepsy and, 139-140
  NMDA and, 31, 139
  stroke and, 13
  synapses and, 133
L-glutamate, 32
Glutamic acid decarboxylase, 134
L-glutamic acid-1-decarboxylase
  (GAD), 24
Glycine, 19, 25, 33t, 111, 133, 139
Glycine receptor, 34
Goldman equation, 17, 99, 100
Golgi apparatus, 12, 96
Golgi cells, 269, 278, 323

Golgi tendon organs, 37, 165, 167,
  169, 322
Golgi type 1, 13
G-protein. *See* Guanosine-5'
  -triphosphate (GTP)-binding
  protein
Granule cells, 278, 323
Granulous cortex, 69
Growth hormone-releasing hormone,
  364
GTP. *See* Guanosine-5'-triphosphate
Guanethidine sulfate, 177
Guanosine-5' triphosphate (GTP), 31, 34
Guanosine-5'-triphosphate (GTP)-
  binding protein (G-protein),
  20, 34, 35, 110, 140
Guanylate cyclase, 31
Guillain-Barré syndrome, 160, 168-169

H

Hallucinations, 279
Haloperidol, 135, 360-361
Heart, 46, 176-177
Hemiballism, 51, 321, 367
Hemiparesis, 241, 372
Herpes simplex, 13
Hexamethonium chloride, 176, 177
Higher functions, 360-380
Hippocampal formation, 6, 26, 55,
  68, 70, 134, 279, 372
Hippocampus, 6, 372, 378
Hips, 159-160
Hirschsprung disease, 50
Histamine, 29-30, 33t
Histamine receptors, 36, 139
Homonymous extrafusal muscle, 167
Homonymous hemianopsia, 243, 270,
  292, 295, 367, 368, 372, 374

Horizontal cells, 277
Horner syndrome, 50, 227, 244, 251, 252
Horseradish peroxidase (HRP), 13
HRP. *See* Horseradish peroxidase
5-HT. *See* 5-hydroxytryptamine
Huntington chorea, 12, 54, 68, 93, 295
    basal ganglia and, 320
    substance P and, 31
Hydrocephalus, 8, 72, 81-82, 377
5-hydroxy-indole-*O*-
        methyltransferase, 134
5-hydroxytryptamine (5-HT, serotonin), 28-29, 33*t*
    depression and, 133
    heart and, 177
    tryptophan and, 130
Hyperacusis, 248
Hypercomplex cells, 278
Hyperpolarization, 11
Hyperreflexia, 56, 163
Hypersomnia, 327
Hypertension, 136-137
Hypertonicity, 56, 163
Hypoglossal nerve, 72, 80-81, 226, 247, 248
Hypoglossal nucleus, 235, 236
Hypothalamus, 10*t*, 26, 30, 55, 177, 227
    Horner syndrome and, 244, 251
    temperature regulation by, 364
Hypotonia, 162

I
IgG, 161
Imidazoleamines, 29-30
IML. *See* Intermediolateral cell column

Indoleamines, 28-29
Inferior cerebellar peduncle, 6-7, 37, 231, 234, 237
Inferior colliculi, 10*t*, 239
Inferior oblique muscle, 243
Inferior olivary nucleus, 10*t*, 231, 234
Inferior recti muscle, 243
Inferior salivatory nucleus, 229, 232
Inferior vestibular nucleus, 236
Inhibitory interneurons, 272-273
Inhibitory postsynaptic potential (IPSP), 21, 102, 110
Initial segment, 101
Inotropic receptors, 21
Intention tremor, 93, 241
Intermediate gray, 167
Intermediolateral cell column (IML), 42, 49
Internal capsule, 40*f*, 56, 67, 243, 293, 318, 367, 370-371, 376
    tongue and, 318
    UMN paralysis and, 317
Internal carotid artery, 270
Interposed nuclei, 54, 236
Interventricular foramen, 72
Intracellular space, 16, 16*t*
Intrafusal muscle, 167
Ion channels, 17, 20-21, 96-97
IP$_3$, 111
Ipsilateral gaze paralysis, 242
IPSP. *See* Inhibitory postsynaptic potential
Iris, 44-45

J
Jacksonian march, 368-369
Jugular foramen, 225
Juxtarestiform body, 54

K

Kainate, 113
Kainate receptor, 33
Kappa (κ) receptors, 36
Kidney, 46
Kinesin, 96
Klumpke palsy, 164
Klüver-Bucy syndrome, 55, 365
Knees, 159-160
Korsakoff syndrome, 366
Krebs cycle, 24

L

Labyrinth organs, 72
Lacrimal glands, 46, 233
Lambert-Eaton syndrome, 22, 131,
    132
Laminas, 165
Large intestine, 46-47
Large molecule neurotransmitters, 22
Larynx, 225, 240
Lateral corticospinal tract, 37, 40*f*,
    162
Lateral cutaneous nerve, 94
Lateral descending pathways, 41*f*
Lateral funiculus, 160, 162, 169
Lateral gaze paralysis, 230
Lateral geniculate nucleus, 69, 269,
    270-271, 273, 277-278, 279,
    292
Lateral inhibition, 277
Lateral medullary syndrome, 50-51
Lateral olfactory stria, 276
Lateral rectus muscle, 229-230, 253,
    255
Lateral reticulospinal tract, 227
Lateral spinothalamic tract, 37, 162,
    166, 171, 241

Lateral vestibulospinal tract, 229
Lead-pipe rigidity, 325
Left ventromedial medulla, 218
Length constant, 98
Lenticular fasciculus, 292-293
Lentiform nucleus, 367
Leucine, 30
Levator palpebrae superioris muscle,
    251
Levodopa, 135
Lidocaine, 97
Ligand-gated channels, 17, 98
Limbic cortex, 6
Lingual nerve, 249
Lipid bilayer, 15
Lipid-soluble substances, 15
Lissauer marginal zone, 165, 171
Lithium, 135, 140-141
LMN. *See* Lower motor neuron
Locked-in syndrome, 250
Loop of Meyer, 51
Lower motor neuron (LMN), 41,
    228, 237
    paralysis, 164, 169, 227
        Brown-Séquard syndrome and,
        168
        internal capsule and, 318
        polio and, 160, 161
        ventral horn and, 159,
        165-166
    ventral horn and, 163
Lower pons, 233
LSD. *See* Lysergic acid diethylamide
Lumbar cord, 42
Lungs, 46
Lysergic acid diethylamide (LSD),
    365
Lysosomes, 12

M

Magnesium, 32-33, 139
Magnetic resonance Imaging (MRI), 1
Magnocellular neurons, 363
Male reproductive system, 47-48
Mammillary bodies, 67, 293, 366
Mammillothalamic tract, 293
MAO. *See* Monoamine oxidase
Mastication, 70, 237
Mechanically gated channels, 17
Medial geniculate nucleus, 239
Medial lemniscus, 237-238, 241, 245, 247
Medial longitudinal fasciculus (MLF), 166, 247
   nucleus cuneatus and, 234
   second-order neurons in, 236
Medial medullary syndrome, 51, 246-247
Medial pallidal segment, 293
Medial rectus, 255
Medial thalamus, 361
Medial vestibulospinal tract, 166, 227, 228
Median nerve, 94
Medical lemniscus, 38*f*
Medical pathways, 41*f*
Mediodorsal nucleus, 293, 379
Medulla, 7, 8, 166, 274
   dorsal columns in, 161, 167
   nTS of, 49, 177
   nucleus ambiguus of, 176, 225
Medullary pyramid, 40*f*, 171
Meissner corpuscles, 169, 272
Meissner plexus, 47
Melatonin, 297
Memantine, 135
Mental retardation, 25

Merkel receptors, 272
Mesencephalic nucleus, 10*t*, 242
Mesencephalon, 10*t*
Mesolimbic pathway, 26
Messenger RNA (mRNA), 95-96
Metabotropic glutamate receptors (mGLURs), 35
Metabotropic receptors, 34-36
Metencephalon, 10*t*
Methamphetamine. *See* 3,4, methylene-deoxy-methamphetamine
Methionine, 30
3,4, methylene-deoxy-methamphetamine (MDMA, ecstasy), 29
Metoprolol, 177
Meyer-Archambault loop, 271-272
mGLURs. *See* Metabotropic glutamate receptors
Microglia, 13
Microtubules, 13
micturition, 47
Midbrain, 8, 137, 162, 178
   Horner syndrome and, 244
   reticular formation of, 228
Middle cerebellar peduncle, 6-7, 237
Middle cerebral artery, 8, 374, 379
Miosis, 252
Mitochondria, 12
Mitral cells, 275-276, 278-279
MLF. *See* Medial longitudinal fasciculus
Monoamine oxidase (MAO), 26, 28, 140
Monosynaptic stretch reflex, 164, 167
Morphine, 139
Motor speech area, 69
Motor systems, 53-55, 160-161, 317-328

MPTP, 322
MRI. *See* Magnetic resonance Imaging
mRNA. *See* Messenger RNA
MS. *See* Multiple sclerosis
Mu (μ) receptors, 36, 139
Multiple sclerosis (MS), 11, 103, 161, 253
Muscarinic receptors, 48
Muscimol, 33
Myasthenia gravis, 22, 131, 132, 159-160
Myelencephalon, 10t
Myelin, 11, 95
Myelination, 14, 43t, 82
Myopia, 269

N

nAChR. *See* Nicotine acetylcholine receptors
Naloxone, 36
Neostriatum, 53, 246, 292, 319, 320. *See also* Caudate nucleus; Putamen
Nernst equation, 17, 100
Nerve growth factor, 82
Neural crest cells, 80
Neural tube, 10t
Neuritis, 269-270
Neurofilaments, 13
Neuroglia, 13-14
Neuromodulators, 176
Neuromuscular junction, 159-160
Neuronal membrane, 15
Neurons, 11-19, 273
Neurotransmitters, 19-36, 23t, 33t, 48, 130-141
  synaptic cleft and, 133

Nicotine acetylcholine receptors (nAChR), 32
Nicotinic receptors, 10, 132, 176
Nissl substance, 12, 95
Nitric oxide (NO), 31-32, 138-139
Nitric oxide synthase (NOS), 31
NMDA. *See* N-methyl-D-aspartic acid
N-methyl-D-aspartic acid (NMDA), 31, 32-33, 111, 113, 137, 139, 140
NO. *See* Nitric oxide
Nociception, 36
Nodes of Ranvier, 11, 14, 19, 95
Nongated channels, 17
Norepinephrine, 27-28, 33t, 48, 130
  β-adrenergic receptors and, 111, 176
  postganglionic neurons and, 252
  prazosin and, 137
  tyrosine and, 134
Normal-pressure hydrocephalus, 376-377
NOS. *See* Nitric oxide synthase
nTS. *See* Solitary nucleus
Nuclear chain fibers, 167-168
Nucleus accumbens, 178
Nucleus ambiguus, 176, 225, 229, 235, 248
Nucleus cuneatus, 234
Nucleus dorsalis of Clarke, 165, 167, 237
Nucleus gracilis, 233-234, 238
Nucleus of Cajal, 242
Nucleus of Darkschewitsch, 242
Nystagmus, 162, 166, 236

O

Obstructive sleep apnea, 379
Occipital cortex, 2, 23, 254
Occipital lobe, 366-367, 368
Oculomotor nerve. *See* Cranial
    nerve III
Olfaction, 243
Olfactory bulb, 23, 275-276, 278
Olfactory cilia, 278
Olfactory glomeruli, 278
Olfactory system, 278-279
Oligodendrocyte, 11, 13, 103
Olivo-cochlear bundle, 241
Opioid peptides, 30-31, 33t, 139, 298
Opioid receptors, 36, 137
Opsin, 269
Optic chiasm, 71-72, 269, 270, 368
Optic disk, 269-270
Optic nerve, 269
Optic tract, 294-295
Orbital prefrontal cortex, 1, 70
Orbitofrontal cortex, 375-376
Organ of Corti, 52, 249
Orientation-sensitive neurons, 273
ORL$_1$, 36
Otic ganglion, 232
Oxygen, 243
Oxytocin, 294

P

Pacemaker current, 177
Pacinian corpuscles, 169, 272
Paleostriatum, 53, 319
Pallidum, 294
Panic disorders, 141
Papez circuit, 70
Papilledema, 296
Paradoxical sleep, 362

Paramedian branch, of basilar artery,
    244-245, 250-251
Paramedian pontine reticular formation,
    242
Parasympathetic nervous system,
    43t-44t, 44, 252
Paraventricular nucleus, 294
Parietal lobe, 1-2, 374, 375
Parinaud syndrome, 253-254
Parkinson disease, 12, 27, 53, 83, 93,
    135, 296, 322, 325
  L-DOPA for, 325
  dopamine and, 68, 294
  dopamine receptors and, 239
Parotid gland, 45, 226, 229
Pars compacta, 239, 246, 325
Passive transport, 16
PCO$_2$. *See* Carbon dioxide partial
    pressure
PCP, 139
Peduncular region, 7
Periaqueductal gray, 177-178, 230,
    240, 297-298
  enkephalin in, 238
  medulla and, 274
Periglomerular cels, 278
Peripheral nerves, 14, 95, 168-169
Peroneal nerve, 94
Petit mal epilepsy, 363
Pharynx, 225, 229, 240
Phenoxybenzamine hydrochloride, 177
Phentolamine, 177
Phenyl-ethanolamine-*N*-
    methyltransferase (PNMT), 28,
    130, 134
Phenylketonuria, 130
Phrenic motor nucleus (PM), 50
Pineal gland, 73

Pituitary gland, 81, 368
microadenoma of, 295-296
Plasma membrane, 11
Plasmapheresis, 169
PM. *See* Phrenic motor nucleus
PNMT. *See* Phenyl ethanolamine *N*-methyltransferase
Polio, 13, 160, 161
Polyprotein, 95
Pons, 7, 8, 68, 227, 243
stroke of, 327
Postcentral gyrus, 1, 37, 272
Posterior cerebral artery, 8, 327-328
Posterior choroidal artery, 368
Posterior communicating artery, 9f
Posterior flocculonodular lobe, 7
Posterior lobe, 55
Posterior median septum, 10f
Posterior spinocerebellar tract, 37, 167
Posterior thalamus, 227
Posterolateral territory, 361
Postganglionic neurons, 46-47, 232
bladder and, 177
Horner syndrome and, 251
norepinephrine and, 252
Postsynaptic receptors, 19, 276
Posttranslational importation, 95
Potassium, 11, 15, 16, 16t, 96, 98-99
action potential and, 176-177
NMDA and, 111
Prazosin, 137
Pre-Botzinger complex, 49
Precentral gyrus, 1, 2, 247, 249, 277, 319
Prefrontal cortex, 1-3, 68, 161, 276, 379
emotion and, 293
olfactory system and, 279
Preganglionic neurons, 46, 251, 252

Premotor areas, 318-319, 320
Premotor cortex, 1, 376
Presynaptic autoreceptors, 141
Presynaptic cleft, 109-110
Pretectal area, 275
Prolactin, 26, 296
Propranolol, 93
Prosencephalon, 10t
Prostaglandins, 111
Prostate gland, 48
Prozac. *See* Fluoxetine
Pruritus, 139
Pseudobulbar palsy, 67
Pseudocoma, 250
Pterygopalatine ganglia, 233
Ptosis, 252
Pupil, 45-46, 251
Pupillary light reflex, 239, 243-244
Purines, 30
Purkinje cells, 109, 231, 234, 324, 326, 327
Putamen, 6, 53, 67, 292
Pyramidal cells, 369
Pyramidal tract, 82, 246
Pyriform cortex, 6, 278-279

Q
Quadrantanopia, 51, 69-70, 272
Quisqualic acid, 33

R
Rabies, 13
Raphe neurons, 133
Rathke pouch, 81
α-receptor blockers, 177
Receptors, 32-36, 33t
in autonomic nervous system, 48
G-protein and, 110

Rectum, 47
Red nucleus, 178, 231, 234, 245, 252
Referred pain, 273-274
REM sleep, 362
Reproductive systems, 47-48
RER. *See* Rough endoplasmic reticulum
Reserpine, 177
Resting membrane potential, 97, 102-103
Reticular formation, 228, 235, 241
Reticulospinal tracts, 37
Retina, 269, 275, 277
Retinitis pigmentosa, 269
Retrograde degeneration, 94-95
Retrograde tracing, 13
Reuptake, 141
Rhodopsin, 269
Rhombencephalon, 10*t*
Ribonucleic acid (RNA), 12
RNA. *See* Ribonucleic acid
Rods, 269
Roof plate, 10*t*
Rostral ventral respiratory group (rVRG), 49
Rostral ventrolateral medullary pressor area (RVLM), 49
Rough endoplasmic reticulum (RER), 12, 30, 96
Rubrospinal tracts, 37, 41*f*, 162, 227, 229
RVLM. *See* Rostral ventrolateral medullary pressor area
rVRG. *See* Rostral ventral respiratory group

S
Salivary glands, 45-46
Salivatory nucleus, 233
Schizophrenia, 12, 141, 365
Schlemm canal, 269
Schwann cells, 11, 14
Scotoma, 51
Second-messenger kinases, 112-113
Second-order neurons, 237
in medulla, 166
in MLF, 236
Seizures, 25, 69, 138
EPSP and, 369-370
temporal lobe and, 372
Senile dementia, 12
Sensory systems, 51-53, 269-279
Septal area, 67
Septum pellucidum, 6, 68, 295
Serine hydroxymethyltransferase, 133
Serotonin. *See* 5-hydroxytryptamine
Serotonin receptors, 34, 35-36
Sex hormones, 297
Sexual behavior, 6, 55
Short-term memory, 55, 67, 292, 372
Simple diffusion, 15
Sinemet. *See* Carbidopa
Sleep apnea, 379
Small cell carcinoma, 131
Small intestine, 46-47
Small molecule neurotransmitters, 22
Sodium, 15, 16, 16*t*, 96, 101, 111, 112
Sodium-potassium pump, 16-17, 101-102
Soft palate, 229
Solitary nucleus (nTS), 49, 177, 229, 236, 244

Solitary nucleus (nTS), (*Cont.*):
  baroreceptor reflex and, 228
  blood pressure and, 229
  taste and, 234, 244
  ventral posterolateral nucleus and, 244
Soma, 11
Special visceral afferents, 51, 243
Special visceral efferents, 51, 71
Sphincter vesicae, 47
Spinal cord, 36-42, 159-171
Spinal trigeminal nucleus, 239
Spindles, 164, 167, 322
Spinothalamic tract, 39*f*, 164, 170-171, 297
Stapedius muscle, 249
Static nuclear bag, 167-168
Stomach, 46-47, 227
Stria terminalis, 293, 372
Stroke, 69, 82, 227-228, 297, 327
  auditory system and, 246
  cerebral artery and, 317-318
  glutamate and, 13
  NMDA and, 137
  posterior cerebral artery of, 327-328
Stylopharyngeus muscle, 232
Subarachnoid hemorrhage, 72, 360
Subcortical structures, 2
Subfornical organ, 73
Subiculum, 372
Sublingual glands, 45
Submandibular ganglia, 233
submandibular glands, 45
Substance P, 19, 31, 139, 165, 274, 319
Substantia gelatinosa, 162, 165, 240
Substantia innominata, 295

Substantia nigra, 10*t*, 26, 53, 246, 294
  dopamine and, 325
  substance P in, 31
Subthalamic fasciculus, 293
Subthalamic nucleus, 53, 321
Sulcus limitans, 8
Sumatriptan, 360
Superior cerebellar artery, 244
Superior cerebellar peduncle, 6-7, 163, 235, 238, 252
Superior colliculi, 10*t*, 239, 245, 254, 275
Superior ganglion, 225
Superior oblique muscle, 253, 254
Superior olivary nucleus, 241
Superior parietal lobes, 1
Superior recti muscle, 243
Superior temporal gyrus, 69, 361
Suprachiasmatic nucleus, 275, 297
Supraoptic nucleus, 364
Supraspinatus muscles, 159
Sustentacular cells, 278
Swallowing, 226, 227, 240
Sympathetic ganglia, 80
Sympathetic nervous system, 42-44, 43*t*-44*t*
Synapses, 19-36, 20, 109-113
  glutamate and, 135
Synaptic boutons, 21
Synaptic cleft, 110
  ACh and, 23
  glutamate and, 24
  neurotransmitters and, 133
  serotonin and, 28
Syndrome of hemineglect, 374-375
Syringomyelia, 42, 81, 82, 160

T

Tabes dorsalis, 42
Tachykinins, 31
Tardive dyskinesia, 321-322
Taste, 225, 243
    chorda tympani nerve and, 249
    cranial nerve IX and, 249
    cranial nerves and, 231
    nTS and, 234, 244
    solitary nucleus and, 229
Taste pathway, 53
Tegmentum, 7, 252
Telecephalic nuclei, 325
Temperature regulation, 55,
        363-364
Temporal gyrus, 23
Temporal lobe, 2
    seizures and, 372
Temporal lobe epilepsy, 55
Tendon reflex, 167
Tetanus, 13
Tethered cord syndrome, 81
Tetraethylammonium, 101, 112
Tetrodotoxin, 101, 112
Thalamic fasciculus, 293
Thalamic pain syndrome, 297
Thalamus, 10t, 178, 229, 269
    lateral spinothalamic tract and, 162
    spinal trigeminal nucleus and, 239
    ventral posterolateral nucleus and,
        279
Thermoreceptors, 296
Thiamine. *See* Vitamin B_1
Thoracic cord, 42
Thyroxine, 363
Tibial nerve, 94
Tongue, 226, 233, 236, 248, 318

Topiramate, 361
Trapezoid body, 246
Tricyclic antidepressants, 298
Trigeminal nerve, 232, 240, 241
Trigger zone, 100-101, 240
Trochlear nerve. *See* Cranial nerve IV
Tryptophan, 130
Tryptophan hydroxylase, 134, 140
Tuberoinfundibular dopaminergic
        system, 296
Tufted cells, 278
Type I synapses, 109
Type II synapses, 109
Tyrosine, 130, 134
Tyrosine hydroxylase, 130, 140

U

UMN. *See* Upper motor neuron
Uncinate fasciculus of Russell, 54
Uncinate fits, 279
Unilateral sensory neglect, 56
Uniports, 15
Upper eyelid, 45
Upper motor neuron (UMN), 41,
        67, 163
    paralysis, 56, 70, 159, 164, 237
        AIDS and, 160
        Brown-Séquard syndrome and,
            168
        crus cerebri and, 245
        internal capsule and, 317
        MLF and, 166
        oculomotor nerve and, 253
Upper pons, 244
Urbach-Wiethe disease, 365
Urethral sphincter, 47
Urinary bladder, 47

V

Vagus nerve, 46, 70, 176, 178, 225
Valium. See Diazepam
Valproic acid, 25
Vasopressin, 139, 294, 363
Velocity detectors, 167
Ventral anterior nucleus, 320
Ventral gray columns, 10t
Ventral horn, 13, 40f, 159, 162, 163,
        165-166, 178
    bladder and, 177
    intermediate gray of, 167
Ventral posterolateral nucleus, 240,
        244, 279
Ventral respiratory group (VRG), 49
Ventral tegmental area, 26, 246
Ventricular system, 6
Ventrolateral nucleus, 178
Ventromedial nucleus, 296-297
Vermal region, 236
Vestibular complex, 320, 324
Vestibular nuclei, 254-255
Vestibular pathway, 52-53

Vestibulospinal tracts, 39
Vigabatrin, 361
Viral encephalitis, 132
Visual system, 51-52, 52f
    damage to, 68
Vitamin B$_1$ (Thiamine), 326, 366
Vitamin B$_{12}$, 42
Voltage gating, 11, 17, 18-19,
        21, 98
Von Hippel-Lindau disease, 318
VPL, 37
VRG. See Ventral respiratory group

W

Wallenberg syndrome, 50-51
α-wave, 362
Weber syndrome, 245, 253, 328
Wernicke aphasia, 56, 69, 292, 367,
        378
White matter, 166

X

X chromosomes, 12

Notes

Notes

Notes